CLINICAL LABORATORY MEDICINE

SELF-ASSESSMENT AND REVIEW

SECOND EDITION

CLINICAL LABORATORY MEDICINE

SELF-ASSESSMENT AND REVIEW

SECOND EDITION

KENNETH D. MCCLATCHEY, D.D.S., M.D.

Chairman, Department Of Pathology
Helen M. and Raymond M. Galvin Professor
Loyola University Medical Center
Maywood, Illinois

HESHAM M. AMIN, M.B., B.CH., M.Sc.

Fellow
Department of Hematopathology
Division of Pathology and Laboratory Medicine
The University of Texas—MD Anderson Cancer Center
Houston, Texas

JONATHAN L. CURRY, M.D.

Resident
Department of Pathology
Loyola University Medical Center
Maywood, Illinois

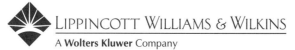

LIPPINCOTT WILLIAMS & WILKINS
A **Wolters Kluwer** Company

Philadelphia · Baltimore · New York · London
Buenos Aires · Hong Kong · Sydney · Tokyo

Acquisitions Editor: Ruth W. Weinberg
Developmental Editor: Raymond E. Reter
Production Editor: Emily Lerman
Manufacturing Manager: Colin J. Warnock
Cover Designer: Patricia Gast
Compositor: Lippincott Williams & Wilkins Desktop Division
Printer: *Victor Graphics*

© 2002 by LIPPINCOTT WILLIAMS & WILKINS
530 Walnut Street
Philadelphia, PA 19106 USA
LWW.com

Printed in the USA

Library of Congress Cataloging-in-Publication Data

McClatchey, Kenneth D.
   Clinical laboratory medicine : self-assessment and review / Kenneth D. McClatchey, Hesham M. Amin, Jonathan L. Curry.—2nd ed.
      p. ; cm.
   Companion v. to Clinical laboratory medicine. 2nd ed. 2001.
   ISBN 0-7817-3150-X (alk. paper)
   1. Diagnosis, Laboratory—Examinations, questions, etc.   I. Amin, Hesham M.
II. Curry, Jonathan L.   III. Title.
   [DNLM: 1. Laboratory Techniques and Procedures—Examination Questions. QY 4
C6414 2001 Suppl. 2002]
   RB37 .C5897 2001 Suppl.
   616.07'56'076—dc21

                                                                  2001038907

Care has been taken to confirm the accuracy of the information presented and to describe generally accepted practices. However, the authors and publisher are not responsible for errors or omissions or for any consequences from application of the information in this book and make no warranty, expressed or implied, with respect to the currency, completeness, or accuracy of the contents of the publication. Application of this information in a particular situation remains the professional responsibility of the practitioner.

The authors and publisher have exerted every effort to ensure that drug selection and dosage set forth in this text are in accordance with current recommendations and practice at the time of publication. However, in view of ongoing research, changes in government regulations, and the constant flow of information relating to drug therapy and drug reactions, the reader is urged to check the package insert for each drug for any change in indications and dosage and for added warnings and precautions. This is particularly important when the recommended agent is a new or infrequently employed drug.

Some drugs and medical devices presented in this publication have Food and Drug Administration (FDA) clearance for limited use in restricted research settings. It is the responsibility of the health care provider to ascertain the FDA status of each drug or device planned for use in their clinical practice.

                              10 9 8 7 6 5 4 3 2 1

CONTENTS

Preface vii

SECTION I: GENERAL LABORATORY

1 Laboratory Management 3

2 Management of the Clinical Laboratory 6

3 Laboratory Safety 8

4 The Interpretation of Laboratory Tests 10

5 Laboratory Information Systems 14

6 Ethics in Laboratory Medicine 15

SECTION II: MOLECULAR PATHOLOGY

7 Introduction to Molecular Diagnostics 19

8 Molecular Biology of Inherited Diseases 21

9 Molecular Biology of Solid Tumors 23

10 Molecular Biology of Infectious Diseases 25

11 Clinical Applications of Molecular Biology of
Hematopoietic Disorders 27

SECTION III: CLINICAL CHEMISTRY

12 Immunochemical Methods 35

13 Plasma Proteins 41

14 Diagnostic Enzymology and Other Biochemical
Markers of Organ Damage 45

15 Lipids and Lipoproteins 49

16 Endocrine Function and Carbohydrate 52

17 Electrolytes and Acid-Base Balance 57

18 Respiration and Measurement of Oxygen and
Hemoglobin 62

19 Nitrogen Metabolites and Renal Function 64

20 Calcium, Magnesium, and Phosphate 67

21 Heme Synthesis and Catabolism 70

22 Toxicology 71

23 Trace Elements, Vitamins, and Nutrition 74

24 Inborn Metabolic Errors 76

25 Point-of-Care Testing 78

26 Tumor Markers 79

SECTION IV: MEDICAL MICROSCOPY AND URINALYSIS

27 Synovial, Pleural, and Peritoneal Fluids 83

28 Urine 86

SECTION V: CYTOGENETICS

29 Basic Cytogenetics 93

30 Clinical Cytogenetics 96

31 Prenatal Cytogenetic Diagnosis 100

32 Cytogenetic Studies in Neoplastic Hematologic
Disorders 103

33 The Chromosome-Breakage Syndromes:
Clinical Features, Cytogenetics, and Molecular
Genetics 106

34 Solid Tumor Cytogenetics 108

SECTION VI: HLA TYPING

35 HLA: Structure, Function, and Methodologies 113

36 Molecular HLA Typing 114

37 HLA: The Major Histocompatability Complex:
Applications 115

38 Bone Marrow Transplantation 117

SECTION VII: HEMATOLOGY

39 Hematopoiesis and the Hematopoietic Growth Factors 121

40 Peripheral Blood and Bone Marrow: Morphology, Counts and Differentials, and Reactive Disorders 122

41 Red Blood Cell Disorders 124

42 Thalassemia and Hemoglobinopathy Syndromes 128

43 Acute Leukemia and Myelodysplastic Syndromes 131

44 Chronic Lymphoproliferative Disorders, Immunoproliferative Disorders, and Malignant Lymphoma 134

45 Chronic Myeloproliferative Disorders 137

SECTION VIII: COAGULATION

46 Overview of Hemostasis 143

47 Laboratory Evaluation of Platelet Disorders 145

48 Coagulation Abnormalities 147

49 Thrombophilia 149

SECTION IX: MICROBIOLOGY

50 Specimen Collection and Processing for Microbiology 153

51 Bacteriology 155

52 Fungi and Fungal Infections 159

53 *Chlamydia, Mycoplasma*, and *Rickettsia* 161

54 Aerobic Actinomycetes 163

55 Antimicrobial Susceptibility Testing 165

56 Molecular Techniques for Diagnosis of Infectious Diseases 168

57 Role of the Clinical Microbiology Laboratory in Hospital Epidemiology and Infection Control 170

58 Autopsy Microbiology 171

59 Diagnostic Virology 172

60 Parasitology 173

SECTION X: IMMUNOPATHOLOGY

61 Basic Principles of Immunodiagnosis 179

62 Flow Cytometry 181

63 Cellular and Humoral Mediators of Inflammation 183

64 Monoclonal Gammopathies 185

65 Primary Immunodeficiency Diseases 187

66 Allergic Conditions 189

67 Receptor Assays of the Clinical Laboratory 191

SECTION XI: BLOOD BANK/TRANSFUSION MEDICINE

68 Organization, Functions, Regulation, and Legal Concerns of Blood Banks 197

69 Blood Collection 199

70 Pretransfusion Testing 201

71 Blood Component Therapy 203

72 Transfusion Therapy 205

73 Neonatal Transfusion 207

74 Complications of Blood Transfusions 209

75 Immune Hemolysis 211

Answers to the Questions 213

PREFACE

This review book is meant to serve as a complement to the Second Edition of *Clinical Laboratory Medicine* by providing the textbook users—medical laboratory technicians, medical technologists, medical students, residents in pathology and internal medicine, clinical laboratory scientists, practicing pathologists, and other physicians—a means of testing their comprehension of the enormous amount of information found therein.

The review book follows the outline of the eleven sections in *Clinical Laboratory Medicine*. Careful attention has been made to guide an individual's study and comprehension of a chapter by using strategic questions. The answers for each chapter are referenced to the textbook.

It is with gratitude that I thank my colleagues Jonathan L. Curry, M.D. and Hesham M. Amin, M.D. for their contributions to the task of question-writing. Their efforts demonstrate their commitment to the art and science of teaching.

I also thank the section editors and contributors to *Clinical Laboratory Medicine*, who made the textbook possible.

Finally, and most importantly, both books have been written to acknowledge the many laboratory professionals who have devoted their lives to better patient care by constantly striving to improve the art and science of clinical laboratory medicine.

Kenneth D. McClatchey, D.D.S., M.D.

CLINICAL LABORATORY MEDICINE

SELF-ASSESSMENT AND REVIEW

SECOND EDITION

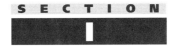

GENERAL LABORATORY

1 Laboratory Management
2 Management of the Clinical Laboratory
3 Laboratory Safety
4 Interpretation of Laboratory Tests
5 Laboratory Information Systems
6 Ethics in Laboratory Medicine

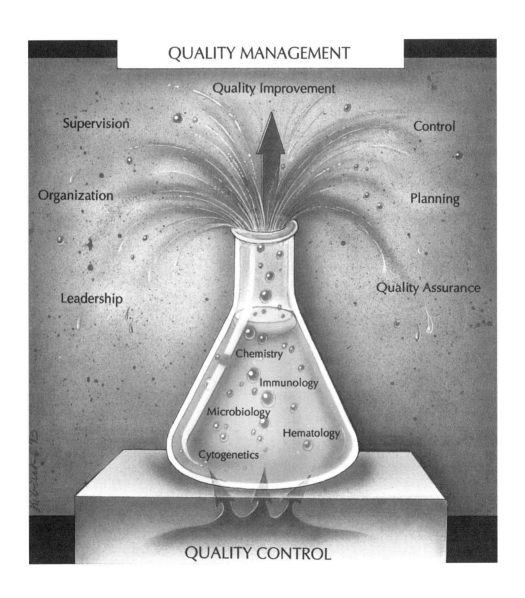

1

LABORATORY MANAGEMENT

QUESTIONS

Select the one best answer of the choices offered.

1. **Medicare, the publicly funded health insurance for all citizens over age 65, and Medicaid, the health insurance for citizens receiving public assistance, began in the**
   A. 1940s
   B. 1950s
   C. 1960s
   D. 1970s

2. **The Clinical Laboratory Improvement Amendments of 1988 (CLIA 88) included all of the following provisions** *except*
   A. proficiency testing
   B. reimbursements
   C. quality assurance
   D. quality control

3. **A leader must first and foremost endorse the concepts of**
   A. accounting
   B. persons
   C. organization
   D. finance

4. **The high-performance manager is all** *except*
   A. strategist
   B. conformist
   C. problem solver
   D. teacher

5. **The essential elements of management include all** *except*
   A. ideas
   B. things
   C. people
   D. action

6. **The management system described as the Juran Trilogy includes all** *except*
   A. quality planning
   B. quality limits
   C. quality control
   D. quality improvement

7. **The Itoh model of workload allocation includes all** *except*
   A. development
   B. finance
   C. improvement
   D. control and maintenance

8. **There is an array of hidden costs in today's service economy outpatient clinical laboratory that includes all** *except*
   A. information services
   B. marketing
   C. laboratory consultation
   D. pricing

9. **The basic entities of a successful quality improvement program include all** *except*
   A. involvement
   B. cooperation
   C. measurement
   D. reward

10. **A key component of the patient health care provider "life cycle" is profoundly associated with**
    A. perceived health care service
    B. insurance
    C. marketing
    D. reward

11. **In today's quality management environment, Douglas McGregor's theory _____ is in vogue.**
    A. Y
    B. X
    C. W
    D. Z

12. **Abraham Maslow describes an ascending order of human needs that includes all *except***
    A. social needs
    B. ego needs
    C. id needs
    D. self-actualization

13. **A key goal of continuous quality improvement is**
    A. compliance
    B. retroactive approach
    C. improved norms
    D. decreased limits

14. **The key variables of business performance include all *except***
    A. price
    B. cost
    C. performance
    D. productivity

15. **The costs most difficult to control in the clinical laboratory are those for**
    A. equipment
    B. labor
    C. reagents
    D. lease

16. **Nonoperating labor costs include all *except***
    A. driver salaries
    B. maintenance personnel salaries
    C. data processing personnel salaries
    D. physician remuneration

17. **Purchase of new or replacement equipment includes all of these categories *except***
    A. depreciable costs development
    B. production volume forecast
    C. depreciation life estimation
    D. future acquisitions forecast

18. **Indirect costs are all test production costs that cannot be directly traced to test production and include all *except***
    A. power
    B. heat
    C. clerk salaries
    D. reagents

19. **The foundation of the financial management system for the clinical laboratory is**
    A. supervisor list
    B. continuous quality improvement (CQI)

    C. chart of accounts
    D. test production

20. **The basic formula for the fundamental laboratory accounting model is**
    A. assets = liabilities + equity
    B. capital = depreciation + earnings
    C. assets = earnings − labor
    D. revenues = labor + materials

21. **Profit is defined as relative ____ for a not-for-profit laboratory.**
    A. investment
    B. efficiency
    C. income
    D. operation

22. **Cost-volume-profit analysis in the clinical laboratory permits the study of the relationships between all *except***
    A. prices
    B. fixed costs
    C. workload volume
    D. depreciation

23. **The technical part of budget preparation includes all *except***
    A. projected workload
    B. calculated indirect costs
    C. adjusting revenue and total costs
    D. converting technical overtime

24. **The basic clinical laboratory budget type includes all *except***
    A. workload
    B. expense
    C. procedure
    D. revenue

25. **Allocated expenses in the clinical laboratory include all *except***
    A. reference laboratory fees
    B. laboratory receptionists
    C. phlebotomy
    D. heat

26. **Variance in the clinical laboratory analysis compares**
    A. direct and indirect costs
    B. deviation of actual costs from budgetal cost
    C. deviation of direct costs from discounted prices
    D. test value and indirect costs

27. **"Make" or "buy" decisions are most often associated with decisions to**

    A. discontinue testing
    B. set indirect cost
    C. increase direct cost
    D. set billing

28. **The most justifiable way to set laboratory test pricing is on the basis of**

    A. price variation
    B. direct costs
    C. actual direct and indirect costs
    D. indirect costs

29. **The charge for a test should most accurately include all *except***

    A. previous losses
    B. a share of all applicable indirect costs
    C. a satisfactory profit
    D. direct costs

30. **"Conversion cost" pricing focuses on**

    A. indirect costs and margin
    B. labor costs and reagents
    C. amount of direct costs in margin
    D. amount of labor and indirect costs required to produce a test

Indicate whether each of the following statements is true (T) or false (F).

31. **"Billable" tests are those clinical laboratory tests that are charged to a patient and create revenue.**

32. **Purchase of clinical laboratory equipment requires analysis that includes forecast of labor costs.**

33. **Reagent rental or "cost-per-test" contracting has all the advantages of maintenance, labor, and shipping.**

34. **Managing laboratory costs is impossible without managing laboratory productivity.**

35. **Operational productivity in the clinical laboratory includes labor, automation, and billing.**

36. **Fiscal productivity in the clinical laboratory does not include health maintenance organization.**

37. **Nonlabor excessive expenses in the clinical laboratory include waste, excessive controls, and improperly sized capital equipment.**

38. **The instrument cost accounting technique method involves labor and material costs and billing services.**

39. **Indirect instrument-related cost calculations include purchase price, life expectancy in years, and annual maintenance cost.**

40. **Preanalytical labor tasks in the clinical laboratory include list gathering, sample cup preparation, and daily quality control.**

MANAGEMENT OF THE CLINICAL LABORATORY

QUESTIONS

Select the one best answer of the choices offered.

1. **Medical diagnostic technologies (MDTs) are the method of choice for health care providers because they**

   A. provide subjective interpretation
   B. furnish fast and judgmental information
   C. are objective and quantifiable
   D. allow hands-on bedside diagnosis

2. **Health care organization (HCO) shift from a centralized inpatient to a decentralized ambulatory care operations is driven mainly by ____.**

   A. Rising cost of inpatient care
   B. Increasing adolescent population
   C. Decreasing technical staff
   D. Growing autopsy rate

3. **Marketing of MDTs includes all *except***

   A. contribute majority of information for patient care data models
   B. largest market segment in the medical technology industry
   C. responsible for 50% of patient care data models
   D. accounts for nearly 10% of hospital costs

4. **The highest percentage of total hospital cost for MDTs is**

   A. transfusion medicine
   B. nuclear medicine (isotopes)
   C. radiology
   D. clinical laboratory

5. **Reimbursement from Medicare or a third-party payer for a new Food and Drug Administration (FDA)-approved, Current Procedural Terminology (CPT-4)-recognized medical diagnostic test requires ____.**

   A. 1–2 years
   B. 2–4 years
   C. 4–6 years
   D. 6–8 years

6. **In an effort to confront challenges of rising clinical laboratory costs, key elements necessary for development of an integrated delivery system include all *except***

   A. require multiskilled personnel
   B. organization should be health insurance company centered
   C. clinical decisions made on evidence-based protocols
   D. operating site communication by information systems

7. **The changes to Medicare and Medicaid programs from the enacted Balance Budget Act of 1997 negatively impacted clinical laboratory operations by all of the following *except***

   A. decreasing laboratory accountability
   B. exposure to new competitive bidding
   C. decreasing reimbursements
   D. enactment of Medical Necessity guidelines

8. **The Medical Necessity legislation instituted in 1996 will increase labor and consumables costs for a test requiring additional efforts in all of the following areas *except***

   A. clerical
   B. legal
   C. supplies
   D. marketing

9. A "provider" who is authorized to use medical diagnostic tests and who may receive reimbursements includes all *except*

    A. institutions (e.g., hospital)
    B. agencies (e.g., public health)
    C. athletic trainers
    D. physicians and nonphysicians

10. High-cost area of the laboratory includes

    A. transfusion medicine
    B. noncomplex, high-volume laboratory medical tests
    C. quality assurance
    D. special chemistry

11. Decisions to "make" or "buy" a laboratory test include knowledge of all *except*

    A. marginal revenue (MR) > marginal cost (MC)
    B. medical specialty requesting the test
    C. projected test volume
    D. rate of reimbursement

Indicate whether each of the following statements is true (T) or false (F).

12. The Balanced Budget Act of 1997 mandated preventive testing for chronic diseases of children.

13. MDTs constitute the single, largest market segment within the medical technology industry.

14. MDTs comprise nearly 1% of hospital costs.

15. A merger and/or acquisition is the same as an integration, in which a parent organization remains intact.

16. Laboratory directors and managers are so frequently required to be involved in matters involving integrations, mergers, acquisitions, and professional and financial survival that it is difficult to realize that they are still the organization's only experts in providing pathology and laboratory services.

17. The federal Health Care Financing Administration (HCFA) has deemed that the clinical diagnostic laboratory should not act as a policing body to assure that providers are accountable for correct medical documentation.

18. Laboratories and hospital administrators must balance the need for patient care and value with the additional variable costs of compliance and regulation created by the Clinical Laboratory Improvement Amendments of 1988 (CLIA 88), Occupational Safety and Health Administration (OSHA), and Medical Necessity guidelines.

19. Data processing in medicine is the method by which a database is transformed into a problem list.

20. Third-party payers are important entities in an HCO's financial management structure because they provide the organization with the minor portion of its revenue from reimbursement.

3

LABORATORY SAFETY

QUESTIONS

Select the one best answer of the choices offered.

1. **Hazard containment is a system to control**

   A. insurance costs
   B. laboratory quality control
   C. maintenance records
   D. accident and injury

2. **Safe work practices include all *except***

   A. avoidance of aerosol formation
   B. segregation of hazardous waste
   C. external quality assessment
   D. proper operation of hazardous equipment

3. **One of the most effective means to minimize personal exposure is**

   A. reusable laboratory coats
   B. gloves
   C. face protection
   D. hand washing

4. **According to the Occupational Safety and Health Administration (OSHA), colored signs in the clinical laboratory that display safety information include all *except***

   A. red
   B. yellow
   C. green
   D. blue

5. **Class IA flammables have**

   A. flash point <22.8°C and boiling point <37.8°C
   B. flash point <22.8°C and boiling point >37.8°C
   C. flash point >22.8°C and boiling point <37.8°C
   D. flash point >35.8°C and boiling point <40.8°C

6. **Corrosives should always be stored**

   A. at eye level
   B. near the floor and below eye level
   C. above eye level
   D. any level in a protective bottle

7. **The U.S. Environmental Protection Agency (EPA) has defined corrosive wastes on the basis of**

   A. color
   B. ion strength
   C. ability to corrode copper
   D. pH or ability to corrode steel

8. **is the standard symbol for**

   A. biohazards
   B. radiation
   C. carcinogens
   D. laser devices

9. **The maximum allowable glass container size of ignitable liquids of class IA is**

   A. 1 pint
   B. 1 gallon
   C. 3 gallons
   D. 5 gallons

10. **Combustible liquids have a flash point that is greater than**

   A. 22.3°C
   B. 37.8°C
   C. 15.4°C
   D. 8.4°C

Indicate whether each of the following statements is true (T) or false (F).

11. A safety can is made of glass and paper.

12. A very simple, commonly used chemical spill containment material is sand and soda ash.

13. At least 10% of hospitalized patients are chronic carriers of hepatitis B.

14. Portable fire extinguishers designated as class C are used for electrical fires.

15. Electrical safety inspections should be performed at least once every 5 years.

16. A cryogenic liquid is any liquid with a boiling point less than −130°F.

17. Modest quantities of radioactive material may be transferred to an offsite location for burial.

18. Telephoned threats of a bomb are to be taken seriously, and the caller should be kept on the line and all the details of the call recorded.

19. All personnel must have documentation in employment records of attendance of safety training programs.

20. The management that work groups must follow sets safety standards.

4

INTERPRETATION OF LABORATORY TESTS

QUESTIONS

Select the one best answer of the choices offered.

1. **The testing cycle begins and ends with a patient who presents with a medical problem and expects to receive a diagnosis or a prognosis and some type of intervention or treatment.**
   A. True
   B. False

2. **The testing cycle is influenced by many factors that increase the uncertainty associated with a test result and thereby decrease the accuracy of the information that it provides.**
   A. True
   B. False

3. **The analytical variation constitutes a major fraction of the overall variability of most laboratory tests.**
   A. True
   B. False
   4. All of the following statements regarding biologic variation are true *except*
   A. Biologic variation in laboratory test results is due to within-subject variation over time and subject-to-subject variation within a population.
   B. The principal cause of the within-subject variation is the existence of endogenous biorhythms for many physiologic parameters.
   C. Biologic variation does not interfere with interpretation of laboratory results when its magnitude is similar to that observed in diseased subjects.
   D. The principal cause of the subject-to-subject variation within a population is the difference among subjects in constitutional factors and/or lifestyle.

5. **All of the following statements regarding biologic rhythms are true *except***
   A. The three types of biologic rhythms that have the most influence on the interpretation of laboratory results are circadian, ultradian, and infradian.
   B. Circadian rhythms usually have a period of <1 day.

C. Ultradian rhythms frequently are observed in the blood levels of various glandular secretions.
   D. The most common example of infradian rhythms is the menstrual cycle.

6. **All of the following analytes demonstrate marked variations related to the circadian rhythm *except***
   A. calcium
   B. sodium
   C. cortisol
   D. melatonin
   E. γ-glutamyltransferase

7. **All of the following statements regarding gender-related differences in test results are true *except***
   A. For analytes for which gender-related differences exist, test results tend to be similar in males and females until after the age of puberty.
   B. The most important mechanism of male/female differences in test results in adults is sex hormone-dependent physiologic processes.
   C. The menstrual cycle is associated with marked changes in the circulating levels of ovarian steroids, which, in turn, influence many physiologic processes.
   D. Most of the male/female differences in test results are clinically significant and require the use of gender-specific reference values.

8. **A significant and rapid change that occurs as children approach the age of puberty is a marked increase in the activity of the hepatic drug-metabolizing enzyme systems.**
   A. True
   B. False

9. **All of the following analytes demonstrate little change with age *except***
   A. potassium
   B. carbon dioxide
   C. liver enzymes
   D. magnesium
   E. phosphate

10. **All of the following analytes show age-related increases *except***

    A. γ-glutamyltransferase
    B. C-peptide
    C. total calcium
    D. Gastrin
    E. copper

11. **All of the following analytes show age-related decreases *except***

    A. lactate dehydrogenase
    B. zinc
    C. androstenedione
    D. platelets
    E. T_3

12. **All of the following statements regarding the effects of genetic heterogeneity on laboratory test results are true *except***

    A. In many instances, racial differences in laboratory values are easily verified.
    B. African Americans tend to have higher serum total protein levels and higher serum levels of γ-globulins, α-globulins, β-globulins, immunoglobulin G (IgG), and immunoglobulin A (IgA) than Caucasians.
    C. Genetic heterogeneity at the molecular level can lead to differences in the reactivity of the subject's DNA, proteins, or cells toward the nucleic acid probes and antibodies that are used as reagents in many diagnostic tests.
    D. Laboratory determination of the *BRCA1* gene can identify individuals at risk for a certain heritable form of breast cancer.

13. **Plasma renin, serum aldosterone, and the catecholamines increase by as much as fourfold with a change from supine to erect posture.**

    A. True   B. False

14. **Exercise-induced increases in blood hormones typically fall to baseline levels within 1 to 2 hours after the end of the exercise period.**

    A. True   B. False

15. **All of the following analytes increase during prolonged fasting or starvation *except***

    A. acetone
    B. creatinine
    C. β-hydroxybutyrate
    D. triglycerides
    E. free fatty acids

16. **All of the following analytes decrease due to alcohol consumption *except***

    A. prolactin
    B. testosterone
    C. cholesterol
    D. cortisol
    E. luteinizing hormone

17. **All of the following analytes increase due to oral contraceptive administration *except***

    A. ferritin
    B. protein S
    C. transcortin
    D. apoprotein B
    E. high-density lipoprotein cholesterol

18. **The accurate interpretation of test results during pregnancy requires the use of reference values derived from a population of healthy pregnant women at a defined stage of gestation.**

    A. True   B. False

19. **All of the following analytes decrease during normal pregnancy *except***

    A. red blood cells
    B. creatinine
    C. iron
    D. alkaline phosphatase
    E. α_1-acid glycoprotein

20. **The reference value that is used most frequently in contemporary laboratory medicine is the reference interval, which is bounded by upper and lower reference limits that are usually chosen to enclose 99% of the values observed in nondiseased subjects.**

    A. True   B. False

21. **All of the following statements regarding the Clinical Laboratory Improvement Act (CLIA) of 1988 regulations related to reference values are true *except***

    A. The reference ranges, as determined by the laboratory performing the tests, must be available to the authorized person who ordered the tests.
    B. In cases where a manufacturer's reference range is available, each individual l'aboratory is still required to establish its own reference values.
    C. Before reporting patient results, the laboratory must establish for each method the specifications for a number of performance characteristics, including the reference range(s).
    D. The reference ranges must be included in the laboratory procedure manual.

22. **All of the following statements regarding the College of American Pathologists standards related to reference values are true *except***

    A. The laboratory should periodically evaluate the appropriateness of its reference intervals and take corrective actions.
    B. There should be a reevaluation of the reference values whenever a laboratory changes an analytical methodology.
    C. Literature references or information from a manufacturer's package insert may not be used as reference values.
    D. The reference values are to be reported with the test results.

23. **All of the following statements regarding the selection of the reference sample to establish the reference interval are true *except***

    A. Ideally, the reference sample should be randomly drawn from the population.
    B. Individuals should be selected based on defined criteria that are independent of the value of the analyte for which the reference values are being determined.
    C. At least 700 reference subjects are required for precise parametric estimates of the 95% reference interval.
    D. Retrospective or prospective selection of reference individuals provides reliable data for the reference interval.

24. **All of the following statements regarding statistical analysis for the establishment of the reference values are true *except***

    A. The nonparametric method is considered difficult to perform.
    B. The nonparametric method requires at least 119 subjects to estimate 90% confidence intervals of reference limits.
    C. The nonparametric method currently is recommended by the National Committee for Clinical Laboratory Standards (NCCLS) for establishing population-based reference values.
    D. In the parametric method, the reference distribution must be tested for "gaussianity" before the estimation of reference limits.

25. **All of the following statements regarding the nonparametric methods are true *except***

    A. The observations for the reference sample are arranged in ascending order and assigned rank numbers.
    B. The limits that enclose 95% of the reference population are estimated by identifying the rank numbers corresponding to the 2.5th and 97.5th percentile.

    C. The confidence intervals are independent of the sample size.
    D. The nonparametric method can be used with non-continuous variables.

26. **Which of the following statements regarding the parametric/nonparametric methods for statistical analysis of reference values is *true*?**

    A. The first step in the nonparametric method is to test the assumption that the distribution of the reference values is gaussian.
    B. Simple test for a gaussian distribution is the comparison of the mean, median, and mode of the distribution.
    C. In the nonparametric method, if the original reference values are not gaussian, they should be transformed.
    D. The biologic variables often are skewed to the left.

27. **Adoption from the literature or from the manufacturer's of instruments and reagent system is the most common practice today to establish the reference values in the laboratory.**

    A. True   B. False

28. **According to recommendation of the NCCLS regarding transference of reference values, if >2 of 20 reference individuals from the receiving laboratory fall outside the 95% reference limits established in the original study, the reference limits of the original study should be rejected.**

    A. True   B. False

29. **The data used to establish the clinical performance of a laboratory test are obtained during the Phase I and Phase II clinical trials that are required for a test to be approved by the U.S. Food and Drug Administration.**

    A. True   B. False

30. **All of the following statements regarding crucial elements essential to the validity of the parameters derived from clinical trials are true except**

    A. The trial should evaluate a broad spectrum of healthy and diseased subjects, and the diseased group should include patients with a narrow range of clinical presentations.
    B. Confidence intervals should be calculated for all parameters that are estimated.
    C. When the diagnostic accuracy of a new test is being compared with that of a previously established test, a large sample of population should be studied.
    D. The clinical status of the subjects in each group should be established using a gold standard method.

31. **The clinical sensitivity of a given test is equivalent to its analytical sensitivity.**

    A. True   B. False

32. **All of the following statements regarding the sensitivity of a test are true except**

    A. The sensitivity of the test is defined as the proportion of diseased subjects who have a test result that is higher than a particular cutoff.
    B. The sensitivity is equivalent to the true positive rate of the test.
    C. The distributions of the test results in healthy and diseased groups usually overlap.
    D. The sensitivity of a test = true positives ÷ (true positives + false positives).

33. **The perfect test in which the sensitivity and specificity are both 1.0 will have a receiver operating characteristic (ROC) curve of a diagonal line with a slope of 1 and an intercept of zero.**

    A. True   B. False

34. **A likelihood ratio expresses the probability that a particular test result will occur in a diseased subject divided by the probability that the same outcome will not occur in a nondiseased subject.**

    A. True   B. False

35. **The discriminatory power of a positive test increases as its likelihood ratio increases above a value of 1.0.**

    A. True   B. False

5

LABORATORY INFORMATION SYSTEMS

QUESTIONS

Select the one best answer of the choices offered.

1. **The ROM stores programs and information only when the computer is operating and can be changed by the user.**

   A. True   B. False

2. **All of the following statements regarding personal computers are true *except***

   A. A modem is a device that allows connection of the personal computer through telephone or fiber-optic lines.
   B. A nibble is a sequence of eight bits.
   C. The modem speed unit is called baud.
   D. A bit is the smallest unit of information.

3. **All of the following statements regarding the laboratory information system project team are true *except***

   A. It is necessary to assign a task force of hospital personnel to coordinate the project.
   B. The working core of the project team must be the hospital clinical director.
   C. The participation of personnel from outside the clinical laboratories is critical to the success of the project.
   D. A clinician can speak to the needs of the physician in terms of test reporting formats and locations of terminals for data retrieval.

4. **Data flow diagrams are the most useful for planning and documenting laboratory operations.**

   A. True   B. False

5. **All of the following statements regarding the advantage of using an outside consultant in the selection of a laboratory information system are true *except***

   A. It allows arbitration of disputes between the various hospital fractions.
   B. It lends an air of credibility to the process.

   C. It saves work for the laboratory director and staff.
   D. It applies a previous successful solution to all future problems.

6. **All of the following statements regarding the test system for the management of a high-quality laboratory information system are true *except***

   A. The reputable vendors can exactly replicate the various computing environments of all their hospital clients.
   B. The test system consists of a copy of the production software and a patient test result database that can be used to stimulate live runs.
   C. The basic idea of the test system is that new releases of software can be tested in the local environment before being brought up live on the production system.
   D. Even the reputable vendors cannot design an error-free software.

7. **Successful collaboration between clinical laboratory managers and expert vendors leads to constructing a test system that can exactly mimic the production environment of the hospital.**

   A. True   B. False

8. **If a hospital does not have a test system, an acceptable alternative is to immediately install the new software on the production system.**

   A. True   B. False

9. **Voice recognition software implementation in the clinical laboratory decreases turnaround time, improves productivity, and gives pathologists more independence.**

   A. True   B. False

10. **In the 1960s, the Federal Bureau of Investigation (FBI) created the Internet as Aparnet to connect different networks at different sites.**

    A. True   B. False

6

ETHICS IN LABORATORY MEDICINE

QUESTIONS

Select the one best answer of the choices offered.

1. **Laboratories must not engage in practices forbidden by law, even in situations in which the law is contrary to the dictates of individual conscience.**

   A. True   B. False

2. **The relationship between a patient and the laboratory has little ethical content.**

   A. True   B. False

3. **With the frequency of third-party payment systems, the opportunities for unethical collusion between the treating doctor and the laboratory are unusual.**

   A. True   B. False

4. **All of the following statements regarding medical ethics in the medical laboratory are true *except***

   A. Medical ethics exist for the protection of the patients, but, in certain circumstances, this protection may be compromised by the need for laboratory testing during medical consultations.
   B. Many of the requirements of medical ethics are common to other professions.
   C. Confidentiality is supported by law.
   D. Adoption of a code of medical ethics increases community confidence that the medical laboratories are part of medicine.

5. **All of the following statements regarding medical ethics in the medical laboratory are true *except***

   A. Medical laboratories frequently are operated as corporate structures.
   B. The market forces applicable in a pure capitalistic model apply to a much lesser extent in medical interactions.
   C. The concept of *caveat emptor* should govern the delivery of medical laboratory service.
   D. Companies that own medical laboratories are required by law to maximize wealth for shareholders.

6. **Which of the following statements regarding the differences between ordinary commercial transactions and medical services is *true*?**

   A. Patients can easily assess the value of the medical services
   B. Symmetry of information between doctor and patient
   C. Effective monopoly of the medical services
   D. Third-party payers of medical services resolve the alarming market signals

7. **The Oath of Geneva, adopted by the World Medical Association in 1948 and subsequently amended in Sydney in 1968, is a modern version of the Hippocratic Oath.**

   A. True   B. False

8. **All of the following are principles derived from the Declaration of Geneva *except***

   A. maleficence
   B. justice
   C. autonomy
   D. beneficence

9. **Nonmaleficence is the duty or obligation to act in the best interest of the patient.**

   A. True   B. False

10. **All of the following are prerequisites in the ethical decision-making tool *except***

    A. stakeholder analysis
    B. testing that autonomy has been upheld
    C. mother/parent test
    D. viewing through the lens of culture

11. **All tests must be carried out to an appropriate standard that should be determined in detail by the medical director of the laboratory.**

    A. True   B. False

12. **All of the following statements regarding reporting test results are true** *except*

    A. Local customs are not to be considered in decisions concerning implying consent for the reporting of results to consultant practitioners.
    B. Test results are confidential unless disclosure is authorized.
    C. Written procedures detailing how various requests are handled should be made available to the patient on request.
    D. It is the responsibility of the clinical laboratory to ensure that transmitting results to the clinicians is secure.

13. **Incompetent patients, such as children and intellectually impaired individuals, have the same right of access to their medical laboratory records as competent adults.**

    A. True   B. False

14. **Parents always have the right of access to their children's medical records.**

    A. True   B. False

15. **Withholding health information from a patient may be justified when disclosure is contrary to the patient's best interests.**

    A. True   B. False

16. **All of the following statements regarding financial arrangement of the medical laboratories are true** *except*

    A. Medical laboratories must always be able to function with professional independence.
    B. Pathologists in private practice can self-refer work.
    C. Under special circumstances, medical laboratories may be subject to nonmedical control.
    D. There is a responsibility of the laboratory to be involved in the equitable allocation of resources.

17. **Hospitals and forensic pathology institutions should have adequate facilities to advise, counsel, and support bereaved relatives.**

    A. True   B. False

18. **All of the following statements regarding consent for autopsies are true** *except*

    A. Rejection by many religions and cultures of autopsies must be accepted.

    B. Consent for autopsies must always be followed meticulously.
    C. In academic institutions, tissues from autopsies may be retained for teaching without explanation to the senior next of kin.
    D. The laboratory should have a clear understanding of the procedures for authorizing an autopsy in the absence of any next of kin.

19. **All of the following statements regarding blood donation are true** *except*

    A. Blood donors should give their blood voluntarily and without expectation of payment.
    B. Blood should be collected under the supervision of a physician.
    C. Confidentiality concerning all personal donor details should be ensured.
    D. The donor has the right to know about results of tests on their blood but not the use to which their blood is put.

20. **In all circumstances, the patient needing blood is free to accept or refuse blood transfusion.**

    A. True   B. False

21. **All of the following statements regarding the regulations of blood donation according to the Code of Ethics for Blood Donation and Transfusion are true** *except*

    A. Suitable testing of each donor must be performed.
    B. Blood must be collected under the responsibility of a physician.
    C. Blood donation shall in all circumstances be voluntary.
    D. Financial profit may be a motive for blood donation.

22. **All of the following statements regarding the regulations of blood donation according to the Code of Ethics for Blood Donation and Transfusion are true** *except*

    A. Every red cell transfusion necessitates preliminary blood grouping testing on the recipient and compatibility testing between the donor and recipient.
    B. A written request signed by a physician must be made before any transfusion of blood or blood products.
    C. The actual transfusion must always be given under the responsibility of a physician.
    D. Regular contact between physicians and those who work in blood transfusion centers is required to ensure the optimal use of blood and blood products.

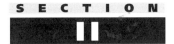

MOLECULAR PATHOLOGY

7 Introduction to Molecular Diagnostics
8 Molecular Biology of Inherited Diseases
9 Molecular Biology of Solid Tumors
10 Molecular Biology of Infectious Diseases
11 Clinical Applications of Molecular Biology of Hematopoietic Disorders

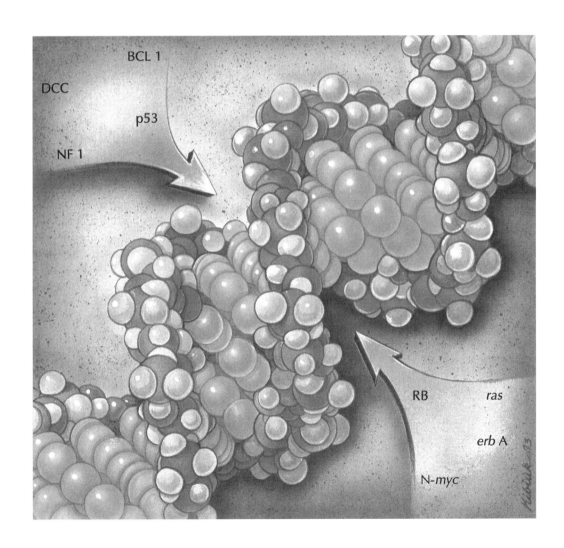

INTRODUCTION TO MOLECULAR DIAGNOSTICS

QUESTIONS

Select the one best answer of the choices offered.

1. **All of the following statements regarding nucleic acid structure are true *except***

   A. The nucleotides consist of a nitrogenous base, a pentose sugar, and phosphate.
   B. On the deoxyribonucleic acid (DNA) strands, the thymine base pairs with the adenine base.
   C. The two strands of DNA are complementary.
   D. The two strands of nucleotides are oriented in a parallel fashion.

2. **All of the following statements regarding DNA replication are true *except***

   A. Helicase enzyme breaks the hydrogen bonds between the base pairs.
   B. The junction between the separated DNA strands and the hydrogen-bounded strands is called the replication fork.
   C. DNA replication of the lagging strand is semidiscontinuous.
   D. DNA ligase enzyme is necessary for replication of the leading strand.

3. **All of the following statements regarding gene structure and expression are true *except***

   A. Exons code for proteins.
   B. Introns govern transcription of a gene.
   C. A codon consists of a triplet of nucleotides that specifies one amino acid.
   D. The process of gene expression involves the translation of messenger ribonucleic acid (mRNA) into protein.

4. **All of the following statements regarding gene structure and expression are true *except***

   A. The TATA box is the most common enhancer sequence.
   B. Enhancers increase the rate of transcription.
   C. Enhancers of immunoglobulin gene expression are only active in B lymphocytes.
   D. All cells within the higher eukaryotic organism contain the same sequence of DNA.

5. **All of the following statements regarding gene structure and expression are true *except***

   A. The *trans*-activator domain mediates the cooperative association of the transcription factors.
   B. There are two different types of transcription factors.
   C. The *trans*-activator is a motif of transcription factors.
   D. The general transcription factors are needed for mRNA initiation or termination.

6. **All of the following statements regarding gene structure and expression are true *except***

   A. Splicing is the process of linking the introns to heterogeneous nuclear RNA (hnRNA).
   B. The cap helps the 40S ribosomal subunit to find and bind to the mRNA in the cytoplasm.
   C. The enzyme adenosine terminal transferase adds a polyadenylate tail to hnRNA.
   D. The introns present in the hnRNA molecule must be removed before translation of mRNA.

7. **All of the following statements regarding protein synthesis are true *except***

   A. The process by which mRNA is decoded into protein is called translation.
   B. Translation requires two different types of RNA, transfer RNA (tRNA) and ribosomal RNA (rRNA).
   C. Translation begins after binding of the 60S ribosomal subunit to mRNA in the cytoplasm.
   D. Protein synthesis begins after assembly of the 80S complex.

8. **All of the following statements regarding the melting temperature (Tm) of the nucleic acid duplex are true *except***

   A. Tm is the temperature at which a specific double-stranded DNA sequence denatures.
   B. The three major factors affecting Tm are the ionic strength of the solution, the presence of specific denaturing agents, and the base composition of the particular nucleic acid sequence.
   C. The maximum rate of hybridization occurs at temperatures approximately 20°C to 25°C below the Tm of the nucleic acid duplex.
   D. Hybridization tends to be fast at temperatures approaching the Tm of the nucleic acid duplex.

Match each of the following definitions with the corresponding process.

9. **Transferring RNA out of the gel onto a filter**

10. **Transferring DNA out of the gel onto a filter**

11. **Transferring protein out of the gel onto a filter**
    A. Southern blotting
    B. Western blotting
    C. Northern blotting

12. **All of the following statements regarding the restriction fragment length polymorphism technique are true except**

    A. It requires highly purified DNA of high molecular weight.
    B. It is not sufficiently sensitive for small deletions or insertions.
    C. It requires 7 to 10 days to obtain a result.
    D. It requires small quantities of DNA.

13. **All of the following statements regarding the different physical and chemical approaches implemented to avoid amplicon contamination in the polymerase chain reaction (PCR) technique are true except**

    A. The PCR technique should be performed in the postamplification area.
    B. Sample preparation should not be performed where biologic amplification has been conducted.
    C. Incorporation of dUTP into the DNA template.
    D. Sample preparation should be confined to the preamplification area.

14. **Signal amplification by branched DNA technology utilizes RNA probes for detection of a DNA target sequence.**

    A. True   B. False

Match each of the following methods for solid support hybridization with the corresponding description (each answer might be used more than once).

15. **Dot-blot**

16. **Slot-blot**

17. **Spot-blot**

18. **Reverse dot-blot**
    A. PCR-amplified fragments are placed in a small well and then drawn under vacuum through the membrane filter.
    B. PCR-amplified fragments are simply spotted onto a nitrocellulose or nylon filter.
    C. Oligo probe is bound to the solid phase support and the denatured amplified product is hybridized to the bound oligo probe.

MOLECULAR BIOLOGY OF INHERITED DISEASES

QUESTIONS

Select the one best answer of the choices offered.

1. **All of the following statements regarding autosomal recessive disorders are true *except***
   A. Individuals with one normal and one mutant gene copy are termed carriers.
   B. Autosomal recessive disorders are close to 100% penetrant.
   C. Autosomal recessive disorders show significant phenotypic variability for identical genotypes.
   D. Neither parent exhibits signs of disease.

2. **All of the following statements regarding X-linked recessive disorders are true *except***
   A. They affect males but never affect females.
   B. Females are similar to carriers of autosomal recessive disorders.
   C. Hypophosphatemic rickets is an X-linked dominant disorder.
   D. Mutant chromosomes never transmit to a male from an affected father.

3. **All of the following statements regarding mitochondrially inherited disorders are true *except***
   A. They are transmitted only by females.
   B. They affect only female offspring.
   C. Heteroplasty leads to significant variability of disease expression.
   D. They are associated with encephalopathies and myopathies.

Match each of the following inherited disorders with the corresponding pattern of inheritance.

4. **β-Thalassemia**

5. **Leber hereditary optic neuropathy**

6. **Glucose-6-phosphate dehydrogenase deficiency**

7. **Hypophosphatemic rickets**

8. **Hereditary breast cancer**
   A. Autosomal dominant
   B. X-linked dominant
   C. Mitochondrial
   D. X-linked recessive
   E. Autosomal recessive

Match each of the following inherited disorders with the corresponding affected gene(s).

9. **Osteogenesis imperfecta**

10. **Neurofibromatosis, type II**

11. **Marfan syndrome**

12. **Hypophosphatemic rickets**

13. **Fragile X syndrome**
   A. PHEX
   B. MERLIN
   C. FMR-1
   D. Fibrillin
   E. Type I collagen

Match each of the following disorders with the corresponding type of genetic mutation (each answer might be used more than once).

14. **Prader-Willi syndrome**

15. **Charcot-Marie-Tooth disease, type 1A**

16. **Gaucher disease**

17. **Autosomal recessive spinal muscular atrophy**

18. **Hypercoagulability—factor V Leiden**
   A. Gene duplication
   B. Imprinted genes
   C. Point mutations
   D. Gene deletion

19. **All of the following statements regarding cystic fibrosis are true *except***
   A. Cystic fibrosis is an autosomal recessive disorder.
   B. Cystic fibrosis is rare in Asians.
   C. The pathogenesis of cystic fibrosis comprises a three-nucleotide deletion of sequences encoding a tyrosine residue at position 508 of the cystic fibrosis transmembrane conductance regulator (CFTR) protein.
   D. >700 different mutations of cystic fibrosis have been identified.

20. **All of the following statements regarding Duchenne/Becker muscular dystrophy are true *except***
   A. The dystrophin gene is the largest of the human genes.
   B. Two phenotypes exist, mild and severe.
   C. Southern blot analysis can be used to identify carrier females.
   D. Approximately two thirds of patients show deletion or duplication of a moderately large region of the dystrophin gene on the short arm of chromosome 1.

21. **Which of the following statements regarding myotonic dystrophy is *true*?**
   A. Transmitting parents of adult patients demonstrate few to no symptoms.
   B. Children of affected adults show five to 30 CTG repeats.
   C. The molecular basis of the disease involves variable expansion of a CTG repeat in the 3′ untranslated region of the tyrosine kinase gene.

   D. Age of onset decreases in successive generations.

22. **All of the following statements regarding hereditary cancer syndromes are true *except***
   A. BRCA1 is located on chromosome 17 and BRCA2 on chromosome 13.
   B. Women who have not inherited a mutant BRCA1/BRCA2 gene have a negligible risk of developing breast cancer.
   C. The c-ret oncogene associated with familial MEN II shows a restricted range of mutations confined to several axons.
   D. Full sequencing of BRCA1/BRCA2 is an option only through a single provider.

23. **All of the following statements regarding hereditary hemochromatosis (HFE) are true except**
   A. The most common variation of the HFE is a point mutation that changes histidine to aspartic acid at residue 63 (H63D).
   B. The HFE gene is located on chromosome 6.
   C. Individuals heterozygous for the C282Y mutation have increased risk of cardiac and cerebrovascular diseases.
   D. Hemochromatosis is the most common autosomal recessive disorder in whites.

24. **All of the following statements regarding activated protein C (APC) resistance are true *except***
   A. Approximately 94% of patients with APC resistance are factor V Leiden heterozygotes.
   B. Approximately 60% of patients with recurrent venous thromboses or thromboembolic events are factor V Leiden heterozygotes.
   C. The genetic basis of APC resistance usually is a deletion in the gene for coagulation factor V.
   D. Direct mutation assays to determine factor V Leiden genotype offer several advantages over the functional APC resistance assay.

9

MOLECULAR BIOLOGY OF SOLID TUMORS

QUESTIONS

Match each of the following oncogenes with its major function.

1. HER2/neu

2. N-myc

3. Sis

4. Raf

5. Bcl-x

6. PRAD1

    A. Inhibitor of apoptosis
    B. Growth factor
    C. Cytoplasmic signal transduction modulator
    D. Cell cycle enhancer
    E. Growth factor receptor
    F. Nuclear transcription factor

Match each of the following oncogenes with the mechanism of inappropriate expression.

7. c-erb B-2

8. ras gene

9. N-myc

10. EWS gene

    A. Amplification
    B. Translocation
    C. Mutation

11. All of the following are among the mechanisms of antitumorigenesis *except*

    A. suppression of deoxyribonucleic acid (DNA) replication
    B. chromosomal stability
    C. loss of heterozygosity
    D. promotion of apoptosis

Match each of the following oncogene translocations with the corresponding disease.

12. EWS-WT1 [t(11;22)]

13. SYT-SSX [t(X;18)]

14. PAX3-FKHR [t(2;13)]

15. EWS-FLI-1 [t(11;22)]

    A. Ewing sarcoma
    B. Desmoplastic small round cell tumor
    C. Alveolar rhabdomyosarcoma
    D. Synovial sarcoma

16. All of the following statements regarding microsatellites are true *except*

    A. Microsatellites are the usual markers for studying loss of heterozygosity.
    B. Changes in microsatellites are detected in 95% of individuals with bladder cancer.
    C. Microsatellites are DNA regions.
    D. Microsatellites are mapped only throughout the autosomes.

Match each of the following prognostic molecular alterations and the corresponding tumor.

17. TRK-A expression

18. Loss of heterozygosity at RB1 locus

19. 22q–

20. Loss of heterozygosity at 17p

21. Loss of heterozygosity at 13q

   A. PNET
   B. Neuroblastoma
   C. Prostate cancer
   D. Retinoblastoma
   E. Gliomas

Match each of the following inherited cancer syndromes with the corresponding predisposition gene.

22. Familial melanoma

23. Li-Fraumeni syndrome

24. Ataxia telangiectasia

25. Ovarian cancer

26. men2a/b

   A. BRCA
   B. ATM
   C. p53
   D. MLM1
   E. RET

27. All of the following statements regarding inherited cancer syndromes are true *except*

   A. Approximately 25% of breast and ovarian cancers have been linked to mutations in the BRCA1/BRCA2 tumor suppressor genes.
   B. Prophylactic colectomy is the treatment of choice for individuals at risk for familial adenomatous polyposis.
   C. Individuals with a 50% risk of inheriting mutations in the RET protooncogene can develop medullary thyroid carcinoma as early as 6 years of age.
   D. Carriers of mutations of MLH1 are at 80% lifetime risk to develop colon cancer.

10

MOLECULAR BIOLOGY OF INFECTIOUS DISEASES

QUESTIONS

Select the one best answer of the choices offered.

1. All of the following are steps of the polymerase chain reaction (PCR) *except*

   A. polymerization
   B. extension
   C. denaturation
   D. annealing

Match each of the following temperatures with the corresponding step of PCR.

2. 72°C

3. 52°C

4. 94°C

   A. Denaturation
   B. Primer annealing
   C. Extension

Match each of the following definitions with the corresponding step of PCR.

5. Double-stranded deoxyribonucleic acid (DNA) is melted

6. Binding to the single-stranded DNA

7. Filling in the gap

   A. Denaturation
   B. Primer annealing
   C. Extension

8. The thermal cyclers used in PCR with the best cost-effectiveness and short assay time utilize

   A. laser
   B. water
   C. metal blocks
   D. air

9. Comparison of air versus heat block thermal cyclers for *Mycobacterium tuberculosis* (MTB)-positive specimens shows high sensitivity for both types of thermal cyclers.

   A. True   B. False

Match each of the following with the corresponding step of extraction of nucleic acids.

10. Phenol-chloroform-isoamyl alcohol

11. *N*-acetyl-L-cysteine

12. Sodium dodecyl sulfate

13. Dialysis

   A. Cell lysis
   B. Digestion-decontamination
   C. Water
   D. Extraction

14. Use of single-copy genes as targets for amplification in PCR is more sensitive than use of targets that constitute repeated DNA or ribonucleic acid (RNA) sequences.

   A. True   B. False

15. All of the following are disadvantages of using IS6110 as a sequence for amplification in the MTB complex except

   A. A few strains have only one copy of IS6110.
   B. Decreased sensitivity of the PCR assay.
   C. Homology might exist with mycobacteria other than MTB.
   D. Rare MTB strains might lack IS6110.

16. Messenger RNA is extremely short-lived and has been used in reverse transcriptase (RT)-PCR formats to detect viable mycobacteria.

   A. True   B. False

17. **All of the following regarding the mtp40 gene used to differentiate MTB from *Mycobacterium bovis* by PCR are true *except***

    A. mtp40 gene is part of the mpcA gene.
    B. mtp40 gene encodes a phospholipase C protein.
    C. mtp40 gene is present in all strains of MTB.
    D. *M. bovis* is more resistant to pyrazinamide.

18. **All of the following are advantages of two-tube nested PCR *except***

    A. decreased false positives
    B. decreased inhibitors of PCR in the clinical samples
    C. increased sensitivity
    D. less risk of contamination

19. **All of the following are advantages of one-tube nested PCR *except***

    A. less expensive than two-tube nested PCR
    B. less contamination risks than two-tube nested PCR
    C. decreased inhibitors of PCR in the clinical samples
    D. increased sensitivity

20. **All of the following regarding methods used to nullify or detect the presence of inhibitors of PCR amplification in clinical specimens are true *except***

    A. column chromatography
    B. two-step nested PCR
    C. centrifugation through a sucrose gradient
    D. one-step nested PCR

21. **All of the following are measures to increase the sensitivity of PCR *except***

    A. use of internal control sequences
    B. adding more lysed specimen to the amplification tube
    C. use of spin columns
    D. use of PCR amplification of samples previously submitted to broth enrichment

Match each of the following definitions with the corresponding amplification method.

22. **Ribosomal RNA substrates are converted to single-stranded DNA substrates that are then transcribed into an RNA amplicon.**

23. **DNA is produced in large quantities from a DNA template.**

24. **RNA templates are converted to single-stranded DNA templates that serve as substrate for the production of multiple DNA particles during amplification.**

    A. RT-PCR
    B. Transcription-mediated amplification (TMA)
    C. PCR

25. **All of the following are advantages of TMA assays *except***

    A. two-tube format
    B. single temperature
    C. results available on the same day
    D. no nucleic acid purification

26. **All of the following are features of the Gen-Probe AMTDT-1 format for the detection of MTB *except***

    A. TMA.
    B. DNA is the amplification product.
    C. Chemiluminescence is the method of detection.
    D. Reverse transcriptase is the enzyme utilized.

27. **All of the following statements regarding versions 1 and 2 of the AMTDT assay for detection of MTB are true *except***

    A. Version 2 is more sensitive with smear negative specimens.
    B. Version 2 is more susceptible to inhibitory substances.
    C. Discrepancy of the results is found in 20% of samples.
    D. Incorporation of internal controls into the two versions would increase confidence in the reliability of the negative results.

28. **All of the following are features of the Roche Amplicor MWP format for detection of MTB *except***

    A. Taq polymerase is the enzyme utilized.
    B. DNA is the amplification product.
    C. Enzyme immunoassay is the method of detection.
    D. Single tube is the format.

11

CLINICAL APPLICATIONS OF MOLECULAR BIOLOGY OF HEMATOPOIETIC DISORDERS

QUESTIONS

Select the one best answer of the choices offered.

1. **The immunoglobulin genes, but not the T-cell receptor genes, are composed of three or four basic gene regions: variable (V), diversity (D), joining (J), and constant (C) regions.**

   A. True   B. False

2. **All of the following statements regarding the immunoglobulin genes are true *except***

   A. The κ light chain gene is located on chromosome 2p12.
   B. The first rearrangement step in the early B-precursor cell begins with the κ light chain gene locus.
   C. The heavy chain gene contains nine C region genes.
   D. Heavy chain gene rearrangement begins with one D region gene recombining with one J region gene.

3. **All of the following statements regarding the immunoglobulin genes are true *except***

   A. If the initial D-J or V-D-J heavy chain gene rearrangement encodes for a termination or non-sense codon, the transcription of the gene becomes "nonproductive."
   B. If the second attempt at heavy chain gene rearrangement is unsuccessful, the B-precursor cell will die.
   C. If the second attempt at κ light chain gene rearrangement is unsuccessful, the B-precursor cell will die.
   D. The κ gene lacks any known D regions.

4. **One mechanism of isotype switching involves the transcription of a long V-D-J-Cm-Cd transcript, which results in the formation of a mixture of V-D-J-Cm and V-D-J-Cd messenger RNA and, consequently, immunoglobulin M and immunoglobulin D.**

   A. True   B. False

5. **All of the following statements regarding T-cell receptor genes are true *except***

   A. The β-positive T cells predominate in epithelial and epidermal locations.
   B. The most common T-cell receptor is composed of α- and β-chains.
   C. The α-chain gene is located on chromosome 14q11.
   D. The δ-chain gene is located on chromosome 14q11.

6. **All of the following statements regarding the T-cell receptor genes are true *except***

   A. The γ-chain gene contains 11 V regions and only two J loci, which leads to limited diversity in this gene subset.
   B. The δ-chain gene is located entirely within the α-chain gene.
   C. The γ-chain gene is located on chromosome 22q11.
   D. A polyclonal mixture of T lymphocytes can demonstrate what appears to be oligoclonal rearrangement of Tγ gene.

7. **Southern blot analysis of clonal rearrangement of either the immunoglobulin or T-cell receptor genes is capable of detecting a clonal proliferation, if the specimen being studied contains 5% monoclonal cells.**

   A. True   B. False

8. **Agarose gel and polyacrylamide gel are equivalent in the evaluation of monoclonality by polymerase chain reaction (PCR).**

   A. True   B. False

9. **All of the following statements regarding laboratory analysis of DNA are true *except***

   A. The most commonly used immunoglobulin heavy chain gene probe is complementary to the JH region.

B. The most commonly used gene probe for T-cell receptor gene rearrangement is complementary to the T-cell receptor β-chain gene.

C. It is essential that multiple restriction enzymes be used when evaluating the T-cell receptor β-chain gene.

D. The limitation of using the *Eco*RI restriction enzyme for T-cell receptor β-chain analysis is its inability to detect rearrangement involving the β1 locus.

10. All of the following statements regarding laboratory analysis of T-cell receptor gene rearrangement are true *except*

A. *Bam*HI restriction enzyme analysis will show rearrangements involving either the β1 or β2 locus.

B. The large size of the germline band seen with *Hind*III restriction enzyme may be difficult to distinguish from rearranged fragments.

C. Analysis with *Eco*RI restriction enzyme will demonstrate rearrangements of the β1 locus.

D. Analysis with *Hind*III restriction enzyme will demonstrate rearrangements of the β2 locus.

11. Apparent loss of T-cell antigen expression is consistent with T-cell malignancy.

A. True   B. False

Match each of the following chromosomal translocations with the corresponding non-Hodgkin lymphoma.

12. t(14;19)(q32;q13.1)

13. t(14;18)(q32;q31)

14. t(2;5)(p23;q35)

15. t(8;22)(q24;q11)

16. t(9;14)(p13;q32)

A. Burkitt lymphoma
B. Anaplastic large cell lymphoma
C. Lymphoplasmacytic lymphoma
D. Small lymphocytic lymphoma
E. Follicular lymphoma

Match each of the following oncogenes with the corresponding non-Hodgkin lymphoma.

17. Bcl-6

18. NPM-ALK

19. Bcl-3

20. Cyclin D1

21. PAX5

A. Mantle cell lymphoma
B. Lymphoplasmacytic lymphoma
C. Diffuse large cell lymphoma
D. Anaplastic large cell lymphoma
E. Small lymphocytic lymphoma

22. All of the following statements regarding chromosomal aberrations in hematopoietic malignancies are true *except*

A. The most common cytogenetic aberrations in chronic lymphocytic leukemia (CLL) are trisomy 12 and structure abnormalities involving the long arm of chromosome 13.

B. The *PAX5* gene is located on the short arm of chromosome 9 and encodes the B-cell–specific activator protein (BSAP).

C. The retinoblastoma gene is located on the long arm of chromosome 13.

D. Deletions of 13q usually are associated with atypical morphology in CLL.

23. All of the following statements regarding chromosomal aberrations in lymphoplasmacytic lymphoma are true *except*

A. t(9;14)(p13;q32) is associated with lymphoplasmacytic lymphoma.

B. Hepatitis C virus infection is highly prevalent in lymphoplasmacytic lymphoma.

C. Functional arrest of the *PAX5* gene causes blastic transformation of B lymphocytes.

D. Overexpression of the *PAX5* gene results in proliferation of splenic B lymphocytes.

24. All of the following statements regarding chromosomal aberrations in hematopoietic malignancies are true *except*

A. PCR analysis is superior to cytogenetics studies in detecting *Bcl-1* translocations.

B. t(11;14)(q13;q32) involves rearrangement of the *Bcl-1* protooncogene from chromosome 11 to the immunoglobulin heavy chain gene on chromosome 14.

C. The *Bcl-1* locus is rearranged in 50% to 80% of mantle cell lymphomas by using Southern blotting.

D. t(11;14)(q13;q32) results in overexpression of cyclin D1.

25. All of the following statements regarding follicular lymphomas are true *except*

A. Expression of the *Bcl-2* protein requires t(14;18) (q32;q31).
B. Follicular lymphoma patients with the major break-point region (MBR) or minor cluster region (mcr) type of translocation involving the *Bcl-2* gene are less likely to show complete remission compared with patients with germline pattern.
C. Expression of the *Bcl-2* protein is seen in follicular lymphomas.
D. *Bcl-2* is an antiapoptotic protein.

26. All of the following statements regarding the *Bcl-2* family are true *except*

A. *Bcl-XL* functions as inhibitor of apoptosis.
B. Overexpression of *Bcl-2* is specific for follicular lymphomas.
C. Detection of *Bcl-2* gene translocation by PCR can be performed on formalin-fixed tissue embedded in paraffin.
D. BAX is a proapoptotic protein.

27. All of the following statements regarding Burkitt lymphoma are true *except*

A. The endemic form of Burkitt lymphoma typically affects children between 5 and 10 years of age.
B. The endemic form of Burkitt lymphoma usually presents with involvement of jaw, abdominal, and extranodal sites.
C. Clonal integration of Epstein-Barr virus is seen in 95% of the nonendemic, sporadic form of Burkitt lymphoma.
D. Presence of the Epstein-Barr virus genome in Burkitt lymphoma has been implicated in neoplastic transformation.

28. All of the following statements regarding Epstein-Barr virus are true *except*

A. Type A Epstein-Barr virus infects immunocompetent individuals more commonly than type B virus.
B. There is a nearly equal mix of type A and type B virus in endemic Burkitt lymphoma.
C. LMP1 is a transforming protein that interacts with tumor necrosis factor receptor (TNFR)-associated factors.
D. Type B Epstein-Barr virus predominates in Hodgkin disease and posttransplant lymphoproliferative disorder.

29. All of the following hematopoietic neoplasms are associated with human herpes virus 8 (HHV-8) *except*

A. posttransplant lymphoproliferative disorders
B. multiple myeloma
C. primary effusion lymphoma

D. angioimmunoblastic lymphadenopathy with dysproteinemia

30. All of the following statements regarding primary effusion lymphoma are true *except*

A. It involves the body cavities secondary to mass lesions.
B. It occurs predominantly in patients infected with human immunodeficiency virus (HIV).
C. It usually is associated with Epstein-Barr virus infection.
D. Primary effusion lymphoma cells are usually of the late B-cell phenotype.

31. All of the following statements regarding Hodgkin disease are true *except*

A. Reed-Sternberg cells represent only 0.1% to 1% of the cells in tissues involved with Hodgkin disease.
B. The lymphocyte-depleted type is biologically different from other categories of Hodgkin disease.
C. The prevalence of Epstein-Barr virus is extremely rare in lymphocyte-predominant Hodgkin disease.
D. Reed-Sternberg cells are derived from germinal center B cells.

32. Sézary cells typically show dual expression of the T-cell markers CD4 and CD8.

A. True   B. False

33. All of the following statements regarding anaplastic large cell lymphoma are true *except*

A. ALK-positive anaplastic large cell lymphoma has a better prognosis.
B. Great majority of cutaneous anaplastic large cell lymphoma is negative for ALK expression.
C. Anaplastic large cell lymphoma is of T- or NK-cell phenotype.
D. Expression of CD30/Ki-1 antigen by anaplastic large cell lymphoma does not correlate with the presence of NPM-ALK.

Match each of the following genes with the corresponding acute leukemia.

34. PML-RARα

35. BCR-ABL

36. CBFβ-MYH

37. MYC-IgH

38. Acute myelogenous leukemia (AML) 1-ETO

A. AML-M3
B. AML-M2
C. Precursor B-acute lymphoblastic leukemia (B-ALL)
D. AML-M4Eo
E. B-ALL

Match each of the following chromosomal aberrations with the corresponding acute leukemia.

39. t(12;21)(p13;q22)

40. inv(16)(p13;q22)

41. t(15;17)(q22;q21)

42. t(8;21)(q22;q22)

43. t(8;14)(q24;q32)

    A. B-ALL
    B. Precursor B-ALL
    C. AML-M4Eo
    D. AML-M3
    E. AML-M2

44. All of the following statements regarding chromosomal aberrations in AML are true except
    A. t(8;21)(q22;q22), which is encountered frequently in AML-M2, is associated with a good prognosis.
    B. The most common translocation in AML-M3 is t(15;17)(q22;q21).
    C. AML-M3 with t(11;17)(q23;q21) is more sensitive to all-*trans* retinoic acid therapy.
    D. t(16;16) is seen in AML-M4Eo.

45. All of the following chromosomal translocations occur in ALL except
    A. t(12;21)(p13;q22)
    B. t(4;11)(q21;q23)
    C. t(15;17)(q22;q21)
    D. t(1;19)(q23;p13)

46. All of the following statements regarding chromosomal aberrations in chronic myelogenous leukemia (CML) are true except
    A. Fluorescence *in situ* hybridization (FISH) and PCR are superior to cytogenetic analysis in detecting the *BCR-ABL* fusion gene in minimal residual disease.
    B. PCR allows identification of a single Ph-positive cell among 10^4 to 10^8 normal cells.
    C. CML is commonly associated with p190 *BCR-ABL* fusion protein.

    D. p190 *BCR-ABL* fusion protein has a more tyrosine kinase activity than p210 *BCR-ABL*.

47. ALL with *BCR-ABL* transcript has a significantly shorter duration of remission, which is associated with shorter survival.
    A. True   B. False

48. All of the following statements regarding chromosomal aberrations in ALL are true except
    A. t(4;11)(q21;q23) is associated with a very poor prognosis.
    B. Myeloid lymphoid leukemia (MLL) gene is located on chromosome 4q21.
    C. The frequency of 11q23 abnormalities reaches 60% to 70% in infant ALL.
    D. The frequency of 11q23 abnormalities is higher in patients treated with topoisomerase II inhibitors.

49. All of the following statements regarding chromosomal aberrations in ALL are true *except*
    A. The most common chromosomal abnormality in pediatric ALL is t(12;21)(p13;q22).
    B. t(12;21)(p13;q22) is associated with a poor prognosis.
    C. The frequency of t(12;21)(p13;q22) is low in adults.
    D. t(12;21)(p13;q22) involves the *TEL-AML1* genes.

50. All of the following statements regarding paroxysmal nocturnal hemoglobinuria (PNH) are true *except*
    A. PNH often arises in patients with aplastic anemia.
    B. PNH is an autosomal recessive genetic disorder.
    C. Decay accelerating protein and CD59 are deficient in PNH.
    D. PNH is a clonal disease.

51. All of the following statements regarding hereditary hemochromatosis (HH) are true *except*
    A. HH is an autosomal recessive genetic disorder.
    B. *HEF* is the gene responsible for HH and it encodes an HLA class II-like protein.
    C. HH is very common among whites.
    D. Investigation of siblings of a homozygote is required.

52. All of the following statements regarding factor V Leiden are true *except*
    A. Factor V Leiden is the most common cause of activated protein C resistance.
    B. The mutation in factor V Leiden gene involves a single point mutation that causes a change in amino acid arginine at position 506 to glutamine.

C. A minority of patients develop abnormalities involving other portions of factor V Leiden.

D. Most of the patients with activated protein C resistance are homozygous for factor V Leiden mutations.

53. All of the following statements regarding von Willebrand disease are true except

A. Next to hemophilia, von Willebrand disease is the second most common inherited bleeding disorder.

B. The role of molecular studies is limited in the diagnosis of von Willebrand disease.

C. The qualitative defects in von Willebrand disease include type 2.

D. von Willebrand factor stabilizes factor VIII.

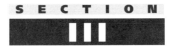
CLINICAL CHEMISTRY

12 Immunochemical Methods

13 Plasma Proteins

14 Diagnostic Enzymology and Other Biochemical Markers of Organ Damage

15 Lipids and Lipoproteins

16 Endocrine Function and Carbohydrate

17 Electrolytes and Acid–Base Balance

18 Respiration and Measurement of Oxygen and Hemoglobin

19 Nitrogen Metabolites and Renal Function

20 Calcium, Magnesium, and Phosphate

21 Heme Synthesis and Catabolism

22 Toxicology

23 Trace Elements, Vitamins, and Nutrition

24 Inborn Metabolic Errors

25 Point-of-Care Testing

26 Tumor Markers

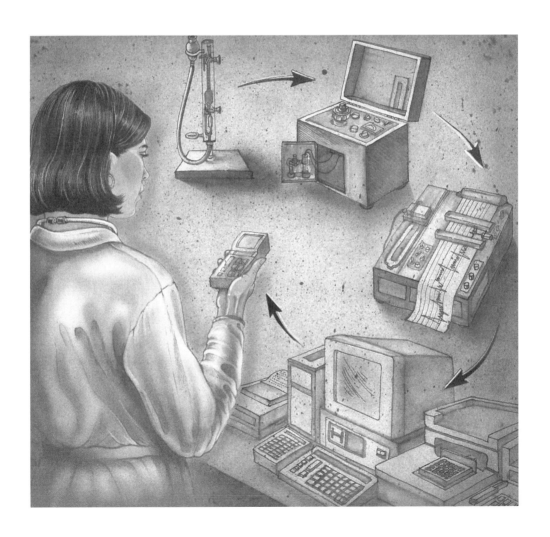

IMMUNOCHEMICAL METHODS

QUESTIONS

Select the one best answer of the choices offered.

1. **All of the following statements regarding immunogens are true *except***

   A. Immunogens usually are large complex molecules.
   B. Immunogens usually differ significantly from normal molecular species found in the host.
   C. Synthetic peptides usually are better immunogens than molecules containing lipid, nucleic acid, or carbohydrate moieties.
   D. Molecules with a complex tertiary structure are better immunogens than linear synthetic peptides.

2. **Figure 12.1 shows a schematic diagram of an immunoglobulin G (IgG) antibody. Which of the following statements is *true*?**

   A. The IgG antibody contains two identical heavy chains.
   B. The heavy chain of the IgG antibody is designated γ and the two light chains either κ or λ.
   C. Digestion of IgG with papain produces three fragments (two Fab and one Fc), whereas digestion with pepsin produces an F(ab′)$_2$ fragment and the body of the IgG is digested to small fragments.
   D. There are three binding sites on the IgG antibody.

3. **Which of the following statements regarding production of antibodies in animals is *true*?**

   A. A broad spectrum of antibodies will be produced.
   B. The antibodies produced are all formed in approximately the same quantity for the immunogen.
   C. Each lymphocyte that is stimulated by the immunogen produces a different type of antibody.
   D. Use of animals challenged with an immunogen rarely produces antibodies in sufficient quantity for *in vitro* use.

4. **All of the following statements regarding monoclonal antibodies (mAbs) are true *except***

   A. mAbs recognize a single antigenic determinant.
   B. mAbs almost always exhibit high affinity.
   C. It may be difficult to produce mAbs of high specificity for small molecules.
   D. The analytical utility of mAbs may be improved by combining the antibodies from multiple clones.

5. **All of the following statements regarding antigen–antibody interactions are true *except***

   A. The antigen–antibody reaction is irreversible.
   B. Antibodies useful for diagnostic assays exhibit high K_a (association constant) values.
   C. Antibodies with low K_d (dissociation constant) bind tightly to the specific antigen.
   D. Assays using antibodies with a small K_a tend to be insensitive.

6. **Intermolecular forces that determine the antigen–antibody complex include all of the following *except***

   A. ionic bonds
   B. hydrogen bonds
   C. covalent bonds
   D. van der Waals forces

7. **Figure 12.2 shows a titration curve for complex formation using a constant quantity of antibody and increasing amounts of antigen. All of the following statements are true *except***

   A. Precipitation increases gradually to a maximum, then decreases.
   B. In the area of antibody excess, each antigen molecule has the maximal complement of antibody but each epitope has a different antibody bound.
   C. With antibody excess, there is maximal cross-linking of antigens forming large complexes.
   D. At the point of antigen–antibody equivalence, there is maximal precipitation.

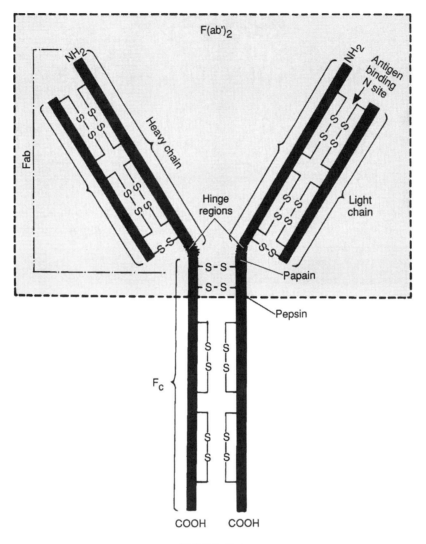

FIGURE 12.1.

8. **Regarding the aggregation inhibition reaction, indicate which of the following statements is *true*.**
   A. The reaction uses antigen-coated particles, such as animal red blood cells or latex beads, as a reagent.
   B. Antigen in the solution to be measured promotes aggregation of free antibodies with the antigen-coated particles.
   C. The concentration of antigen in the test solution is directly proportional to the amount of aggregation.
   D. Agglutination inhibition assays can be titered with a series of standard solutions to produce a precise measurement of the antigen in the test solution.

9. **All of the following statements regarding radial immunodiffusion are true *except***

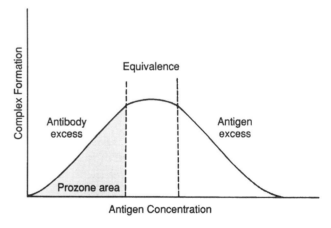

FIGURE 12.2.

A. Radial immunodiffusion utilizes a gel support medium such as agar or agarose.

B. The rate of diffusion of antigen and antibody through the gel depends on the concentration and molecular size of the antigen and antibody and on the lattice structure of the gel.

C. Precipitation occurs at the point where the antigen and antibody are in equivalence.

D. Antigens or antibodies of higher concentration diffuse more slowly than those of lower concentration.

10. Figure 12.4 shows four radial immunodiffusion plates. All of the following statements are true *except*

A. The precipitation line shown in plate A exhibits no spurs or cross-lines indicating an arc of identity.

B. Plate C shows a line of partial identity (PID) and a line of identity (ID).

C. A double precipitin line (DB) seen in plate B occurs only with immunoglobulin M (IgM) antibodies.

D. The plates in Fig. 12.4 show examples of the Ouchterlony technique.

11. All of the following statements regarding the Ouchterlony technique are true *except*

A. The technique is inexpensive.

B. The technique is highly sensitive.

C. If the concentrations of antigen and antibody are not in a reasonable relationship, no precipitin line may form.

D. The technique is useful to identify antigens.

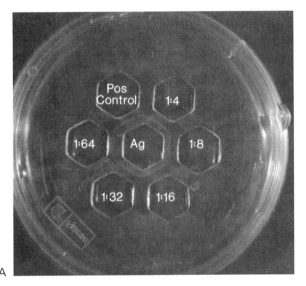
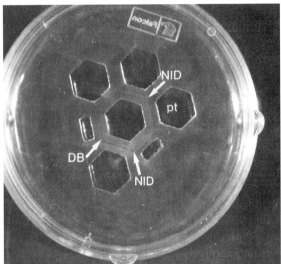
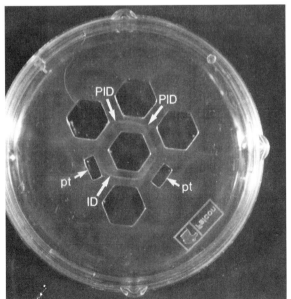
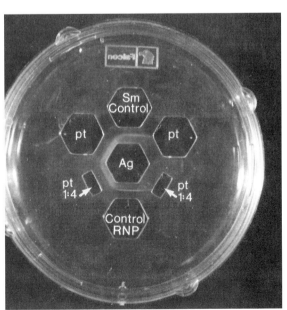

FIGURE 12.4.

12. The Mancini technique for gel diffusion _____.

A. uses antibody in a liquid support medium
B. uses antibody incorporated directly into an agarose gel that is poured onto a solid support, forming a plate
C. shows significant antibody denaturation if the gel is heated above 50°C
D. does not provide a quantitative estimate of the amount of antigen in the test solution

13. All of the following statements regarding immuno-electrophoretic techniques are true *except*

A. They are useful for analyzing test solutions with a simple number of components.
B. They are useful for analyzing test solutions with multiple components of very similar chemical characters.
C. They separate components in a solution based on size and charge.
D. They can efficiently separate very similar molecules, which can be quantitated using immunotechniques.

14. All of the following statements regarding Laurell rocket immunoelectrophoresis are true *except*

A. It uses antibody dispersed into an agarose gel.
B. the pH of the gel is set at 8.6 and the isoelectric point of most IgG antibodies.
C. Under an electric field, the antibodies migrate through a gel, forming a triangular spike-shaped precipitin arc.
D. The area inside the triangular precipitation front is directly proportional to antigen concentration.

15. Which of the following statements regarding crossed immunoelectrophoresis is *true*?

A. Other names for this technique include double crossed immunoelectrophoresis and two-dimensional immunoelectrophoresis.
B. The technique can analyze only two antigens at the same time.
C. The technique is not useful for metabolic studies involving interconversion of initial reactant and product.
D. It should use a high antibody concentration and a high electric field strength.

16. All of the following statements regarding immuno-electrophoresis are true *except*

A. It is rarely used in the clinical laboratory.
B. It can be used to process large numbers of specimens and can be automated.
C. It is mainly utilized for identifying serum proteins, especially monoclonal gammopathies, light chains, and protein deficiencies.

D. It may use antiserum directed against multiple proteins or be specific for a single protein.

17. Figure 12.6 shows an immunofixation electrophoresis and immunoelectrophoresis on a patient serum sample. Which of the following statements is *correct*?

A. The patient exhibits a diffuse hypergammaglobulinemia.
B. The control specimen on the immunoelectrophoresis failed to reach with the IgM antibody.
C. The patient exhibits an IgG κ monoclonal gammopathy.
D. The patient's κ arc shown on immunoelectrophoresis exhibits a normal shape but an increased concentration.

18. All of the following statements regarding immunofixation electrophoresis are true *except*

A. It may be performed on serum, urine, or cerebrospinal fluid.
B. Individual globulins and light chains can be directly compared with the corresponding bands seen on the electrophoresis pattern of whole serum.
C. It is easier to interpret than immunoelectrophoresis.
D. Cost per test is lower than immunoelectrophoresis.

19. All of the following statements regarding nephelometry are true *except*

A. It measures light scattering.
B. It is capable of detecting antibody or antigen in low concentrations.
C. It uses a detector at zero angle (180 degrees) with the incident source.
D. It measures scattered signal against no signal of incident light because the scattered light is out of line from the incident radiation.

20. All of the following statements regarding labels for antigens and antibodies are true *except*

A. Labeled antigens and antibodies have made turbidimetric methods obsolete.
B. Labels may include radioisotopes, and fluorescent, luminescent, and phosphorescent compounds.
C. For small molecules, labels should not significantly alter the environment of the binding site.
D. For small molecules, the integrity of the binding site may be preserved by attaching the label with a carbon space arm or incorporating carbon-14 or tritium directly into the molecule.

21. Which of the following statements regarding competitive assay is *true*?

A. It uses a fixed concentration of antibody at a level that is insufficient to bind all antigen present.

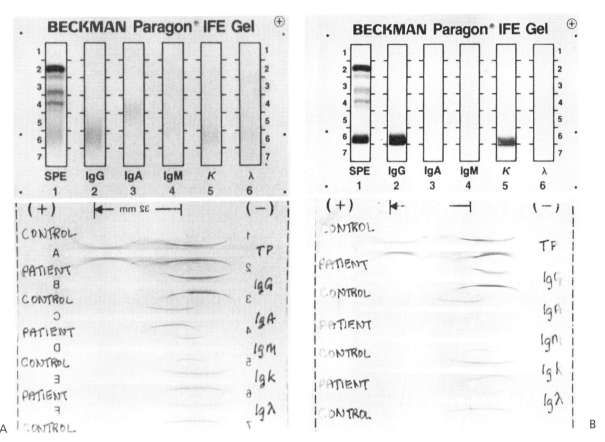

FIGURE 12.6.

B. It does not require separation of antigen–antibody complexes from unbound label.

C. It uses sufficient antibody to bind all antigen present in solution.

D. It requires separation of antigen–antibody complexes from unbound label.

22. **All of the following statements regarding γ emitter are true *except***

   A. Rate of decay of the isotope is unaffected by the environment of the immunoassay reaction.

   B. It requires a scintillation cocktail to measure emission.

   C. It can be measured directly without using a scintillation cocktail.

   D. It always utilizes a heterogeneous immunoassay system.

23. **The radioisotope ^3H characteristic emission is _____.**

   A. β

   B. α

   C. γ

   D. δ

24. **All of the following statements regarding enzyme immunoassays (EIAs) are true *except***

   A. The enzyme label functions as an amplifier, producing many molecules of substrate for each antigen–antibody complex formed.

   B. The enzyme multiplied immunoassay technique (EMIT) is a homogeneous assay commonly used for therapeutic drug monitoring.

   C. The enzyme-linked immunoabsorbent assay (ELISA) is a heterogeneous assay system.

   D. ELISAs are always competitive immunoassays.

25. **Glucose-6-phosphate/NADP⁺ is a substrate for which of the following enzymes?**

   A. Alkaline phosphatase

   B. Glucose-6-phosphate dehydrogenase

   C. Glucose oxidase

   D. Peroxidase

26. **Which of the following statements regarding ELISA is *true*?**

   A. solid-phase "sandwich" ELISA may use antibody bound to a solid phase to which a patient specimen is added, followed by a second enzyme-labeled antibody.

B. "Sandwich" ELISA is best suited for larger molecules, such as peptides.

C. "Sandwich" ELISA is best suited for smaller molecules, such as drugs or steroids.

D. ELISA is not quantitative.

27. **Regarding fluorescence immunoassay, all of the following statements are true** *except*

A. The absorbing and emitting wavelengths of the fluorophore are different.

B. Performance of fluorescent immunoassays can be improved by placing the detector in direct line with the exciting light.

C. Molecules that fluoresce typically are ringed compounds that are extensively conjugated and exhibit molecular rigidity and planarity.

D. Fluoroimmunoassays are designed similar to EIAs.

28. **All of the following statements regarding fluorescent immunoassay are true** *except*

A. Fluorescence is insensitive to temperature and viscosity.

B. Naturally fluorescent molecules, such as bilirubin and protein, may interfere with the assays.

C. Internal filtering arising from absorption of emitted light by molecules in the specimen may interfere with the assay.

D. Time-resolved fluorescence uses fluorophores with a large Stokes shift and an extended decay time, such as lanthanide chelate, to minimize background and nonspecific fluorescence.

29. **All of the following statements regarding bioluminescence and chemiluminescence assays are true** *except*

A. Bioluminescence-based assays have found only limited use due to reagent expense.

B. Chemiluminescence-based assays use luminals, acridinium esters, and dioxetanes.

C. Luminals emit light when they are oxidized by a catalytic agent such as peroxidase.

D. Acridinium esters require a catalyst for oxidation.

30. **All of the following statements about data reduction methods for immunoassays are true** *except*

A. Data reduction methods include point-to-point and regression methods.

B. Point-to-point methods attempts to draw a smooth line through the data points progressing from one point to the next.

C. Regression methods fit a line through the data points such that each point is a minimal distance from the line.

D. Standard regression analysis recognizes outliers and treats these points differently.

Indicate whether each of the following statements is true (T) or false (F).

31. **The sensitivity and specificity of a radioimmunoassay (RIA) is dependent on the antibody and the amplification system, respectively.**

32. **In the Mancini diffusion technique the formation of asymmetrical rings usually means that the antibody is recognizing >1 antigen.**

33. **RIAs are advantageous because of the high sensitivity and ease of batch specimen processing.**

34. **Fluorescence is a property where light energy is absorbed and reemitted as a light of shorter wavelength.**

35. **Chemiluminescent reactions are less expensive and more user friendly than immunoassays.**

13

PLASMA PROTEINS

QUESTIONS

Select the one best answer of the choices offered.

1. **All of the following statements regarding plasma proteins are true** *except*

    A. Most plasma proteins are synthesized by the liver.
    B. Some plasma proteins cross the blood–brain barrier and enter the cerebrospinal fluid (CSF).
    C. Historically, albumin was separated from globulins based on its greater solubility in water.
    D. Most plasma proteins function mainly to maintain the colloid oncotic pressure of plasma.

2. **Figure 13.1 shows a densitometric scan of a normal serum electrophoresis pattern. Match the following regions on protein electrophoresis with the principal protein(s) found in each region.**

    A. Albumin   _____ Antitrypsin
    B. α1   _____ Macroglobulin/haptoglobin
    C. α2   _____ Immunoglobulins
    D. β   _____ Albumin
    E. γ   _____ Low-density lipoprotein/
                        transferrin/C3

3. **All of the following plasma proteins are synthesized by the liver** *except*

    A. albumin
    B. haptoglobin
    C. ceruloplasmin (CER)
    D. immunoglobulins

4. **All of the following statements regarding the total plasma protein are true** *except*

    A. Plasma total protein is 3% to 5% higher than serum protein.
    B. Prolonged tourniquet application may increase the measured total protein.
    C. Most of the total plasma protein arises from the globulins.

D. Albumin is responsible for 80% of the plasma colloid oncotic pressure.

5. **All of the following pathologic conditions will decrease the total plasma protein values** *except*

    A. pregnancy
    B. dehydration
    C. salt retention syndromes
    D. chronic liver disease

6. **Which of the following pathologic conditions will most likely increase the albumin to globulin (A:G) ratio?**

    A. Multiple myeloma
    B. Dehydration
    C. Nephrotic syndrome
    D. Humoral-mediated immune deficiency

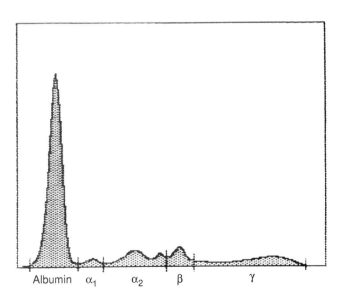

FIGURE 13.1.

7. **All of the following proteins increase during acute phase response** *except*

   A. albumin
   B. fibrinogen
   C. C-reactive protein (CRP)
   D. α_1-antitrypsin (AAT)

8. **Regarding the acute phase response, all of the following statements are true** *except*

   A. Acute phase response may be detected by the erythrocyte sedimentation rate (ESR).
   B. Increase in CRP, an acute phase reactant, typically occurs within days.
   C. Acute phase response may occur following inflammation, surgery, myocardial infarction, malignancy, and other conditions.
   D. CRP may increase by 3,000-fold during an acute phase response.

9. **Figure 13.2 shows selected serum protein electrophoresis patterns in various diseases. Match the following patterns with the most likely condition.**

   A. Pattern C   ____ Cirrhosis
   B. Pattern D   ____ Nonselective protein loss
   C. Pattern E   ____ Acute inflammation
   D. Pattern F   ____ Nephrotic syndrome
   E. Pattern G   ____ Iron deficiency
   F. Pattern H   ____ Chronic inflammation
   G. Pattern I   ____ Hyperbetalipoproteinemia

10. **All of the following statements regarding prealbumin are true** *except*

    A. It is a synthetic precursor of albumin.
    B. Its synonyms include transthyretin and thyroid-binding prealbumin.
    C. It binds small amounts of thyroxine.
    D. It may be useful to assess nutritional status.

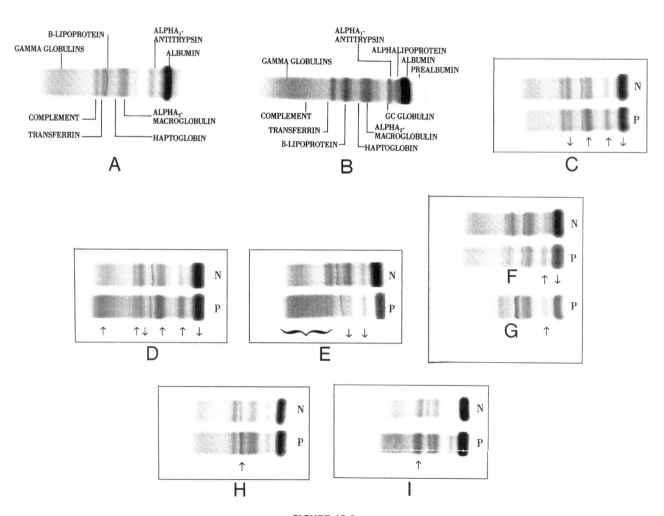

FIGURE 13.2.

11. **All of the following statements regarding albumin are true *except***

    A. It is the most abundant plasma protein.
    B. It contains no carbohydrate.
    C. It is composed of an α and a β subunit.
    D. It may form dimers, producing an extra band on electrophoresis.

12. **All of the following exhibit significant binding to albumin *except***

    A. catecholamines
    B. unconjugated bilirubin
    C. penicillin
    D. free fatty acids

13. **Which of following pathologic conditions will show hyperalbuminemia?**

    A. Malignancy
    B. Dehydration
    C. Third spacing (ascites, effusion)
    D. Inflammatory bowel disease

14. **All of the following methods can be used to measure albumin *except***

    A. dye binding
    B. densitometry
    C. immunoassay
    D. reaction with glyoxylic acid

15. **All of the following statements regarding AAT are true *except***

    A. It functions as a proteinase inhibitor.
    B. Deficiency is associated with emphysema and cirrhosis.
    C. The most common phenotype is PiMM.
    D. The phenotype PiMZ produces severe deficiency.

16. **All of the following statements regarding AAT deficiency are true *except***

    A. It may present as neonatal hepatitis.
    B. Low levels of AAT may be congenital or acquired.
    C. The phenotype PiZZ is the only phenotype associated with disease.
    D. Cigarette smoking accelerates the progression to emphysema.

17. **Which of the following statements regarding α₂-macroglobulin (AMG) is *true*?**

    A. It is one of the largest serum proteins.
    B. It rarely is measured in the clinical laboratory.
    C. It is an important acute phase reactant.
    D. Its levels are increased in nephrotic syndrome.

18. **All of the following statements regarding CER are true *except***

    A. Hypoceruloplasminemia produces copper deficiency.
    B. It exhibits oxidase activity.
    C. About 90% of plasma copper is bound to CER.
    D. It is synthesized by the liver.

19. **All of the following statements regarding Wilson disease are true *except***

    A. It is associated with decreased plasma CER.
    B. It is associated with decreased serum and urine copper.
    C. The defect in Wilson disease is not due to an abnormal CER molecule.
    D. It is associated with cirrhosis and lenticular degeneration.

20. **Which of the following diseases is associated with both emphysema and cirrhosis?**

    A. Wilson disease
    B. AAT deficiency
    C. Analbuminemia
    D. AMG deficiency

21. **Which of the following statements regarding haptoglobin is *true*?**

    A. It exhibits many abnormal phenotypes associated with disease.
    B. Its principal function is to bind free hemoglobin.
    C. Hemolysis results in increased haptoglobin level.
    D. Hemoglobin–haptoglobin complexes are cleared by the kidney and excreted in the urine.

22. **All of the following statements regarding transferrin are true *except***

    A. Most plasma iron is bound to transferrin.
    B. Total iron binding capacity is principally an index of the serum transferrin level.
    C. Normally, 95% of the iron binding sites on transferrin are saturated.
    D. Iron deficiency anemia is associated with increased transferrin.

23. **Match the following lipoproteins with the electrophoretic zone in which they are found on serum protein electrophoresis.**

    A. High-density lipoprotein _____ Albumin/ α region
    B. Low-density lipoprotein _____ Pre-β region
    C. Very low-density lipoprotein _____ β Region

24. All of the following statements regarding β₂-microglobulin (B2M) are true *except*

A. It is the common light chain of the class I major histocompatibility complex (MHC) antigen.
B. It is present on all nucleated cells.
C. Plasma B2M may be decreased in multiple myeloma.
D. It is filtered by the glomerulus and degraded by renal tubular cells.

25. All of the following statements regarding CRP are true *except*

A. It binds the C-polysaccharide of *Streptococcus pneumoniae*.
B. It may be measured to assess the acute phase response.
C. Elevated levels may produce a band in the β or γ region on serum protein electrophoresis.
D. It usually is measured by isoelectric focusing.

26. All of the following statements regarding measurement of total protein are true *except*

A. The biuret method is based on the reaction of copper ions with the imidazole groups of histidine.
B. The Lowry method uses a biuret reaction followed by reaction with Folin-Ciocalteu reagent.
C. Dye binding methods for total protein include Coomassie brilliant blue and amido black.
D. Turbidimetric assays are based on the precipitation of proteins with sulfosalicylic or trichloroacetic acid.

27. All of the following statements regarding electrophoresis of proteins are true *except*

A. A protein at its isoelectric point will not migrate in an electric field.
B. The net charge on a protein is largely due to the ionic properties of its peptide bonds.
C. A protein is a buffer at a pH above its isoelectric point will have a net negative charge and will migrate toward the anode.
D. A protein is a buffer at a pH below its isoelectric point will have a net positive charge and will migrate toward the cathode.

28. Which of the following electrophoretic methods is used to separate proteins based on size and charge?

A. Paper
B. Polyacrylamide
C. Cellulose acetate
D. Agarose

29. All of the following statements regarding routine serum protein electrophoresis are true *except*

A. Agarose is a purified form of agar.
B. γ-Globulins migrate cathodal to the origin due to the electroendosmotic effect.
C. Most proteins have enough negative charge to overcome the electroendosmotic effect and migrate toward the anode.
D. Proper interpretation of the electrophoresis pattern requires densitometric scanning.

30. Protein bands in the γ zone on routine serum protein electrophoresis may be due to all of the following proteins *except*

A. CER dimers
B. CRP
C. Fibrinogen
D. Immunoglobulins

Indicate whether each of the following statements is true (T) or false (F).

31. Marked hyperproteinemia in the absence of dehydration usually reflects increased synthesis of γ-globulins.

32. Increased ESR is not related to increased levels of fibrinogen.

33. AAT mainly functions to inhibit trypsin proteinases.

34. Free hemoglobin not bound to haptoglobin or processed by the kidneys is methemoglobin.

35. Transferrin, albumin, and β-lipoprotein are positive acute phase reactants.

36. Elevation in B2M may reflect increased lymphocyte turnover.

37. ESR is a more sensitive and faster indicator of inflammation than CRP.

38. Capillary electrophoresis is comparable with conventional electrophoresis in addition to providing high separation efficiency and ease of automation.

39. Ion exchange chromatography uses a charged support medium to separate molecules based on their acid–base properties.

40. Isoelectric focusing is a powerful method to separate proteins and is a commonly used laboratory technique used in a majority of clinical laboratories.

14

DIAGNOSTIC ENZYMOLOGY AND OTHER BIOCHEMICAL MARKERS OF ORGAN DAMAGE

QUESTIONS

Select the one best answer of the choices offered.

1. **All of the following statements regarding serum enzymes are true *except***

   A. Most serum enzymes used for diagnostic purposes have a direct physiologic role in the blood.
   B. Most serum enzymes are cleared from the blood by the reticuloendothelial system.
   C. Some serum enzymes, such as amylase, are cleared by the kidneys.
   D. The half-life of serum enzymes varies from hours to days.

2. **Figure 14.1 shows the relationship between substrate concentration and the velocity of an enzyme-catalyzed reaction. All of the following statements are true *except***

   A. In the region of first-order kinetics, the reaction velocity is directly proportional to the substrate concentration.

   B. In the region of zero-order kinetics, the reaction is independent of the substrate concentration.
   C. The Michaelis-Menten constant K_m is the substrate concentration that corresponds to one half the maximal reaction rate.
   D. When developing an enzyme assay, it is optimal to use a substrate concentration equal to K_m.

3. **Regarding enzyme reactions, which of the following statements is *true*?**

   A. Most enzymes operate optimally within a wide pH range.
   B. pH can influence the direction of an enzyme reaction.
   C. By convention, most enzymes are assayed at 25°C.
   D. As a general rule, doubling the temperature will quadruple the rate of an enzyme reaction.

4. **All of the following statements regarding enzyme inhibitors are true *except***

   A. Competitive inhibitors compete with substrate for binding to the active site of the enzyme.

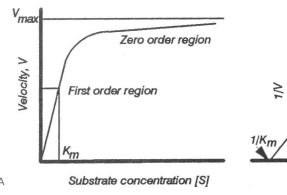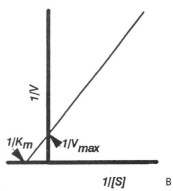

FIGURE 14.1.

B. Competitive inhibitors increase K_m but do not affect V_{max}.

C. Noncompetitive inhibitors decrease V_{max} and increase K_m.

D. Noncompetitive inhibitors interact with the enzyme–substrate complex, prohibiting the formation of a product.

5. **Figure 14.2 shows a typical enzyme-catalyzed reaction for a single-reagent kinetic assay. Which of the following statements is *true*?**

   A. The lag phase represents the time necessary to inactivate enzyme inhibitors.

   B. The linear phase is characterized by a constant rate of change in absorbance.

   C. At the first-order phase, the reaction is proceeding at maximal velocity.

   D. A delay of 5 minutes usually is necessary before absorbance readings become meaningful because of the lag phase.

6. **All of the following statements regarding enzyme assays are true *except***

   A. An international unit (IU) is defined as the amount of enzyme necessary to catalyze the conversion of 1 μmol of substrate per minute.

   B. A Système Internationale (SI) unit is the amount of enzyme that will catalyze the conversion of 1 nmol of substrate per second (nanokatal).

   C. Immunoassays measure enzyme activity using monoclonal or polyclonal antibodies.

   D. Immunoassays are especially useful for measuring isoenzymes.

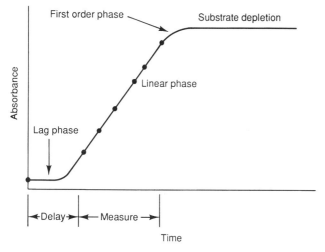

FIGURE 14.2.

7. **Enzymes commonly measured to assess hepatic dysfunction include all of the following *except***

   A. amylase

   B. alanine aminotransferase (ALT)

   C. aspartate aminotransferase (AST)

   D. γ-glutamyltransferase (GGT)

8. **Enzyme markers indicating cholestatic liver disease include all of the following *except***

   A. alkaline phosphatase (ALP)

   B. ALT

   C. 5′-nucleotidase (5′-NT)

   D. GGT

9. **All of the following are causes of toxic hepatitis *except***

   A. carbon tetrachloride

   B. acetaminophen toxicity

   C. hemochromatosis

   D. halothane

10. **Which of the following statements regarding cirrhosis is *true*?**

    A. Liver enzyme levels can be normal in patients with cirrhosis.

    B. Cirrhosis is characterized by hepatocellular necrosis and inflammation.

    C. Primary biliary cirrhosis typically exhibits elevations in ALP and antimitochondrial antibody.

    D. Primary hepatocellular carcinoma more commonly occurs in patients with chronic hepatitis B and cirrhosis than in those with normal livers.

11. **All of the following statements regarding ALP are true *except***

    A. ALP is a cell membrane enzyme.

    B. No single physiologic substrate for ALP has been identified.

    C. Reference ranges for ALP are higher in children and the elderly than in adults.

    D. The most common substrate for measuring ALP is NADPH.

12. **Which of the following statements regarding ALP isoenzymes is *true*?**

    A. The clinical need for ALP isoenzymes measurement is rare.

    B. The most prevalent isoenzymes in normal serum are kidney and bone.

    C. The most commonly used method for measuring ALP isoenzyme is immunoassay.

    D. The tissues with the highest ALP activity include the liver and bone, which have the same isoenzyme.

13. **All of the following statements regarding GGT are true *except***
    A. GGT is a cell membrane enzyme present on nearly all cells.
    B. GGT has no isoenzymes but does exhibit isoforms.
    C. Most serum GGT arises from the liver and a small amount from the prostate.
    D. An elevated GGT level in a patient with low ALP indicates that the hepatobiliary system is the source of the ALP.

14. **All of the following statements regarding 5′-NT are true *except***
    A. 5′-NT is a membrane-bound cytosolic enzyme.
    B. Osteoblastic bone diseases may cause marked elevations in 5′-NT.
    C. 5′-NT is commonly measured using adenosine-5-monophosphate as a substrate.
    D. The assay of 5′-NT is run with and without nickel ions to differentiate 5′-NT from ALP.

15. **All of the following statements regarding ALT and AST are true *except***
    A. ALT is mainly useful to assess liver disease, whereas AST may be useful to assess liver and skeletal muscle diseases and myocardial infarction.
    B. Patients with vitamin B_6 deficiency may show false elevations in ALT and AST unless pyridoxal 5′-phosphate is added to the assay.
    C. AST has both a cytosolic and a mitochondrial isoenzyme.
    D. Assays for ALT use lactic dehydrogenase and those for AST use malate dehydrogenase as indicator reactions.

16. **All of the following enzyme markers are used for obstructive liver diseases *except***
    A. 5′-NT
    B. GGT
    C. α-fetoprotein
    D. ALP

17. **All of the following statements regarding acute hepatocellular injury are true *except***
    A. The transaminases ALT and AST are the most useful markers of hepatocellular injury.
    B. The extent of ALT and AST elevations correlate with both the severity of disease and the prognosis.
    C. In end-stage liver disease, transaminase levels may be normal.
    D. The highest levels of transaminases are observed in acute viral and toxic hepatitis.

18. **All of the following diseases are associated with a de Ritis ratio greater that 1 *except***
    A. myocardial or skeletal muscle disease
    B. alcoholic liver disease
    C. Reye syndrome
    D. chronic active hepatitis

19. **All of the following statements regarding alcoholic liver disease are true *except***
    A. AST often is disproportionately elevated relative to ALT.
    B. ALT is less elevated than AST partly due to a dietary deficiency of pyridoxal phosphate.
    C. GGT synthesis is induced by alcohol and is a sensitive marker of recent alcohol intake.
    D. Patients with alcoholic liver disease may exhibit a de Ritis ratio <1.

20. **All of the following statements regarding creatine kinase are true *except***
    A. Cytoplasmic creatine kinase (CK) consists of two subunits producing three isoenzymes (MM, MB, BB) with three MM and two MB isoforms.
    B. Mitochondrial CK catalyzes the transfer of a high-energy phosphate bond from ATP to creatine and cytoplasmic CK catalyzes the reverse reaction at physiologic pH.
    C. CK usually is assayed directly by measuring the hydrolysis of creatine phosphate.
    D. Adenylate kinase interferes with CK assays but may be eliminated with inhibitors.

21. **Which of the following statements regarding CK isoenzymes and variants is *true*?**
    A. CK-MM is the predominant isoenzyme in both skeletal muscle and myocardium.
    B. Myocardium contains a higher percentage of CK-MB than skeletal muscle.
    C. Macro CK type 1 represents CK-BB linked to immunoglobulin and has no clinical significance, whereas macro CK type 2 is a polymeric aggregate of mitochondrial CK and may be seen in metastatic cancer.
    D. Normal serum contains predominately KC isoforms MM3 and MB2.

22. **All of the following statements regarding CK isoenzyme assays are true *except***
    A. Immunoinhibition is useful because it is inexpensive and can be used on automated chemistry analyzers as a screening method.
    B. Electrophoresis is less sensitive than immunoassay but permits all CK isoenzymes to be visualized.

C. Nonisotopic immunoassay methods measure enzyme concentration instead of activity.

D. Immunoassays are rapid but insensitive.

23. All of the following statements regarding lactate dehydrogenase (LDH) are true *except*

A. LDH isoenzyme assays use electrophoresis or measurement of LD_1, immunoprecipitation or chemical inhibition.

B. LDH is a tetramer consisting of H and M subunits with five isoenzymes.

C. LDH is present primarily in skeletal muscle and myocardium.

D. The myocardium contains the most LD_1 isoenzyme.

24. All of the following statements about troponin are true *except*

A. Troponin is a regulatory protein complex located on the thin filament of striated muscles.

B. Troponin consists of four isotypes designated T, I, C, and D.

C. Troponin T and troponin I are better markers for myocardial infarction than CK-MB.

D. Cardiac troponin T and troponin I isotypes are different from skeletal muscle isotypes.

25. Criteria of the World Health Organization (WHO) for diagnosis of acute myocardial infarction (AMI) include all of the following *except*

A. elevated troponin T or troponin I

B. clinical signs and symptoms

C. specific changes in the electrocardiograph

D. elevations in serum CK, CK-MB, LDH, and LDH isoenzymes

26. All of the following statements regarding amylase are true *except*

A. Amylase can pass through the glomerulus into the urine.

B. Normal serum amylase consists exclusively of the pancreatic isoenzyme.

C. Macroamylase is usually the salivary isoenzyme bound to immunoglobulin and it accounts for 2% to 5% of hyperamylasemia.

D. Most currently used assays for amylase use saccharogenic or chromogenic methods.

27. All of the following statements regarding pancreatitis are true *except*

A. Acute pancreatitis typically presents with an elevated serum amylase, amylase clearance, and lipase.

B. The sensitivity of amylase and lipase for acute pancreatitis is high (90%), but the specificity of either enzyme alone is low.

C. In chronic pancreatitis, amylase and lipase levels may be normal or low.

D. Acute pancreatitis virtually always is caused by alcoholism.

Indicate whether each of the following statements is true (T) or false (F).

28. Phenobarbital induces microsomal enzyme production that leads to increased synthesis of GGT.

29. Substrate concentrations for test conditions should be in the first-order region and all other factors that influence the reaction rate should be optimized and controlled.

30. Samples with high enzyme activity can deplete the substrate before the first analytical reading is taken.

31. Beer's law allows enzyme activity to be determined from the change in absorbance per unit of time.

32. Restoring glutathione stores with administration of *N*-acetyl-L-cysteine to prevent liver damage is the treatment for acute acetaminophen overdose.

33. Mallory bodies are suggestive of cytomegalovirus infection.

34. Primary biliary cirrhosis affects men more often than women and is histologically characterized by inflammation and destruction of bile ducts.

35. Patients with vitamin B$_6$ deficiency will produce falsely low serum aminotransferase levels unless pyridoxal 5′-phosphate is added to the reagent formulation.

15

LIPIDS AND LIPOPROTEINS

QUESTIONS

Select the one best answer of the choices offered.

1. **Which of the following statements regarding free fatty acids (FFAs) is** *true*?

   A. Naturally occurring form of double bonds in FFA is in the *trans* isomer.
   B. Omega-3 FFAs are unhealthy.
   C. Palmitate, stearate, oleate, linoleate, and arachidonate are the most abundant animal fatty acids.
   D. Saturated fatty acids have multiple double bonds.

2. **All of the following statements about fatty acids are true** *except*

   A. Unsaturated fatty acids refer to double bonds.
   B. Rotation of the fatty acid molecule is restricted at the site of the double bond.
   C. Polyunsaturated fatty acids contain two or more double bonds.
   D. Double bonds in fatty acids always exist in the *cis* isomer.

3. **All of the following statements regarding the structure of phospholipids are true** *except*

   A. They may contain ethanolamine, choline, serine, or inositol.
   B. They contain glycerol, fatty acids, phophate group, and alcohol.
   C. They are the principal component of cell membranes.
   D. They are routinely measured as part of a comprehensive cardiovascular risk assessment.

4. **All of the following statements regarding lipoproteins are true** *except*

   A. They function to transport lipids in the body.
   B. They are composites of lipids and protein.
   C. They are insoluble in aqueous media.

   D. They contain a core of cholesterol esters and triglycerides surrounded by cholesterol, phospholipid, and proteins.

5. **Which of the following shows the correct order for the size of lipoproteins from largest to smallest?**

   A. Chylomicron, high-density lipoprotein (HDL), low-density lipoprotein (LDL), very low-density lipoprotein (VLDL)
   B. Chylomicron, VLDL, LDL, HDL
   C. HDL, chylomicron, VLDL, LDL
   D. LDL, HDL, VLDL, chylomicron

6. **All of the following statements regarding lipoproteins are true** *except*

   A. Lower density is mainly due to the relative proportion of lipid and water in the lipoprotein.
   B. Triglyceride-rich lipoproteins include chylomicrons and VLDL.
   C. Lower density is associated with increasing triglyceride content.
   D. Lower density is associated with decreasing protein content.

7. **Which of the following statements regarding apolipoprotein B (apo B) is** *true*?

   A. Apo B-100 is synthesized by the liver.
   B. Apo B-100 is the major protein of VLDL and HDL.
   C. Apo B-48 is derived from the intestines.
   D. Apo B-48 is associated with chylomicrons.

8. **All of the following statements regarding familial hyperlipidemia are true** *except*

   A. Type I is associated with increased chylomicrons.
   B. Types IIa and IIb are associated with increased LDL or LDL/VLDL, respectively.
   C. Type V is associated with increased chylomicrons and VLDL.
   D. All types are associated with elevated cholesterol and triglyceride levels.

9. **Which of the following statements regarding triglycerides is *true*?**

    A. Triglycerides are composed of three long-chain fatty acids esterified to phosphatidylcholine.
    B. Triglycerides are composed of only short-chain fatty acids esterified to glycerol.
    C. Serum or plasma triglyceride measurement is greatly affected by fasting.
    D. Triglycerides are stored in adipose tissue, predominately as large polymers.

10. **Which of the following statements is *true*?**

    A. A 12-hour fast is necessary for standardization of triglyceride measurements.
    B. Serum triglyceride level is only minimally affected by recent food consumption.
    C. Triglyceride levels show little intraindividual variation.
    D. A reliable triglyceride level in any given patient can be obtained by a single random measurement.

11. **Which of the following statements regarding specimens for cholesterol measurement is *true*?**

    A. Either fasting or nonfasting samples are acceptable.
    B. The fasting status of the patient has a significant effect on cholesterol levels when screening healthy subjects.
    C. Nonfasting specimens typically show high cholesterol levels, even in healthy subjects.
    D. Plasma values are generally higher than serum levels.

12. **All of the following are risk factors for development of atherosclerotic vascular disease according to the National Cholesterol Education Panel *except***

    A. male older than 45 years of age
    B. low HDL (<35 mg/dL)
    C. alcoholism
    D. family history of coronary artery disease

13. **Which of the following LDL cholesterol values has a borderline high LDL risk assessment category?**

    A. <130 mg/dL
    B. 130–159 mg/dL
    C. <200 mg/dL
    D. ≥200 mg/dL

14. **Which of the following statements regarding the National Cholesterol Education Program (NCEP) is *true*?**

    A. NCEP has identified risk factors, including obesity, for development of atherosclerotic vascular disease.

B. NCEP interpretive guidelines include desirable, borderline, and high-risk ranges.
    C. NCEP does not provide interpretive guidelines but reports cholesterol values along a continuous range.
    D. According to the NCEP, the desirable blood cholesterol level is 239 to 240 mg/dL.

15. **All of the following are cardiovascular risk ranges for cholesterol according to NCEP guidelines *except***

    A. HDL <35 mg/dL
    B. total cholesterol 200–239 mg/dL
    C. total cholesterol 180–220 mg/dL
    D. total cholesterol ≥240 mg/dL

16. **All of the following statements about triglyceride measurement are true *except***

    A. Enzymatic tag methods also measure phospholipids and glucose levels.
    B. Glycerol contamination may give falsely elevated levels of triglyceride with some assays.
    C. Most commercial procedures for triglyceride assay use enzymatic methods.
    D. Most enzymatic methods are based on measurement of liberated glycerol.

17. **All of the following statements regarding enzymatic assays for triglycerides are true *except***

    A. Enzymatic methods use lipolytic enzymes to hydrolyze triglyceride to FFAs and glycerol.
    B. Free glycerol interference can be from deficient glycerol kinase enzyme.
    C. Enzymatic assays are easily automated.
    D. Enzymatic assays require prior extraction of samples with solvents.

18. **All of the following statements regarding cholesterol are true *except***

    A. The reference method of cholesterol measurement is highly accurate but is not suitable for automation.
    B. Plant sterols also are reactive in enzymatic methods, but their concentration in clinical specimens is negligible.
    C. The reference method for cholesterol uses an enzymatic procedure.
    D. Enzymatic methods are popular because they are easy to automate, use small sample volumes, and avoid caustic reagents.

19. **All of the following statements regarding enzymatic cholesterol methods are true *except***

    A. Most laboratories use enzymatic methods.

B. Enzymatic methods use cholesterol esterase to hydrolyze cholesterol esters.

C. Enzymatic methods use cholesterol oxidase to produce hydrogen peroxide, which then is quantitated.

D. Enzymatic methods use cholesterol reductase to convert cholesterol to a colored product.

20. **Which of the following statements regarding ultra-centrifugation for lipoproteins is *true*?**

A. It requires short spin times.

B. It is suitable for automation.

C. It is the most commonly used method for measuring lipoproteins in the clinical laboratory.

D. It separates chylomicrons, VLDL, and β-VLDL from plasma.

21. **With respect to electrophoretic mobility, which of the following lipoproteins migrates with β-globulins?**

A. Chylomicrons

B. VLDL

C. LDL

D. HDL

22. **All of the following statements regarding apolipoprotein A-I (apo A-I) are true *except***

A. It is measured by immunoturbidimetry or immunonephelometry.

B. It is the major protein constituent of LDL.

C. It is the major protein constituent of HDL.

D. Apo A-I levels reflect the HDL content of serum or plasma.

Indicate whether each of the following statements is true (T) or false (F).

23. **Fatty acids that have no double bonds, such as palmitate, are unsaturated fatty acids.**

24. **Saturated and *trans* double-bond fatty acids both elevate serum cholesterol.**

25. **Cholesterol is only present in animals and cannot be derived from plant products.**

26. **Elevated plasma lipoprotein (a) [Lp(a)] has been associated with an increased risk of coronary artery disease and development of myocardial infarction.**

27. **High plasma levels of LDL will be removed from the circulation by the scavenger pathway, producing "foam cells."**

28. **According to NCEP guidelines, dietary and pharmacologic therapy should be initiated in patients without clinically evident atherosclerotic disease, who have <2 two risk factors and LDL cholesterol >160 mg/dL.**

29. **LDL cholesterol can be calculated by the equation: LDL cholesterol = total cholesterol − triglycerides/5.**

30. **Apo B-100 is present in HDL and VLDL.**

16

ENDOCRINE FUNCTION AND CARBOHYDRATE

QUESTIONS

Select the one best answer of the choices offered.

1. **Cyclic secretions are the only mechanism of hormonal release.**

   A. True
   B. False

2. **All of the following statements regarding hormonal receptors are true *except***

   A. Receptors are highly selective and bind only to certain specific hormones.
   B. Plasma membrane receptors interact with molecules that are unable to diffuse through the membrane.
   C. Binding to intracellular receptors allows the hormone to be translocated to the nucleus.
   D. Hormone–receptor binding follows the laws of mass action.

3. **All of the following statements regarding hormonal receptors are true *except***

   A. The number of hormonal receptors on the cell membrane varies depending on the level of the circulating hormone.
   B. The calcium–calmodulin complex is an activated complex that can stimulate intracellular enzymes.
   C. After removing the entire receptor–hormone complex from the cell membrane to the inside of the cell, the receptors are invariably degraded and new receptors are produced.
   D. Amine hormones use a complex system to affect cellular function, including the guanine-nucleotide binding proteins (G proteins).

4. **All of the following statements regarding second messengers are true *except***

   A. Cyclic AMP is a second intracellular messenger responsible for direct alterations of cellular functions.
   B. Ionic calcium is a second intracellular messenger, and its levels are very rigidly controlled.

   C. Ionic calcium induces its intracellular effects via activation of phospholipase C.
   D. Inositol 1,4,5-triphosphate liberates calcium from bound stores within the cell.

5. **All of the following statements regarding the hypothalamic–pituitary axis are true *except***

   A. Pituitary hormones show both pulsatile and diurnal variations.
   B. All the anterior pituitary hormones are synthesized in the pars distalis.
   C. Blood and hormones from the hypothalamus communicate with the anterior pituitary through the portal venous complex.
   D. The anterior pituitary comprises approximately 50% of the total pituitary mass.

6. **All of the following statements regarding growth hormone (GH) are true *except***

   A. GH is the most abundant of the anterior pituitary hormones.
   B. Somatostatin stimulates secretion of GH.
   C. The neuropeptide cells of the hypothalamus secrete somatostatin.
   D. GH is not a true growth factor.

7. **Excessive production of GH causes gigantism in children, whereas it produces acromegaly in adults.**

   A. True
   B. False

8. **All of the following can cause stimulation of GH production *except***

   A. arginine
   B. Dopa
   C. exercise
   D. glucose

9. **All of the following statements regarding prolactin (hPrL) are true *except***

   A. hPrL can occur in three forms, monomeric, dimeric (big hPrL), and polymeric (big big hPrL).

B. The polymeric form constitutes <2% of the total circulating hPrL.

C. The polymeric form is biologically and pharmacologically more active.

D. Secretion of hPrL is episodic.

10. **All of the following can cause stimulation of hPrL secretion** *except*

   A. dopamine
   B. levodopa
   C. thyrotropin-releasing hormone (TRH)
   D. suckling

11. **All of the following statements regarding hormonal changes during pregnancy and lactation are true** *except*

   A. Suckling stimulates production of hPrL.
   B. Suckling stimulates production of gonadotropin-releasing hormone (GnRH).
   C. Suckling stimulates production of oxytocin.
   D. Luteinizing hormone (LH) decreases during lactation.

12. **All of the following can cause increased hPrL secretion** *except*

   A. estrogens
   B. renal insufficiency
   C. tricyclic antidepressants
   D. hyperthyroidism

13. **All of the following statements regarding follicle-stimulating hormone (FSH) and LH are true** *except*

   A. FSH and LH are released in response to the stimulatory effect of GnRH, which is synthesized in the median eminence of the hypothalamus.
   B. Recent immunoassay techniques, which are very specific and very sensitive for FSH or LH, utilize monoclonal antibodies highly specific to the β subunit.
   C. The β subunit of FSH and LH shows great homology to the β subunit of human chorionic gonadotropin (hCG) and thyroid-stimulating hormone (TSH).
   D. Specificity and hormone effect of FSH and LH are conferred by the β subunit.

14. **All of the following statements regarding FSH and LH are true** *except*

   A. FSH stimulates receptors for LH binding.
   B. In men, LH stimulates testosterone secretion.
   C. Gonadal failure is a late symptom of pituitary insufficiency.
   D. In men, FSH stimulates Sertoli cell development.

15. **Both pituitary gonadotropins and testosterone levels are depressed in Klinefelter syndrome.**

   A. True   B. False

16. **Fasting is a requirement for accurate laboratory measurement of pituitary gonadotropins.**

   A. True   B. False

17. **All of the following statements regarding the antidiuretic hormone (ADH) are true** *except*

   A. The effect of ADH is to increase water permeability of the distal tubule collecting duct.
   B. The osmoreceptors responsible for ADH release are located in the juxtaglomerular apparatus.
   C. Secretion of ADH is suppressed below plasma osmolality of 280 mOsm/kg.
   D. Alcohol decreases the threshold for ADH secretion.

18. **All of the following stimulate the release of ADH** *except*

   A. hypocalcemia
   B. pain
   C. carbamazepine
   D. nausea

19. **All of the following statements regarding diabetes insipidus are true** *except*

   A. The dehydration test differentiates between the different clinical types of diabetes insipidus.
   B. Central diabetes insipidus can be either familial or acquired.
   C. Nephrogenic diabetes insipidus can exist as a familial X-linked recessive disease.
   D. Administration of des-amino-D-arginine vasopressin (DDAVP) produces a urine concentration increase of 50% in nephrogenic diabetes insipidus.

Match each of the following laboratory tests with the appropriate result in neurogenic diabetes insipidus (each answer might be used more than once).

20. **Random plasma osmolality**

21. **Random urine osmolality**

22. **Urine osmolality during mild water deprivation**

23. **Urine osmolality after ADH administration**

24. **Plasma level of ADH**

   A. Increased
   B. Decreased
   C. No change

Match each of the following laboratory tests with the appropriate result in psychogenic polydipsia (each answer might be used more than once).

25. Urine osmolality during mild water deprivation

26. Random plasma osmolality

27. Plasma level of ADH

28. Random urine osmolality

29. Urine osmolality after ADH administration

    A. Increased
    B. Decreased
    C. No change

30. All of the following statements regarding T_3 and T_4 are true *except*

    A. The fraction of free T_4 determines hyperthyroidism and hypothyroidism.
    B. Only approximately 0.03% of T_4 is biologically active.
    C. Use of oral contraceptives causes the most common abnormalities in thyroid hormone studies.
    D. Approximately 85% of the increase in serum T_3 arises from direct thyroid gland secretion.

31. The *most* common cause of hyperthyroidism is

    A. TSH-secreting pituitary adenoma
    B. toxic multinodular goiter
    C. excess exogenous thyroid hormone administration
    D. Graves disease

32. All of the following statements regarding Graves disease are true *except*

    A. Graves disease is an autoimmune disorder.
    B. Patients with Graves disease have circulating thyroid-stimulating immunoglobulins.
    C. Patients with Graves disease usually respond to therapeutic measures directed at TSH or TRH control.
    D. Patients with Graves disease have circulating long-acting thyroid stimulators.

33. Hyperthyroidism should be ruled out in all of the following *except*

    A. cardiac disease
    B. sexual dysfunction
    C. generalized weakness
    D. weight gain

34. All of the following statements regarding congenital hypothyroidism are true *except*

    A. The disorder usually is familial.
    B. Initial screening is performed using serum T_4 determination.
    C. False-positive results may occur in premature infants.
    D. Elevated TSH levels are strong evidence for primary hypothyroidism.

35. All of the following statements regarding thyroid function tests are true *except*

    A. Increased T_3 uptake is seen in pregnant women.
    B. Increased T_3 uptake is seen in hepatic failure.
    C. Elevated serum thyroglobulin levels are seen in follicular thyroid carcinoma.
    D. Elevated serum thyroglobulin levels are seen in subacute thyroiditis.

Match each of the following with the corresponding anatomical layer of the adrenal cortex (each answer might be used more than once).

36. Adrenocorticotropic hormone (ACTH)

37. Renin–angiotensin system

38. Mineralocorticoids

39. Estrogen

    A. Zona glomerulosa
    B. Zona fasciculata
    C. Zona reticularis

40. All of the following statements regarding Cushing syndrome are true *except*

    A. The most common cause of Cushing syndrome is pituitary-dependent bilateral adrenal hyperplasia.
    B. Cushing disease is the most common clinical presentation of Cushing syndrome.
    C. Both urinary 17-hydroxysteroid and 17-ketosteroid are elevated in Cushing syndrome.
    D. Dexamethasone administration increases urinary cortisol levels in Cushing syndrome.

Match each of the following conditions with the typical response to the dexamethasone suppression test (each answer might be used more than once).

41. Paraendocrine neoplasm of the lung

42. Bilateral adrenal hyperplasia

43. Normal individuals

44. Adrenal adenoma

A. Suppression of urinary cortisol levels with 0.5 dexamethasone every 6 hours for 48 hours
B. Suppression of urinary cortisol levels with 2.0 dexamethasone every 6 hours for 48 hours
C. Failure to suppress urinary cortisol levels

45. All of the following are included in the polyglandular autoimmune syndrome type I *except*

A. mucocutaneous moniliasis
B. diabetes mellitus
C. adrenal insufficiency
D. hypoparathyroidism

Match each of the following with the corresponding polyglandular autoimmune syndrome (each answer might be used more than once).

46. Hypoparathyroidism

47. Thyroid dysfunction

48. Adrenal insufficiency

49. Diabetes mellitus

50. Mucocutaneous moniliasis

A. Polyglandular autoimmune syndrome type I
B. Polyglandular autoimmune syndrome type II
C. Polyglandular autoimmune syndrome type I and type II

51. The most common cause of congenital adrenal hyperplasia is 21-hydroxylase deficiency.

A. True   B. False

Match each of the following laboratory diagnostic measurements with the corresponding adrenal cortical enzyme (each answer might be used more than once).

52. 17-hydroxypregnenolone:17-hydroxyprogesterone

53. 17-hydroxyprogesterone

54. 11-deoxycortisol

55. Dehydroepiandrosterone:androstenedione

A. 21-hydroxylase
B. 11-hydroxylase
C. 3β-dehydrogenase

56. All of the following are included in the management of an adrenal incidentaloma (>5 cm in diameter) *except*

A. urinary vanillylmandelic acid level

B. watch and repeat imaging in 6 months
C. serum cortisol level
D. serum dehydroepiandrosterone sulfate level

57. All of the following statements regarding type I insulin-dependent diabetes mellitus (IDDM) are true *except*

A. There is progressive loss of pancreatic β-cell function.
B. Antibodies to islet cells are present in a high percentage of cases at time of clinical onset.
C. A relationship exists between IDDM and the DR3 and DR4 loci on the sixth chromosome.
D. It accounts for approximately 30% of patients with diabetes.

58. All of the following statements regarding the diagnosis of diabetes mellitus and gestational diabetes are true *except*

A. Normal fasting blood sugar is >110 mg/dl.
B. Screening for gestational diabetes requires administration of 100 g of glucose between weeks 24 and 28 of pregnancy.
C. Fasting blood sugar >105 mg/dL is diagnostic of gestational diabetes.
D. Individuals with impaired fasting glucose demonstrate fasting blood sugar of 110 to 126 mg/dL.

59. All of the following statements regarding glycosylated hemoglobin (hemoglobin A_{1c}) are true *except*

A. Hemoglobin A_{1c} should be monitored every 3 to 6 months at the onset of therapy.
B. Hemoglobin A_{1c} gives an integrated estimate of blood sugar over approximately 3-month lifespan of the red blood cell.
C. A target level of hemoglobin A_{1c} <7.0% is sought.
D. Hemoglobin A_{1c} undergoes nonenzymatic glycation as a function of integrated blood sugar levels.

60. All of the following statements regarding hypoglycemia are true *except*

A. Antibodies to insulin are helpful in identifying exogenous insulin administration.
B. Ten percent of normal subjects have blood sugar levels <47 mg/dL.
C. The ratio of serum insulin to blood glucose should be <0.3 after an overnight fast.
D. The glucose tolerance test should be part of the workup of patients with hypoglycemia.

Match each of the following peptides with the corresponding clinical finding.

61. Gastrin

62. Glucagon

63. Vasoactive peptide

64. Serotonin

65. Somatostatin

  A. Verner-Morrison syndrome
  B. Gallstones
  C. Migratory necrotizing skin rash
  D. Zollinger-Ellison syndrome
  E. Right-sided endocardial valvular thickening

Match each of the following substances with its effect on the serum calcium regulation.

66. Vitamin D

67. Parathyroid hormone

68. Calcitonin

  A. Decreases resorption of calcium and phosphate in bone
  B. Increases conversion of 25-OHD$_3$ to 1,25(OH)$_2$D$_3$ in the kidney
  C. Increases absorption of calcium and phosphate in the intestine

69. All of the following statements regarding hypercalcemia are true *except*

  A. Parathyroid adenoma causes approximately 90% of the cases of hypercalcemia.
  B. Restlessness and hyperactivity are common symptoms of hypercalcemia.
  C. Hyperparathyroidism is a component of both multiple endocrine neoplasia (MEN) 1 and MEN 2 syndromes.
  D. Sarcoidosis is associated with increased dietary calcium absorption.

70. All of the following statements regarding the syndrome of familial hypocalciuric hypercalcemia are true *except*

  A. The ratio of urinary calcium clearance to urinary creatinine clearance is <0.01.
  B. Inactivating mutation of a transmembrane calcium transporter is present.
  C. The pathogenesis is similar to that seen in patients with lithium-associated hypercalcemia.
  D. Serum parathormone concentrations are decreased.

71. All of the following statements regarding hypoparathyroidism and pseudohypoparathyroidism are true *except*

  A. There is blunted parathormone receptor activity in pseudohypoparathyroidism.
  B. There is marked increase in urinary cyclic AMP excretion after parathormone administration in pseudohypoparathyroidism.
  C. Replacement of magnesium corrects the hypocalcemia in hypoparathyroidism.
  D. There is a defect in the guanidine-nucleotide coupling protein in pseudohypoparathyroidism.

72. Which of the following statements regarding demineralizing bone disorders is *true*?

  A. The residual bone is qualitatively abnormal in osteoporosis.
  B. Osteomalacia is characterized by increased osteoclastic bone resorption.
  C. Calcium levels are normal in osteomalacia.
  D. Osteoporosis can arise secondary to hypothyroidism.

Match each of the following with the corresponding pituitary gonadotropin (each answer might be used more than once).

73. Interstitial Leydig cells

74. Granulosa cells

75. Inhibin

76. Androgen-binding protein

77. Interstitial cells of the ovary

78. Sertoli cells

  A. FSH
  B. LH

79. All of the following statements regarding pheochromocytoma are true *except*

  A. Measurement of plasma catecholamines and their metabolites is more reliable than the urinary levels for diagnosis of pheochromocytoma.
  B. Urine collections should include urinary creatinine to ensure adequacy of collection.
  C. Initial anatomic localization should be attempted before using abdominal computed tomographic imaging.
  D. Pheochromocytoma may present as a component of MEN 2A and MEN 2B.

17

ELECTROLYTES AND ACID–BASE BALANCE

QUESTIONS

Select the one best answer of the choices offered.

1. **All of the following statements regarding fluid distribution in the body are true *except***

   A. Total body water comprises 60% of lean body mass.
   B. In a 70-kg person, 66% of body water is in the extracellular compartment.
   C. Effective circulating volume (ECV) may be decreased despite increased extracellular fluid volume (ECF).
   D. Decrease in ECV results in renal sodium and water retention.

2. **All of the following are primarily regulated by changes in water balance *except***

   A. plasma sodium
   B. osmolality
   C. volume
   D. antidiuretic hormone (ADH)

3. **Which of the following statements about the physiologic effect of aldosterone is *true*?**

   A. Increases potassium excretion
   B. Promotes renal water conservation
   C. Promotes sodium excretion
   D. Enhances potassium absorption

4. **All of the following sensors monitor fluid volume *except***

   A. hypothalamus
   B. carotid sinuses
   C. aortic arch
   D. afferent juxtaglomerular arterioles

5. **All of the following statements regarding potassium are true *except***

   A. Obligatory potassium losses occur through urine and the gastrointestinal tract.
   B. Potassium is the major extracellular solute.
   C. Only 2% of the total body potassium is extracellular.
   D. Plasma potassium losses often are partially compensated by redistribution from cellular potassium.

6. **Which of the following reference method measures serum sodium?**

   A. Flame photometry
   B. Ion-selective electrode
   C. Coulometry
   D. Spectrophotometry

7. **All of the following statements regarding methods for electrolyte analysis are true *except***

   A. Flame photometry uses a high-temperature flame to excite atoms, which emit a characteristic wavelength of light when they return to the ground state.
   B. Ion-selective electrodes use a thin membrane capable of binding a selected ion species more than other ions in the sample.
   C. Coulometry measures the voltage transferred in an electrochemical reaction.
   D. Spectrophotometric methods for sodium use cyclic organic molecules to bind the ion, resulting in a color change.

8. **All of the following statements regarding the spectrophotometric method for chloride measurement are true *except***

   A. Sensitivity of the method is improved by adding mercuric nitrate to the reagent.
   B. Reagent for the method contains mercuric thiocyanate and ferric ion.
   C. Color change is measured when mercuric chloride is formed.

D. Color change is measured when ferric ion combines with free thiocyanate.

9. **Which of the following statements regarding ion activity versus ion concentration is *true*?**

   A. Activity coefficient of an ion is independent of the total ionic strength of the solution.
   B. Activity coefficient of an ion in plasma may vary widely.
   C. Activity of an ion equals the activity coefficient times the concentration of the ion.
   D. Distinction between activity and concentration is important clinically.

10. **All of the following statements regarding plasma volume versus water volume are true *except***

    A. Normal plasma contains 93% water by volume.
    B. Nonwater volume of plasma is largely due to proteins.
    C. Water content of plasma may be significantly increased by hyperlipidemia or hyperproteinemia.
    D. Pseudohyponatremia may occur with flame photometric methods and ion-selective electrodes that use a diluted sample.

11. **All of the following are true of calculated osmolality *except***

    A. Multiplying the sodium by 2 gives an approximation of total cations and anions in plasma.
    B. Dividing glucose by 18 converts mg/dL to mOsm/kg.
    C. Dividing urea by 2.8 converts mg/dL to mmol/L.
    D. In patients with renal failure, calculating the effective plasma osmolality by dropping the term for urea.

12. **All of the following statements regarding hyponatremia are true *except***

    A. Most cases are associated with hypoosmolality.
    B. The most prominent effects of hyponatremia are renal failure and pulmonary edema.
    C. Chronic hyponatremia that develops slowly is better tolerated than acute hyponatremia.
    D. Almost all cases of hyponatremia are associated with a defect in renal water excretion.

13. **Which of following causes of hyponatremia demonstrates an increase in serum osmoles, hypovolemia, and a low urinary sodium concentration?**

    A. Hyperglycemia
    B. Pseudohypernatremia
    C. Syndrome of inappropriate antidiuretic hormone (SIADH) secretion
    D. Renal failure with hypervolemia

14. **All of the following statements regarding SIADH secretion are true *except***

    A. It is a common cause of hyponatremia.
    B. Its causes include ectopic production of ADH by tumor, pulmonary diseases, central nervous system disorders, and drugs.
    C. The diagnosis is suggested by demonstrating hyponatremia, hypoosmolality, and normal extracellular volume status.
    D. Urine sodium usually is low.

15. **All of the following statements regarding hypernatremia are true *except***

    A. Hypernatremia is generally associated with increased osmolality.
    B. Symptoms are mainly cardiac, including arrhythmia and cardiac arrest.
    C. Symptoms of hypernatremia are mainly neurologic.
    D. Significant hypernatremia is always associated with a defect in the thirst response or occurs in patients who cannot access or drink water (coma, infants).

16. **Which of the following conditions of hypernatremia demonstrates hypervolemia, urine osmolality >700 mOsm/kg, and urine sodium >20 mEq/L?**

    A. Hyperaldosteronism
    B. Insensible losses
    C. Osmotic diuresis
    D. Diabetes insipidus

17. **All of the following statements regarding diabetes insipidus are true *except***

    A. It is classified as either central (CDI) or nephrogenic (NDI).
    B. CDI is due to a defect in ADH secretion, whereas NDI is due to impaired renal response to ADH.
    C. Characteristics include hypernatremia, normovolemia, urine osmolality <700, and variable urinary sodium concentration.
    D. Differentiation of NDI from CDI is based on urine electrolyte levels.

18. **Which of the following statements regarding hypokalemia is *true*?**

    A. Signs and symptoms typically begin to occur at a plasma potassium of 4.0 mmol/L.
    B. Manifestations include neuromuscular findings, impaired renal concentrating ability, cardiac arrhythmia, and increased digitalis sensitivity.
    C. Electrocardiographic findings are similar to hyponatremia.
    D. It is classified based on plasma osmolality.

19. **All of the following conditions are associated with hypokalemia *except***

    A. alkalosis
    B. rhabdomyolysis
    C. insulin
    D. catecholamines

20. **All of the following statements regarding hyperkalemia are true *except***

    A. Signs and symptoms include muscle weakness and cardiac conduction abnormalities.
    B. Symptoms of muscle weakness generally do not occur until serum potassium is >7 mmol/L.
    C. Electrocardiographic changes generally do not occur below a serum level of 7.5 mmol/L.
    D. Chronic hyperkalemia virtually always is associated with impaired urinary potassium excretion.

21. **Which of the following statements regarding pseudohyperkalemia is *true*?**

    A. It occurs in samples with hemolysis or leukocytosis.
    B. It is due to increased plasma lipids or proteins.
    C. It is the result of pseudohypoaldosteronism.
    D. It is secondary to adrenal insufficiency.

22. **All of the following are causes of hypochloremia *except***

    A. bromism
    B. vomiting
    C. metabolic alkalosis
    D. hyperaldosteronism

23. **Which of the following statements regarding acid–base regulation is *true*?**

    A. The major factors determining the rate of alveolar ventilation are the arterial pH and PO_2.
    B. Acidemia stimulates respiration and alkalemia induces hypoventilation.
    C. Ammonia formation is the main mechanism by which kidneys augment hydrogen ion excretion in states of acidosis.
    D. Excretion of free hydrogen ion by the kidney is significant to acid–base balance.

24. **All of the following statements regarding β_2-microglobulin (B2M) are true *except***

    A. It is the common light chain of the class I major histocompatibility (MHC) antigen.
    B. It is present on all nucleated cells.
    C. Plasma B2M may be decreased in multiple myeloma.
    D. It is filtered by the glomerulus and degraded by renal tubular cells.

25. **All of the following acid–base parameters usually are measured directly by blood gas instruments *except***

    A. bicarbonate
    B. pH
    C. PO_2
    D. PCO_2

26. **All of the following statements regarding blood pH measurements are true *except***

    A. pH meters use a glass electrode that is selective for hydrogen ions.
    B. By convention, measurements are made at 25°C.
    C. Blood pH measurements are temperature sensitive.
    D. "Suspension effect" is a systematic bias resulting from red blood cells at the interface with a concentrated KCl bridge solution.

27. **All of the following statements regarding blood carbon dioxide measurements are true *except***

    A. PCO_2 is measured using a modified pH electrode.
    B. The electrode for measuring PCO_2 uses a gas-permeable membrane.
    C. Total CO_2 includes dissolved CO_2, carbonic acid, bicarbonate ion, carbonate ion, and carbamates.
    D. Unlike PO_2, measurement of PCO_2 is not temperature dependent.

28. **All of the following statements regarding specimens for blood gas analysis are true *except***

    A. Arterial blood is the preferred specimen.
    B. Capillary blood sampling requires that the skin be warmed so the PO_2 will be close to the arterial level.
    C. Correlation of capillary PCO_2 to arterial PCO_2 is not very good.
    D. Correlation of capillary PO_2 to arterial PO_2 is not very good.

29. **All of the following statements regarding specimens for blood gas analysis are true *except***

    A. Both glass and plastic syringes may be used, but glass is technically superior.
    B. Specimens in both glass and plastic syringes should be chilled in ice water.
    C. Plastic syringes can alter PO_2 and PCO_2 due to room air dissolved in plastic.
    D. Heparin is the preferred anticoagulant.

30. **All of the following are acceptable quality control materials for blood gas analysis *except***

    A. aqueous controls
    B. stabilized whole blood or hemolysate
    C. whole blood matrix
    D. perfluorocarbon emulsion

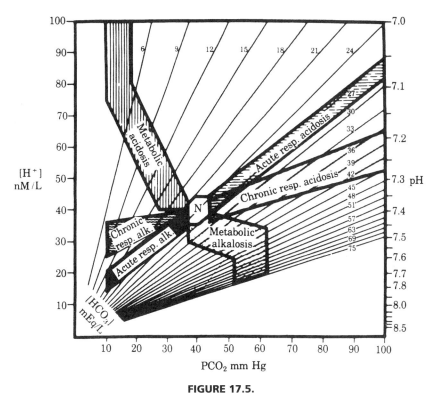

FIGURE 17.5.

31. Which laboratory values correspond with a primary metabolic acidosis?

A. Decreased pH, decreased HCO_3^-
B. Decreased pH, increased P_{CO_2}
C. Increased pH, increased HCO_3^-
D. Increased pH, decreased P_{CO_2}

32. Figure 17.5 shows a nomogram for interpreting acid–base disorders. What is the acid–base disorder for pH 7.35, P_{CO_2} 55?

A. etabolic acidosis
B. Acute respiratory alkalosis
C. Chronic respiratory acidosis
D. Metabolic alkalosis

33. According to the simplified set of rules of acid–base disorders in Table 17.6, pH of 7.35 and P_{CO_2} of 52

TABLE 17.6. SIMPLIFIED RULES FOR INTERPRETATION OF ACID-BASE DISORDERS

Rule 1	A change in P_{CO_2} of 10 mm Hg will change the pH by 0.08.
Rule 2	A change in bicarbonate of 10 mmol/L will change the pH by 0.15.

*a*Adapted from Cornella L, Braen R, Olding M. Blood gases and acid-base disorders. In: *Clinician's pocket reference*, 4th ed. Laguna Niguel, CA: Capistrano Press, 1983:157–168.

mm Hg will classify into which of the following acid–base disorders?

A. Reparatory acidosis
B. Metabolic acidosis
C. Compensated metabolic acidosis
D. Compensated reparatory acidosis

34. All of the following are associated with respiratory acidosis *except*

A. botulism
B. brainstem injury
C. fever
D. cardiac arrest

35. All of the following are associated with respiratory alkalosis *except*

A. aspirin overdose (early)
B. central nervous system infection
C. liver failure
D. aspirin overdose (late)

36. All of the following statements regarding metabolic alkalosis are true *except*

A. It includes chloride-responsive and chloride-resistant types that are distinguished by measuring urine chloride.
B. Contraction alkalosis results from depletion of salt and water without a concomitant loss of bicarbonate.

C. During contraction alkalosis, the kidney cannot excrete the excess bicarbonate due to conservation of sodium.

D. Hyperkalemia promotes development of metabolic alkalosis.

37. **Which of the following is a major cause of chloride-responsive metabolic alkalosis?**

    A. Vomiting
    B. Hyperaldosteronism
    C. Cushing syndrome
    D. Bartter syndrome

38. **All of the following are associated with an anion gap metabolic acidosis *except***

    A. rhabdomyolysis
    B. ketoacidosis
    C. renal tubular acidosis (RTA), type I
    D. ethylene glycol

39. **What is the anion gap in a patient with serum sodium of 140, serum chloride of 105, and bicarbonate of 24?**

    A. 11 (abnormal)
    B. 59 (abnormal)
    C. 11 (normal)
    D. Not enough data available

40. **Which type of RTA is due to a defect in the inability to secrete hydrogen ions in the distal tubules?**

    A. RTA, type I
    B. RTA, type II
    C. RTA, type III
    D. RTA, type IV

Indicate whether each of the following statements is true (T) or false (F).

41. **Potassium salts are the major component of plasma osmolality.**

42. **Flame photometry is the reference method for measurement of serum chloride.**

43. **Measurement of serum potassium concentration with a potassium ion-selective electrode that responds slightly to sodium can be tolerated.**

44. **Urea freely crosses cell membranes and does not influence the distribution of water in the body.**

45. **Obtaining arterial blood gas (ABG) samples in a plastic syringe should be chilled on ice and analyzed within 20 minutes.**

46. **Ingestion of large quantities of licorice may cause a metabolic alkalosis secondary to weak mineralocorticoid activity.**

47. **Salicylate overdose initially causes a respiratory alkalosis because of a stimulatory effect on the central respiratory center.**

48. **A high osmol gap with a high anion gap metabolic acidosis is suggestive of methanol or ethylene glycol poisoning.**

49. **RTA, type II results from deficiency of aldosterone.**

50. **RTA, type III results from renal bicarbonate wasting.**

RESPIRATION AND MEASUREMENT OF OXYGEN AND HEMOGLOBIN

QUESTIONS

Select the one best answer of the choices offered.

1. **Compliance is a measure of the stretchability of the lung and is inversely proportional to elasticity.**

    A. True   B. False

2. **Assuming the surface tension is the same, the smaller the alveolar radius, the lesser the pressure required to maintain the alveolar volume.**

    A. True   B. False

3. **All of the following statements regarding ventilation-perfusion matching (V/Q ratio) are true *except***

    A. Most of the total lung ventilation is directed to the apices.
    B. V/Q mismatch is the most common cause of hypoxemia in disease states.
    C. Ventilation and perfusion are unevenly distributed in the normal lung.
    D. Overall V/Q ratio is normally approximately 0.8.

4. **All of the following statements regarding the regulation of respiration are true *except***

    A. Changes in PCO_2 affect the rate and depth of respiration.
    B. Decrease in pH stimulates both the central and peripheral chemoreceptors.
    C. Juxtaproximal tubular cells in the kidney sense hypoxia and respond by increasing erythropoietin levels.
    D. Central chemoreceptors respond to the changes in pH and PO_2.

5. **Hemoglobin-oxygen affinity is reduced by all of the following *except***

    A. increase in PCO_2
    B. increase in erythrocyte 2,3-diphosphoglycerate concentration

C. increase in pH
D. increase in temperature

6. **All of the following statements regarding the oxygen electrode method are true *except***

    A. One molecule of oxygen is reduced to $2OH^-$ at a platinum wire cathode.
    B. Current depends on the number of oxygen molecules reaching the cathode per unit time.
    C. The method is based on potentiometry.
    D. Calibration is done with two different gas mixtures.

7. **All of the following statements regarding specimen and specimen handling for measurement of different hemoglobin species are true *except***

    A. For measurement of only carboxyhemoglobin (COHb) or methemoglobin (metHb), venous blood is preferred.
    B. Heparin or ethylenediaminetetraacetic acid can be used as anticoagulants for measurement of COHb or metHb.
    C. Heparinized arterial blood is required for measurement of oxyhemoglobin (O_2Hb).
    D. The specimen should be stored on ice for measurement of metHb.

8. **O_2Hb and oxygen saturation measurements are interchangeable.**

    A. True   B. False

9. **All of the following statements regarding quality control (QC) and proficiency testing of the oximetry measurements are true *except***

    A. different readings of dye mixtures usually are obtained on various makes of oximeters.
    B. Stabilized hemolysates is the ideal material for QC of oximetry measurements.

C. Stabilized erythrocytes may be more resistant to lysis than normal red cells.

D. Total hemoglobin measured by an oximeter can be checked by using fresh whole blood together with the cyanmethemoglobin reference method for the total hemoglobin.

Match each of the following optical-based methods used in point-of-care testing instruments with the corresponding analyte.

10. Colorimetric measurement of pseudoperoxidase activity

11. Optode based on fluorescence quenching

12. Optode based on absorbance measurement of immobilized pH indicator

13. Optode based on pH sensor and gas permeable membrane

A. P_{CO_2}
B. pH
C. Total hemoglobin
D. P_{O_2}

14. All of the following statements regarding hypoxia and hypoxemia are true *except*

A. Hypoxia implies that inadequate amounts of oxygen are available to the tissues.
B. Hypoxemia refers to decreased blood P_{O_2}.
C. Hypoxemia is one cause of hypoxia.
D. Hypoxia does not exist with normal P_{O_2}.

Match each of the following mechanisms of respiratory failure with the corresponding blood gas findings (each answer might be used more than once).

15. Diffusion impairment

16. Low inspired oxygen

17. V/Q mismatch

18. Hypoventilation

19. Right to left shunt

A. Low P_{O_2} and normal P_{CO_2}
B. Low P_{O_2} and elevated P_{CO_2}
C. Low P_{O_2} and normal/low P_{CO_2}
D. Low P_{O_2} and elevated P_{CO_2} when severe

Match each of the following clinical findings with the corresponding abnormal pattern of breathing (each answer might be used more than once).

20. Regular, deep, and rapid breathing

21. Cerebrovascular accidents

22. Alternating hyperventilation and hypoventilation with periods of apnea

23. Diabetic ketoacidosis

A. Cheyne-Stokes breathing
B. Kussmaul breathing

Match each of the following pathophysiologic/clinical findings with the corresponding respiratory disease.

24. Normal respiratory cycles but with reduced volumes

25. The interstitial compartment is the initial site of fluid accumulation

26. Derangement of alveolar-capillary permeability

27. Two types of patients: "fighters" and "nonfighters"

A. Adult respiratory distress syndrome (diffuse alveolar damage)
B. Diffuse interstitial lung diseases
C. Chronic obstructive pulmonary disease
D. Pulmonary edema

28. All of the following statements regarding metHb are true *except*

A. Homozygous metHb reductase deficiency produces elevated metHb levels with cyanosis.
B. Methemoglobinemia can be treated by the administration of oxygen.
C. The normal concentration of metHb is <1.5% of total hemoglobin.
D. Increased metHb levels can result from sulfonamide ingestion.

29. All of the following statements regarding COHb are true *except*

A. The affinity of hemoglobin to CO is 210 times that of oxygen.
B. Smokers may exhibit COHb levels of 8% of total hemoglobin.
C. The half-life of COHb is 4 to 5 hours while breathing 100% oxygen.
D. The interaction between CO and hemoglobin is reversible.

NITROGEN METABOLITES AND RENAL FUNCTION

QUESTIONS

Select the one best answer of the choices offered.

1. **All of the following are important endocrine functions performed by the kidney** *except*

    A. It produces erythropoietin.
    B. It produces renin.
    C. It metabolizes (activates) vitamin D.
    D. It activates aldosterone.

2. **All of the following statements regarding normal renal anatomy are true** *except*

    A. A nephron is composed of glomerulus, proximal convoluted tubule, loop of Henle, distal convoluted tubule, and collecting tubule.
    B. An afferent arteriole enters the glomerulus and an efferent arteriole exits the glomerulus.
    C. The loop of Henle is responsible for countercurrent multiplication.
    D. The proximal convoluted tubule is the primary site for action of antidiuretic hormone (ADH).

3. **Which of the following statements regarding normal renal physiology is** *true?*

    A. Normal glomerular filtration rate (GFR) is 50 mL/min or 72 L/day.
    B. Concentration of urine is greatest in the inner medullary zone of the kidney.
    C. Tubular secretion always requires an active carrier-mediated mechanism.
    D. Only 5% of the glomerular filtrate ultimately reaches the renal pelvis as urine.

4. **All of the following statements regarding renal regulation of acid–base balance are true** *except*

    A. Hydrogen ion can combine with ammonia to form ammonium ion.
    B. In the tubular cell, carbon dioxide is used as a source of hydrogen ion and bicarbonate.
    C. Hydrogen ion excretion requires resorption of cations, particularly potassium.
    D. Hydrogen ion secretion in the proximal tubule is almost entirely used in reabsorbing bicarbonate.

5. **All of the following statements regarding urine specific gravity (SG) are true** *except*

    A. Urine SG is defined as the ratio of the weight of a volume of urine to the weight of an equal volume of water.
    B. Random urine samples exhibit a wider range of normal SG values than 24-hour urine samples.
    C. Urine SG and urine osmolality are comparable measurements of renal concentrating ability.
    D. Urine SG is related to the concentration of dissolved solutes.

6. **All of the following statements regarding methods for measuring urine SG are true** *except*

    A. The colligative properties most commonly used in the laboratory to measure osmolality are based on osmotic pressure.
    B. Dipstick test strips use a polymer with repeating carboxylic acid groups and detect a pH change with an indicator.
    C. Nonionic species, such as glucose, produce falsely low estimations of SG using test strips.
    D. Urine SG can be determined by refractometry.

7. **All of the following statements regarding urine osmolality are true** *except*

    A. Osmolality is determined by the sum of the active concentration of all species dissolved in a solution.
    B. Measurement is independent of colligative properties.
    C. Osmolality measurements may differ from SG, especially when the urine contains high levels of protein, glucose, or radiopaque dyes.
    D. The most commonly used methods are based on freezing point depression or vapor pressure.

8. **All of the following are colligative properties** *except*

   A. freezing point depression
   B. vapor pressure depression
   C. boiling point elevation
   D. refractive index

9. **All of the following conditions typically are associated with low urine osmolality** *except*

   A. central diabetes insipidus
   B. water loading
   C. nephrogenic diabetes insipidus
   D. dehydration

10. **Which of the following statements regarding urea is** *true*?

    A. Urea is the major nitrogen-containing metabolite from the degradation of protein.
    B. The major organs responsible for urea formation include the lungs, pancreas, and brain.
    C. Urea levels are exquisitely sensitive to minor changes in GFR.
    D. Urea is freely filtered by the glomerulus and approximately 25% is reabsorbed into extracellular fluid.

11. **All of the following may be associated with a low serum urea level** *except*

    A. low-protein diet
    B. congestive heart failure
    C. pregnancy
    D. androgen administration

12. **All of the following prerenal causes of an elevated serum urea are due to increased synthesis** *except*

    A. Cushing syndrome
    B. cirrhosis
    C. hemolysis
    D. gastrointestinal bleeding

13. **The most commonly used method for assay of urea is**

    A. urease with glutamate dehydrogenase
    B. conductometric urease
    C. diacetyl
    D. O-phthalaldehyde

14. **All of the following statements regarding urease/ glutamate dehydrogenase methods for urea are true** *except*

    A. The urease reaction is coupled to glutamate dehydrogenase to produce NAD^+.
    B. Urease with glutamate dehydrogenase coupled reaction is the most common analytic method.
    C. Urease converts urea to ammonia.
    D. The reaction is difficult to automate.

15. **All of the following statements regarding creatinine metabolism are true** *except*

    A. Creatinine is formed by nonenzymatic degradation of creatine.
    B. Approximately 0.1% of total body creatine is degraded per day.
    C. Creatinine is excreted by glomerular filtration and a lesser amount (10% to 20%) by tubular secretion.
    D. Creatinine is not reabsorbed by the renal tubules.

16. **All of the following conditions are associated with an increase in serum creatinine** *except*

    A. myopathic muscle disease (e.g., dermatomyositis)
    B. muscle atrophy
    C. congestive heart failure
    D. cirrhosis

17. **All of the following statements regarding urea nitrogen to creatinine ratio are true** *except*

    A. Normal ratio is 10:1 to 20:1.
    B. Prerenal azotemia is associated with an increased ratio.
    C. Postrenal azotemia is associated with a decreased ratio.
    D. Intrinsic renal disease is associated with a normal ratio.

18. **Which of the following statements regarding urine creatinine level is** *true*?

    A. It depends mainly on the muscle mass of the subject.
    B. It is quite variable in an individual.
    C. It is generally higher in females.
    D. It provides accurate measurement of the completeness of a timed urine collection.

19. **All of the following conditions are true of the Jaffe reaction for creatine analysis** *except*

    A. It utilizes creatininase to produce ammonium ion.
    B. It is based on the reaction of creatinine with picrate.
    C. The rate of reaction is dependent on the alkali concentration.
    D. It is not specific for creatinine.

20. **All of the following are noncreatinine chromogens that cause positive interference in the Jaffe reaction** *except*

    A. protein
    B. glucose
    C. ascorbic acid
    D. bilirubin

21. **All of the following may be used to decrease interference by noncreatinine chromogens in the Jaffe reaction** *except*

A. pretreatment with Lloyd's reagent
B. use of endpoint as opposed to kinetic assays
C. precipitation of proteins
D. addition of buffers to complex glucose

22. All of the following may be used to assay creatinine *except*

A. creatininase methods
B. creatinine hydrolase
C. creatinine reductase
D. high-pressure liquid chromatography

23. All of the following statements regarding creatinine clearance are true *except*

A. It provides similar information as the inulin clearance and practical to perform.
B. It is greater in males than females.
C. It overestimates the GFR.
D. The coefficient of variation for creatinine clearance is small (<3%).

24. Which of the following indicators measures renal plasma flow?

A. Creatine clearance
B. *p*-Aminohippurate
C. Sodium clearance
D. Inulin clearance

25. Which of the following statements regarding uric acid metabolism is *true*?

A. Uric acid is the major end product of purine metabolism.
B. Virtually all uric acid in the body arises from the liver.
C. Of the filtered uric acid, 60% is actively reabsorbed in the proximal tubules of the kidney.
D. Uric acid is excreted primarily through the gastrointestinal tract.

26. All of the following are associated with hyper-uricemia *except*

A. gout
B. lymphoma
C. Lesch-Nyhan syndrome
D. Fanconi syndrome

27. All of the following statements regarding gout are true *except*

A. It is characterized by hyperuricemia and uric acid crystal deposition in and around the joints.
B. It is associated with nephrolithiasis.
C. Most patients have a positive family history.
D. Approximately 90% of patients are male.

28. All of the following statements regarding methods for assay of uric acid are true *except*

A. Phosphotungstic acid methods are based on the oxidation of uric acid to allantoin with the production of a colored product.
B. Phosphotungstic acid methods are specific, but nonsensitive.
C. Uricase methods are based on the oxidation of uric acid to allantoin and hydrogen peroxide.
D. Phosphotungstic acid method give plasma uric acid values 0.2 to 0.4 mg/dL higher than uricase methods.

29. All of the following statements regarding ammonium are true *except*

A. The major source of ammonia is the gastrointestinal tract.
B. Ammonia is metabolized to urea in the liver.
C. Elevated ammonia levels are observed in enzyme deficiencies of the urea cycle, Reye syndrome, and severe liver disease.
D. Blood ammonia levels closely correlate with the severity of hepatic encephalopathy.

30. The most common cause of acute renal failure is

A. malignancy
B. intrinsic renal disease
C. urinary tract obstruction
D. acute tubular necrosis

20

CALCIUM, MAGNESIUM, AND PHOSPHATE

QUESTIONS

Select the one best answer of the choices offered.

1. **All of the following statements regarding calcium are true** *except*

   A. Calcium is required for many enzyme functions, for normal muscle and cardiac function, as a structural component of bone, and as a second messenger controlling secretion of many hormones.
   B. Hypocalcemia may be associated with cardiac arrhythmia, neuromuscular irritability, and tetany.
   C. The major role of calcium is intracellular, although measurements in the clinical laboratory use blood specimens.
   D. Reliable measurements of ionized calcium currently are not practical.

2. **All of the following statements regarding parathyroid hormone (PTH) are true** *except*

   A. PTH secretion is stimulated by a decreased ionized calcium.
   B. PTH acts on bone by activating osteoclasts.
   C. PTH acts on the kidney by stimulating tubular calcium resorption.
   D. PTH acts on the liver to promote vitamin D hydroxylation.

3. **All of the following statements regarding vitamin D metabolism are true** *except*

   A. Vitamin D may be obtained from either the diet or skin exposure to sunlight.
   B. Vitamin D increases calcium and decreases phosphate resorption in the intestine.
   C. Vitamin D_3 is activated by hydroxylation at the 25 position in the liver and at the 1 position in the kidney.
   D. Vitamin D enhances the effect of PTH on bone and kidney.

4. **All of the following statements regarding calcitonin are true** *except*

   A. It is secreted by medullary cells in the parathyroid.
   B. It is secreted in response to increased ionized calcium.
   C. It inhibits bone osteoclasts.
   D. It inhibits the action of PTH and vitamin D.

5. **Which of the following statements regarding calcium homeostasis is** *false*?

   A. Only 1% of the total body calcium is in the extracellular fluid.
   B. Intracellular calcium levels are much higher than plasma concentrations.
   C. Approximately 45% of calcium is ionized in the blood.
   D. Approximately 40% of calcium is bound to albumin.

6. **Calcium in blood exists in all of the following forms** *except*

   A. ionized
   B. protein bound
   C. bound to inorganic anions
   D. complexed to calmodulin

7. **All of the following statements regarding ionized calcium are true** *except*

   A. Ionized calcium is the active form.
   B. Ionized calcium can be calculated from the total calcium.
   C. Ionized calcium concentration is increased at lower pH.
   D. Ionized calcium should be measured on aerobically collected blood.

8. **The differential diagnosis of hypocalcemia includes all of the following** *except*

   A. autoimmune hypoparathyroidism

B. malignancy

C. magnesium deficiency

D. after thyroid or parathyroid surgery

9. **Which of the following statements is associated with hypocalcemia?**

    A. Hypermagnesemia

    B. Primary hyperparathyroidism

    C. Neonates 1 to 3 days after birth

    D. Lung cancer

10. **Which of the following statements regarding hypercalcemia secondary to pseudohypoparathyroidism is *true*?**

    A. Serum magnesium normal, PTH low

    B. Serum magnesium normal, PTH high, serum phosphate high

    C. Serum magnesium normal, PTH high, serum phosphate low

    D. Serum magnesium normal, PTH high, serum phosphate normal

11. **All of the following statements regarding hypocalcemia are true *except***

    A. Neonatal hypocalcemia is always abnormal.

    B. Hypocalcemia may occur in patients receiving citrated blood products.

    C. Hypoparathyroidism may be caused by autoimmune disease or after surgical procedures of the neck.

    D. Pseudohypoparathyroidism results from defective renal response to PTH.

12. **All of the following may contribute to altered ionized calcium levels in patients with renal failure *except***

    A. altered vitamin D metabolism

    B. altered serum magnesium levels

    C. acidosis

    D. secondary hypoparathyroidism

13. **Hypomagnesemia may induce hypocalcemia by all of the following mechanisms *except***

    A. impaired action of calcitonin

    B. inhibition of PTH secretion

    C. inhibition of PTH action at its receptor on bone

    D. interference with the action of vitamin D

14. **All of the following statements regarding hypercalcemia are true *except***

    A. Total calcium level may be normal.

    B. Primary hyperparathyroidism and malignancy are the most common causes.

    C. Hypercalcemia may be asymptomatic.

D. PTH-like protein has PTH-like activity on the kidney but not on bone.

15. **Tumors commonly associated with hypercalcemia include all of the following *except***

    A. bronchogenic carcinoma

    B. breast carcinoma

    C. astrocytoma

    D. head and neck cancers

16. **All of the following statements regarding specimens for calcium measurement are true *except***

    A. Total calcium should only be performed on serum.

    B. Specimens for ionized calcium must be collected anaerobically.

    C. Anticoagulants that bind calcium interfere with all methods of measurement, including atomic absorption.

    D. Metabolic activity of cells affects pH and, therefore, ionized calcium.

17. **Which of the following statement regarding atomic absorption for measuring calcium is *true*?**

    A. Atomic absorption spectroscopy is the reference method for total calcium.

    B. Many automated methods of measuring serum calcium are based on atomic absorption.

    C. Atomic absorption is based on the reaction between calcium and the dye ortho-cresolphthalein complexone.

    D. Anticoagulants that bind calcium do not interfere with ion-selective electrodes.

18. **All of the following methods are used to measure calcium *except***

    A. ortho-cresolphthalein

    B. bromocresol green

    C. ion-selective electrodes

    D. atomic absorption

19. **Which of the following statements regarding magnesium metabolism is *true*?**

    A. Renal magnesium resorption competes with calcium resorption.

    B. PTH increases renal magnesium resorption and enhances intestinal absorption.

    C. Aldosterone has the opposite effect on magnesium as PTH.

    D. Most magnesium in serum is protein bound.

20. **All of the following are associated with hypomagnesemia *except***

    A. diarrhea

B. diuretics

C. renal insufficiency

D. cisplatin

21. **All of the following anticoagulants exhibit significant magnesium binding and should not be used for sample collection** *except*

   A. heparin

   B. EDTA (ethylenediaminetetraacetic acid)

   C. citrate

   D. oxalate

22. **All of the following statements regarding methods for measuring magnesium are true** *except*

   A. Serum total magnesium levels may not reflect physiologically active magnesium.

   B. Serum concentration accurately reflects intracellular magnesium.

   C. Ion-selective electrodes for magnesium have become available only recently.

   D. Hemolysis during phlebotomy may significantly elevate magnesium levels.

23. **All of the following are acceptable methods for measuring serum magnesium** *except*

   A. arsenazo III (colorimetric)

   B. atomic absorption spectroscopy

   C. calmagite (colorimetric)

   D. methylthymoblue (colorimetric)

24. **All of the following are causes of hyperphosphatemia** *except*

   A. renal failure

   B. lymphoblastic leukemia

   C. rhabdomyolysis

   D. hyperparathyroidism

25. **A patient has high serum phosphate, glomerular filtration rate of 60 mL/min, and increased urinary phosphate concentration. Which of the following diagnosis is most likely?**

   A. Rhabdomyolysis

   B. Chronic renal failure

   C. Acute renal failure

   D. Hypoparathyroidism

21

HEME SYNTHESIS AND CATABOLISM

QUESTIONS

Select the one best answer of the choices offered.

1. **The primary sites of heme synthesis are the bone marrow and the spleen.**

   A. True   B. False

2. **Porphyrins are the oxidized forms of porphyrinogens.**

   A. True   B. False

3. **Porphyrins with cutaneous manifestations include**

   A. variegate porphyria
   B. porphyria cutanea tarda
   C. erythropoietic porphyria
   D. A and B
   E. A, B, and C

4. **Acute intermittent porphyria is an autosomal dominant disease.**

   A. True   B. False

5. **Acute porphyrias, inherited in an autosomal dominant manner, are**

   A. acute intermittent porphyria
   B. variegate porphyria
   C. hereditary coproporphyria
   D. A and B
   E. A, B, and C

22

TOXICOLOGY

QUESTIONS

Select the one best answer of the choices offered.

1. **All of the following statements regarding clinical toxicology are true** *except*
   A. Drug history frequently is unreliable or unavailable.
   B. For some intoxications, measurement of serum drug levels may be useful to gauge the severity of intoxication, the prognosis, and to evaluate therapy.
   C. Screening for drugs of abuse usually tests for a broad panel of drugs.
   D. The traditional mission of the clinical toxicology laboratory is analysis of drugs for the purpose of patient care.

2. **Specific treatments are available for all of the following drugs** *except*
   A. acetaminophen
   B. barbiturates
   C. methanol
   D. ethanol

3. **All of the following statements regarding drug testing during pregnancy or on infants are true** *except*
   A. Screening usually focuses on a small panel of the most frequently abused drugs.
   B. Urine testing during pregnancy may be useful to diagnose dependency and to monitor drug use during pregnancy.
   C. Urine screening of infants underestimates the number of babies at risk.
   D. Identification of an illicit drug in an infant's urine constitutes medical, not legal, information and should never be reported to government agencies.

4. **A basic stat clinical toxicology service should include all of the following** *except*
   A. phenothiazines
   B. salicylate/acetaminophen
   C. barbiturates

   D. tricyclic antidepressants

5. **All of the following statements regarding drug screens are true** *except*
   A. They represent a compromise between turnaround time, specificity, and sensitivity.
   B. They include only qualitative assays.
   C. Turnaround time increases as the number of drug assays increases.
   D. They should be designed to detect a shorter list of drugs based on the prevalence of drugs in the population and clinical usefulness of detection.

6. **All of the following statements regarding drug screens are true** *except*
   A. They usually are performed on urine.
   B. Urine samples permit analysis of drugs in low concentration.
   C. Urine tests are only qualitative.
   D. Plasma samples are preferred because urine contains a mixture of drugs and metabolites.

7. **All of the following statements regarding quantitative toxicology testing are true** *except*
   A. Quantitative tests are more time consuming.
   B. Quantitative levels can be misleading for drugs to which tolerance can develop.
   C. Quantitative testing typically is performed on blood as opposed to urine samples.
   D. Quantitative results are always confirmed.

8. **Toxicology tests in which quantitative information is generally useful to patient management include all of the following** *except*
   A. alcohols
   B. acetaminophen
   C. barbiturates
   D. theophylline

9. **All of the following statements regarding toxicologic methods are true** *except*

A. Drug screen methods, including colorimetry, immunoassay, thin-layer chromatography (TLC), and gas chromatography (GC), do not necessarily give unequivocal drug identification.

B. Confirmation of a positive result should always be performed on the original specimen aliquot and not a new aliquot.

C. Some toxicology assays are drug group specific rather than analyte specific for a particular drug.

D. Confirmation testing is mandatory in forensic toxicology.

10. **All of the following statements regarding spot tests for drugs are true *except***

A. Only urine is appropriate as a specimen.

B. They may identify a class of drugs or a particular drug.

C. They are rapid, inexpensive screening tests.

D. A positive test should prompt more definitive testing.

11. **Which of the following is a spot test for volatiles?**

A. Trinder

B. Cresol-ammonia

C. Dichromate

D. Forrest

12. **All of the following statements regarding TLC for drug testing are true *except***

A. It is not widely used because the method is labor intensive.

B. It requires highly trained personnel.

C. It has lower resolution compared with GC or high-pressure liquid chromatography (HPLC).

D. The ability to perform simultaneous analyses of several specimens is an advantage.

13. **All of the following statements regarding GC for drug testing are true *except***

A. It is useful for separating a mixture of drugs.

B. It is the method of choice for volatile compounds.

C. No single column is sufficient for a drug screen.

D. The high sensitivity of electron capture detector (ECD) makes this method suitable for drug screening.

14. **All of the following statements regarding HPLC for drug testing are true *except***

A. HPLC can separate complex mixtures of drugs.

B. It is unsuitable for analysis of nonvolatile or thermally labile drugs.

C. It is used most often in the analysis of targeted groups of drugs rather than as a broad-spectrum drug screen.

D. An automated liquid chromatography system suitable for routine drug screens has recently been developed.

15. **All of the following statements regarding ethanol are true *except***

A. Test obtained for medical reasons may be used for legal purposes.

B. It is metabolized by liver alcohol dehydrogenase at a rate that follows zero-order kinetics, regardless of concentration.

C. Death may occur at blood levels of 400 to 600 mg/dL.

D. "Proof" means two times the percent of ethanol by volume.

16. **All of the following statements regarding specimens for ethanol analysis are true *except***

A. Urine is not a suitable specimen.

B. Whole blood levels are lower than plasma or serum.

C. Most state laws define alcohol concentration in terms of whole blood, not plasma or serum.

D. For legal purposes, it is acceptable to convert plasma or serum levels to whole blood values using a conversion factor of 1.18.

17. **Breath alcohol test is based on what law of physics?**

A. Beer Lambert

B. Henry

C. Ohm

D. Faraday

18. **Which volatile alcohol is metabolized by alcohol dehydrogenase to acetone?**

A. Methanol

B. Isopropanol

C. Ethanol

D. Ethylene glycol

19. **A patient arrives to the emergency department obtunded. The following laboratory values were obtained: Na = 140 mm/L, K = 3.5 mm/L, Cl = 108 mm/L, HCO₃ = 8 mmol/L, BUN = 10 mg/dL, creatine = 0.9 mg/dL. What is the anion gap?**

A. 24

B. 20

C. 16

D. 10

20. **An infant arrives in the emergency department with abdominal pains and nausea. Accidental ingestion of acetaminophen was suspected. Twelve hours after ingestion, the plasma concentration of aceta-**

minophen was 30 μg/μL. **Which of the following statements is most accurate?**

A. There is a high potential for liver toxicity.
B. Immediate treatment with *N*-acetylcysteine is required.
C. Liver toxicity is unlikely.
D. Procedures for liver transplantation should be initiated.

21. **Which of the following acid–base abnormalities is classically seen in salicylate overdose?**

A. Respiratory acidosis and metabolic alkalosis
B. Respiratory alkalosis and metabolic acidosis
C. Respiratory alkalosis and metabolic alkalosis
D. Respiratory acidosis and metabolic acidosis

22. **All of the following statements regarding cyclic antidepressants are true *except***

A. They are responsible for 25% of all fatal drug exposures.
B. They include tricyclic, tetracyclic, and bicyclic drugs.
C. Toxicity includes anticholinergic and cardiotoxic effects.
D. Hemoperfusion is effective therapy, and drug levels correlate closely with clinical severity.

23. **All of the following statements regarding acute iron toxicity are true *except***

A. It is particularly common in children younger than 6 years.
B. Estimation of ingested elemental iron is important to assessing toxicity.
C. Severe toxicity is manifested mainly by pancreatitis and adrenal insufficiency.
D. Ingestion can be documented by abdominal x-ray for nonchewable tablets.

24. **Which drug has the street name "roofies," rochies," and "rophies"?**

A. Rohipnol

B. γ-Hydroxybutyrate
C. Cocaine
D. Marijuana

25. **Which illicit drug has gained popularity among "rave" party participants?**

A. Gibson (martini with an olive)
B. Marijuana
C. γ-Hydroxybutyrate
D. Opium

Indicate whether each of the following statements is true (T) or false (F).

26. **The main disadvantage of mass spectrometer is cost of instrumentation.**

27. **Alcohol concentration in whole blood is lower than in plasma.**

28. **Methanol is metabolized formaldehyde by aldehyde dehydrogenase.**

29. **The method of choice for identification and measurement of methanol and isopropanol is GC.**

30. **The most common volatile alcohol that causes an increase in serum osmolality is ethylene glycol .**

31. **Barbiturate intoxication is treated with gastric lavage and charcoal.**

32. **Levels of plasma benzodiazepine correlate well with severity of intoxication.**

33. **Deferoxamine interferes with dye-binding calorimetric assays and give falsely low results.**

34. **Benzoylecgonine is the major metabolite of cocaine.**

35. **Dehydration, hyperthermia, and cardiac arrhythmias are seen in "ecstasy" overdose.**

23

TRACE ELEMENTS, VITAMINS, AND NUTRITION

QUESTIONS

Select the one best answer of the choices offered.

1. **All of the following statements regarding malnutrition are true** *except*

   A. Approximately 40% of hospitalized patients have some degree of nutritional deficiency.
   B. Approximately 15% of hospitalized patients have clinically significant protein-calorie malnutrition.
   C. The most common nutritional deficiency in hospitalized patients is deficiency of various vitamins.
   D. It predominately affects infants and children in developing countries.

2. **All of the following statements regarding kwashiorkor are true** *except*

   A. protein deficiency
   B. hepatomegaly
   C. calorie deficiency
   D. hyperpigmentation ("flaky paint" dermatitis)

3. **All of the following statements regarding marasmus are true** *except*

   A. subcutaneous fat near normal
   B. severe muscle wasting
   C. calorie deficiency
   D. protein deficiency

4. **All of the following statements regarding obesity are true** *except*

   A. It is defined in men as having >20% of body weight as fat and in women >30%.
   B. There are no routine laboratory tests available to assess total body fat.
   C. Fenfluramine is an effective and safe therapy for obesity.
   D. Dieting that produces a net negative calorie balance is associated with early weight loss of up to 2 kg due to diuresis resulting from urea depletion.

5. **All of the following tests are useful for routine monitoring of adults on total parenteral nutrition (TPN)** *except*

   A. albumin
   B. prealbumin
   C. triglycerides
   D. magnesium

6. **All of the following laboratory values are the most accurate reflection of nutritional status** *except*

   A. albumin
   B. prealbumin
   C. transferrin
   D. retinol binding protein

7. **The correct order in which various serum proteins respond to changes in nutritional status from fastest to slowest is**

   A. retinol binding protein, transferrin, prealbumin, albumin
   B. transferrin, retinol binding protein, albumin, prealbumin
   C. albumin, prealbumin, retinol binding protein, transferrin
   D. retinol binding protein, prealbumin, transferrin, albumin

8. **Urinary hydroxyproline has been used to assess**

   A. collagen catabolism
   B. glucose metabolism
   C. protein status
   D. triglyceride metabolism

9. **Vitamin A deficiency is associated with which disorder?**

   A. Coagulopathy
   B. Pellagra
   C. Scurvy
   D. Night blindness

10. The most active form of vitamin D is
    A. ergocalciferol
    B. 1,25-(OH)D (calcitriol)
    C. cholecalciferol
    D. 25-(OH)D (calcidiol)

11. **Assessment of vitamin D status is best determined by measurement of serum**
    A. 1,25-(OH)D
    B. 25-(OH)D
    C. calcium
    D. parathyroid hormone (PTH)

12. **Manifestation of thiamine deficiency takes**
    A. years
    B. months
    C. weeks
    D. *in utero*

13. **All of the following are characteristic of niacin deficiency *except***
    A. dermatitis
    B. delirium
    C. diarrhea
    D. dementia

14. **All of the following are considered trace elements *except***
    A. Mg
    B. Fe
    C. Zn
    D. Mn

15. **The most popular analytical method used in detection of trace elements is**
    A. mass spectrometry
    B. atomic absorption spectrophotometry
    C. emission spectrometry
    D. x-ray fluorescence spectrometry

16. **Menkes kinky hair syndrome (trichopoliodystrophy) is characterized by functional deficiency in which element?**
    A. Co
    B. Mg
    C. Zn
    D. Cu

17. **The toxic forms of arsenic is**
    A. arsenobetain
    B. arsenocholin
    C. metallic arsenic
    D. arsine gas

18. **According to Centers for Disease Control (CDC) guidelines, children with lead levels 10 to 14 mg/dL**
    A. are not considered to have lead poisoning
    B. have a poor prognosis
    C. are rescanned frequently
    D. should have chelation therapy initiated

19. **Inhalation of mercury results in a triad that includes all the following *except***
    A. gingivitis
    B. diarrhea
    C. tremor
    D. psychiatric changes

20. **Ingestion of elemental mercury is associated with which of the following?**
    A. It does not cause poisoning
    B. Esophageal erosions
    C. Cancer
    D. Renal failure

Indicate whether each of the following statements is true (T) or false (F).

21. **Parenteral nutrition is indicated for patients who cannot be fed orally or enterally for >3 days.**

22. **Administration of solutions <5,000 mOsm by peripheral parenteral nutrition will prevent phlebitis.**

23. **Serum carotene is not a good indicator of vitamin A status.**

24. **Vitamin C deficiency is defined by a concentration of <50 mg of ascorbic acid in the second 24-hour urine collection.**

25. **Silicon, tin, and vanadium are crucial components of many different tissues and enzyme systems.**

26. **Selenium is the most abundant and least toxic of all the essential elements.**

27. **High levels of aluminum are found in the neurofibrillary tangles in the hippocampus in patients with Alzheimer disease.**

28. **Carbon monoxide is a colorless gas with a garlic-like odor.**

29. **A random urine is a reliable specimen for assessment of arsenic poisoning.**

30. **Gold toxicity is independent of dose, and serum or urine measurement of gold provides no additional information on severity or efficacy of therapy.**

24

INBORN METABOLIC ERRORS

QUESTIONS

Select the one best answer of the choices offered.

1. **All of the following statements regarding primary disorders of amino acid metabolism are true** *except*

   A. All are fatal if untreated.
   B. Primary aminoacidemia results from blocks in the first or second step of amino acid catabolism.
   C. Free amino acids are normally present in all body fluids, including plasma and urine.
   D. Circulating amino acids are the product of protein catabolism.

2. **All of the following statements regarding hyperphenylalaninemia syndrome are true** *except*

   A. Newborn screening is not necessary.
   B. Mental retardation, microcephaly, and eczema are clinical characteristics.
   C. Infants have a typical musty odor.
   D. Disorder is treated by dietary restriction.

3. **All of the following are considered primary disorders of amino acid metabolism** *except*

   A. homocystinuria
   B. tyrosinemia
   C. hyperornithinemia
   D. cystinuria

4. **Urea cycle defects include all of the following** *except*

   A. Hartnup disorder
   B. arginase deficiency
   C. ornithine carbamoyltransferase (OTC) deficiency
   D. carbamoyl phosphate deficiency

5. **Nephrolithiasis, mental retardation, and renal disease classically are associated with which amino acid disorder?**

   A. Phenylketonuria (PKU)
   B. Cystinuria

   C. Tyrosinemia
   D. Homocystinuria

6. **The ferric chloride test is the most commonly used urine spot test for**

   A. homocystinuria
   B. Lowe syndrome
   C. PKU
   D. OTC deficiency

7. **All of the following statements regarding amino acid analysis are true** *except*

   A. Thin-layer chromatography is the most sensitive technique.
   B. Quantitative analysis by high-pressure liquid chromatography (HPLC) with spectrometric detection is the most accurate method to assess amino acid abnormalities.
   C. Thin-layer chromatography provides semiquantitative assessment of amino acid levels.
   D. Patient specimens are compared with age-matched normal controls.

8. **All of the following are organic acidurias arising from blocks in amino acid metabolism** *except*

   A. propionic acidemia
   B. isovaleric acidemia
   C. methylmalonic acidemia
   D. argininemia

9. **Maple syrup urine disease (MSUD) is a disorder resulting in the accumulation of _____ in the urine.**

   A. glycine
   B. branched-chain α-keto acids
   C. homocysteine
   D. pyruvate

10. **All of the following are organic acidurias arising from blocks in fatty acid metabolism** *except*

    A. systemic carnitine deficiency

B. medium-chain acyl-CoA dehydrogenase deficiency
C. glutaric aciduria
D. propionic acidemia

11. **A neonate with severe hypoglycemia, lactic acidosis, hepatomegaly, and doll-like facies has which type of inborn metabolic disorder?**

A. McArdle disease
B. von Gierke disease
C. Pompe disease
D. PKU

12. **All of the following statements regarding mucopolysaccharidoses (MPS) are true *except***

A. Examples of MPS include Gaucher disease, Sandhoff disease, and metachromatic leukodystrophy.
B. MPS result from defects in degradative enzymes for keratin sulfate, dermatan sulfate, and heparin sulfate.
C. MPS typically exhibit a chronic progressive course with hepatosplenomegaly, dysostosis multiplex, coarse facies, and, in some cases, metal retardation.
D. Treatment by enzyme replacement with bone marrow transplantation is promising.

13. **All of the following are oligosaccharidoses *except***

A. fucosidosis
B. mannosidosis
C. Niemann-Pick disease
D. sialidosis

14. **All of the following statements regarding sphingolipidoses are true *except***

A. Sphingolipids are a group of molecules containing sphingosine linked to a fatty acid side chain to form a ceramide.
B. Sphingolipids are particularly abundant in the liver and kidney.
C. Diagnosis is confirmed by enzyme assays.
D. Typically, they are characterized by a progressive neurodegenerative course or severe visceral involvement.

15. **Deficiency in β-glucosidase is seen in**

A. Niemann-Pick disease
B. Tay-Sachs disease
C. Gaucher disease
D. Krabbe disease

Indicate whether each of the following statements is true (T) or false (F).

16. **Nonketotic hyperglycinemia is successfully treated with a low-glycine diet.**

17. **Abnormal elevations in histidine, sarcosine, and proline are clinically benign.**

18. **Clinical abnormalities associated with carnitine deficiency resemble those of Reye syndrome, including hepatic dysfunction, encephalopathy, hypoglycemia, and hyperammonemia.**

19. **Gas chromatography provides a positive identification of organic acids and gives a characteristic mass/charge ratio for each ionizable species.**

20. **Classic galactosemia displays a high incidence of ovarian failure and hypogonadotropic hypogonadism.**

21. **Galactosemia is screened in most states in the United States.**

22. **von Gierke disease results in severe hyperglycemia and lactic acidosis with ketosis.**

23. **Patients with McArdle disease characteristically present in their third or fourth decade with muscle cramps following vigorous exercise.**

24. **Niemann-Pick disease most commonly occurs in Ashkenazi Jews.**

25. **Newborn screening for PKU, homocystinuria, and tyrosinemia are routinely performed.**

25

POINT-OF-CARE TESTING

QUESTIONS

Select the one best answer of the choices offered.

1. **All of the following are the three laboratory services clinical pathologists may provide to clinicians** *except*

   A. point-of care
   B. research laboratory
   C. centralized laboratory
   D. reference laboratory

2. **All of the following statements have influenced the evolution of point-of-care testing (POCT)** *except*

   A. movement toward centralized laboratory testing
   B. expanding menu
   C. improvement of analytical technologies
   D. necessity for rapid turnaround time

3. **Clinical utility of POCT includes all of the following** *except*

   A. detection of translocations
   B. screening
   C. management
   D. diagnosis

4. **When evaluating and validating POCT devices, factors to consider include all of the following** *except*

   A. ease of use
   B. data management
   C. accuracy and precision
   D. leasing agreement

5. **All of the following statements regarding waived testing are true** *except*

   A. It is simple and accurate.
   B. Errors pose no significant risk to the patient.

   C. It does not require a Clinical Laboratory Improvement Amendment (CLIA) 88 certificate.
   D. It is a subcategory of POCT under CLIA 88.

6. **All of the following are examples of CLIA-waived POCTs** *except*

   A. dipstick microalbumin
   B. group A streptococcus antigen
   C. bedside glucose
   D. blood pH

7. **All of the following statements regarding nonwaived testing are true** *except*

   A. It requires a CLIA 88 certificate.
   B. It is noncomplex and easy to perform.
   C. It requires specific training for testing personnel.
   D. Proficiency testing standards available.

Indicate whether each of the following statements is true (T) or false (F).

8. **The unit cost of POCT tends to be lower than other alternatives.**

9. **Eventually, most of the high-volume and critical turnaround time-dependent tests will be available by POCT.**

10. **Home testing is a growing application for POCT.**

11. **All POCT devices currently available and approved by the Food and Drug Administration are reliable.**

12. **It is recommended that the POCT management team control the CLIA certificates.**

13. **A CLIA certificate is not required for waived testing.**

TUMOR MARKERS

QUESTIONS

Select the one best answer of the choices offered.

1. **All of the following statements regarding carcinoembryonic antigen (CEA) are true *except***

   A. Well-differentiated tumors produce CEA, whereas poorly differentiated produce little, if any, CEA.
   B. CEA currently is used to screen for colorectal cancer.
   C. CEA is useful in monitoring cancer of the breast, ovary, and pancreas.
   D. CEA is elevated in all solid-tissue tumors.

2. **All of the following statements regarding CA19-9 are true *except***

   A. It is a more sensitive and specific marker than CEA for adenocarcinoma of the pancreas.
   B. It is not elevated in islet cell carcinoma of the pancreas.
   C. It is only found in serum of Lewis antigen secretors.
   D. It is not elevated in acute pancreatitis.

3. **All of the following statements regarding α-fetoprotein (AFP) are true *except***

   A. AFP screening is not useful in detecting cirrhotic patients who will develop hepatocellular carcinoma.
   B. AFP is an important marker in germ cell tumor, but only when used with the β-subunit of chorionic gonadotropin.
   C. Lectin binding of AFP in yolk sac tumors has been documented.
   D. The method utilized to measure AFP can significantly affect the results.

4. **All of the following statements regarding CA-125 are true *except***

   A. The assay is only approved by the Food and Drug Administration for monitoring second-look opera-

tions in women who have been treated for ovarian cancer.
   B. Elevations of CA-125 are not seen in nonmalignant conditions.
   C. Elevated CA-125 is highly suggestive of residual ovarian tumors.
   D. CA-125 cannot be used for early diagnosis of ovarian cancers.

5. **All of the following statements regarding prostate-specific antigen (PSA) are true *except***

   A. PSA cannot be used to screen for prostatic adenocarcinoma.
   B. PSA is used to monitor patients with prostatic adenocarcinoma.
   C. The meaningful change in PSA between successive specimens is ±30%.
   D. Hormone therapy may reduce PSA concentrations by as much as 50% without any effect on the cancer.

6. **All of the following statements regarding alkaline phosphatase (ALP) are true *except***

   A. Elevations of ALP are greater with osteolytic bone lesions than osteoblastic lesions.
   B. Elevations in metastatic bone lesions in prostate cancer are much higher than metastatic bone lesions in breast cancer.
   C. ALP can be used to differentiate malignant involvement of liver and bone.
   D. Serum ALP is elevated in primary bone cancer.

7. **All of the following statements regarding neuron-specific enolase (NSE) are true *except***

   A. The γγ isomer is the predominant form in the brain.
   B. In serum, it is a nonspecific marker for neuroendocrine tumors.
   C. Elevations of NSE are not found in patients with non-small cell lung carcinoma.
   D. Decreases in NSE reflect response to therapy.

MEDICAL MICROSCOPY AND URINALYSIS

27 Synovial, Pleural, and Peritoneal Fluids

28 Urine

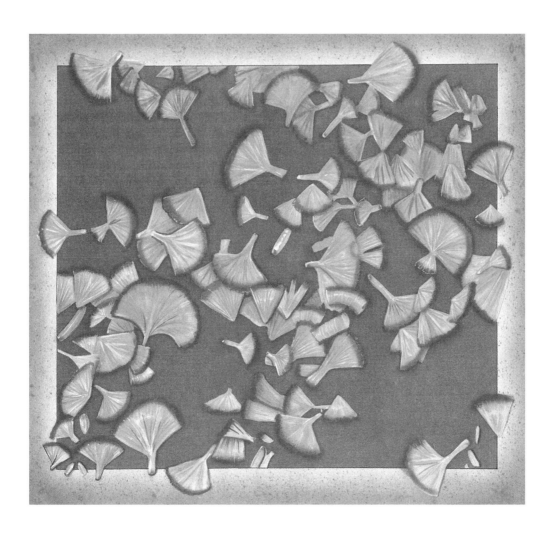

SYNOVIAL, PLEURAL, AND PERITONEAL FLUIDS

QUESTIONS

Select the one best answer of the choices offered.

1. **Which of the following statements regarding normal synovial fluid is *true*?**

    A. It is nonviscous.
    B. It clots easily.
    C. It is an ultrafiltrate of plasma.
    D. It contains abundant amounts of lipids.

2. **The viscosity of synovial fluid is**

    A. dependent on the composition of the ultrafiltrate
    B. due to the presence of the high-molecular-weight glycosaminoglycan, hyaluronic acid
    C. due to the high concentration of β_2-microglobulin
    D. low because of lubricin secretion by synovial cells

3. **Septic arthritis is most likely caused by**

    A. hematogenous spread
    B. trauma
    C. surgical procedure
    D. iatrogenic

4. **The most common cause of septic arthritis in young adults is**

    A. *Salmonella* sp
    B. *Streptococcus pneumoniae*
    C. *Escherichia coli*
    D. *Neisseria gonorrhoeae*

5. **Gram-negative septic arthritis occurs commonly in which of the following patients?**

    A. Adolescent females
    B. Intravenous drug users
    C. Neonates
    D. Geriatric patients

6. **All of the following statements regarding gouty arthritis are true *except***

    A. It is induced by calcium pyrophosphate dihydrate (CPPD) crystals.
    B. It occurs predominately in males.
    C. It presents clinically as a monoarticular arthritis.
    D. It involves most commonly lower extremity joints.

7. **CPPD-induced arthritis**

    A. commonly occurs in teenagers
    B. may be clinically indistinguishable from gout
    C. is treated by lowering serum uric acid levels
    D. is due to deposition of monosodium urate (MSU) crystals

8. **All of the following statements regarding rheumatoid arthritis are true *except***

    A. It affects women three times more frequently.
    B. Most patients develop the disease at 50 years of age or older.
    C. Joints are symmetrically involved.
    D. Proximal interphalangeal joints commonly are involved.

9. **Pathologic evaluation of rheumatoid joints demonstrate all of the following *except***

    A. synovium infiltrated with macrophages and T lymphocytes
    B. vascular proliferation
    C. soft tissue edema
    D. atrophy and hypoplasia of synovial lining cells

10. **Which laboratory method of evaluation should receive top priority when there is a limited amount of synovial fluid available for analysis?**

    A. Chemical examination
    B. Erythrocyte count
    C. Gram stain and culture
    D. Immunologic studies

11. **Causes for low viscosity of joint fluid include all of the following *except***

    A. inflammation
    B. edema
    C. trauma
    D. hypothyroidism

12. **Grossly bloody synovial fluid can be seen in all of the following conditions *except***

    A. septic arthritis
    B. hemophilia
    C. chondrocalcinosis
    D. pigmented villonodular tenosynovitis

13. **Total cell count of synovial fluid may be obtained best by**

    A. hemacytometer chamber
    B. electronic counters
    C. microscopic count at 400×
    D. automated counters

14. **Ragocytes or RA cells are**

    A. platelet clumps
    B. hemosiderin-laden macrophages
    C. neutrophils with refractile round cytoplasmic inclusions
    D. histiocytes containing red blood cells in their cytoplasm

15. **All of the following statements regarding birefringence are true *except***

    A. It is a property of material that has two optical axes.
    B. Crystals can be positively or negatively birefringent.
    C. Optical axes correspond to the path lengths at which light is transmitted.
    D. MSU crystals are negatively birefringent.

16. **Which of the following statements regarding CPPD is *true*?**

    A. It consists of needle-shaped, 5- to 20-μm long crystals.
    B. The fast ray bisects the acute angle of the optical axis.
    C. It has a characteristic "Maltese cross" appearance.
    D. They consist of rhomboidal-shaped, 1- to 20-μm long crystals.

17. **Which of the following statements regarding chemical examination of synovial fluid is *true*?**

    A. Chemical test contributes valuable information in establishing a diagnosis.
    B. Synovial fluid protein does not distinguish transudates from exudates.

C. Synovial uric acid level is clinically valuable in diagnosis of gouty arthritis.
D. Increased levels of pentosidine or ectonucleotide phyorphosphohydrolase are diagnostic of rheumatoid arthritis.

18. **All of the following statements regarding immunologic examination of synovial fluid are true *except***

    A. Normal immunoglobulin concentrations are about 10% that of serum.
    B. Immunoglobulins are increased in rheumatoid arthritis.
    C. Increases in both serum and synovial complement are found in systemic lupus erythematosus.
    D. Normal total hemolytic complement activity (CH_{50}) is 33% to 50% of the serum value.

19. **Which of the following statements regarding preanalytical processing of pleural fluid is true?**

    A. Heparin is the anticoagulant of choice.
    B. Store at room temperature for 48 hours.
    C. Aerobic collection for pH measurement.
    D. Use heparinized containers for cell counts (1,000 units of heparin/100 mL of fluid).

20. **All of the following statements regarding peritoneal fluid analysis are correct *except***

    A. It normally is <100 mL in volume.
    B. Exudate is a protein-poor fluid.
    C. Transudate is characterized by a serum/ascites albumin gradient (SAAG) >1.1 g/dL.
    D. Measuring pH, lactate, γ-interferon, and adenosine deaminase activity (ADA) may aid in differentiating sterile cirrhotic ascots from tuberculous peritoneal effusion.

Indicate whether each of the following statements is true (T) or false (F).

21. **Diagnosis of viral arthritis usually is established with culture of the synovial fluid.**

22. **Synovial fluid HIV p24 antigen has been demonstrated even when peripheral blood was negative for the antigen.**

23. **MSU crystals can persist in synovial fluid for months in patients following treatment.**

24. **Mucin clot test is a qualitative test to estimate the amount of fibrinogen and prothrombin.**

25. Normal joint fluid lacks fibrinogen, prothrombin, factors V and VII, antithrombin, and tissue thromboplastin.

26. Tart cells are neutrophils containing phagocytized homogenized nucleus.

27. Synovial fluid eosinophilia is seen in metastatic adenocarcinoma.

28. Charcot-Leyden crystals have been described in allergic reaction to intraarticular injection of steroids.

29. The strength of birefringence is determined by the thickness of the object and the difference in the degree of refraction between the fast and slow rays.

30. Not all crystals are birefringent; however, all birefringent objects are crystals.

31. Calcium oxalate crystals are bipyramidal, 1 to 2 μm in size, and positively birefringent.

32. Group II inflammatory differential diagnosis of joint fluid includes psoriasis, rheumatoid arthritis, lupus erythematosus, and pigmented villonodular tenosynovitis.

33. The two most common malignant tumors causing pleural effusions are lymphomas and malignant mesotheliomas.

34. Exudates can be categorized into catarrhal, fibrinous, hemorrhagic, purulent, or serous.

35. Peritoneal fluid total erythrocyte count greater than 100,000 cells/μL is visually diagnostic of hemoperitoneum.

URINE

QUESTIONS

Select the one best answer of the choices offered.

1. **Urinalysis request forms should include all of following information** *except*
   A. name, gender, age, and race
   B. clinical impression
   C. cost per test
   D. time and date of collection

2. **All of the following statements regarding refractometers are true** *except*
   A. Acetone is used as the standard and is given the value of 1.50.
   B. They provide a quantitative estimate of the specific gravity of urine.
   C. Instrument calibration should be performed daily in a high-volume laboratory.
   D. They measure the total solids in solution.

3. **All of the following statements regarding the appearance of freshly voided normal urine are true** *except*
   A. It is clear and pale yellow to amber in color.
   B. The yellow color is due to the synthesis of urochrome pigment.
   C. Foods such as beets may cause abnormally colored red urine.
   D. Color intensity may vary with the concentration of the urine.

4. **The preferred time to obtain a urine specimen for analysis is**
   A. before bed time
   B. early morning
   C. late afternoon
   D. early evening

5. **All of the following statements regarding collection of urine are true** *except*

A. Urinalysis should be performed within 2 hours of voiding.
B. Refrigeration of urine sample is not necessary.
C. It may be preferable in some instances to allow the urine to stand at room temperature.
D. Addition of antibacterial agents, such as formaldehyde or thymol crystals, is recommended.

6. **A false-negative reaction with the urine dipstick can occur with all of the following** *except*
   A. low doses of aspirin
   B. high concentration of ascorbic acid (vitamin C)
   C. urine exposed to long periods of light
   D. residual oxidizing detergents in the container

7. **All of the following statements regarding urine glucose are true** *except*
   A. Glucose is freely filtered by the glomerulus and almost entirely reabsorbed by the renal tubules.
   B. Clinically it is the most important reducing substance found in the urine.
   C. Glycosuria generally occurs when blood levels of glucose equal or exceed 125 mg/dL.
   D. Renal threshold varies in the range from 160 to 200 mg/dL in individuals.

8. **All of the following statements regarding urine protein are true** *except*
   A. Albumin is the predominant protein present in urine.
   B. Albumin is filtered by the glomerulus and secreted by the tubules and collecting ducts.
   C. Tamm-Horsfall mucoprotein (THM) is secreted by the distal tubules.
   D. Standing will increase quantities of protein in the urine.

9. **Which of the following statements regarding urine microalbumin is** *true*?
   A. It represents one fourth of the molecular size of albumin.

B. It is screened for in patients newly diagnosed with diabetes.

C. It provides information on reversible glomerular injury.

D. It describes undetectable levels of urine albumin by dipstick.

10. **All of the following are ketone bodies** *except*

A. acetone

B. phenylpyruvic acid

C. acetoacetic acid

D. β-hydroxybutyric acid

11. **Which of the following is a cause of low specific gravity?**

A. Dehydration

B. End-stage renal disease

C. Diabetes insipidus

D. Nephrotic syndrome

12. **All of the following statements regarding phenylketonuria (PKU) are true** *except*

A. Early diagnosis by urine screening is an important preventive measure.

B. Treatment is diet free of phenylalanine.

C. It is an acquired metabolic disorder in which phenylalanine hydroxylase activity is decreased.

D. Accumulation of phenylpyruvic acid causes brain damage.

13. **All of the following statements regarding uric acid crystals are true** *except*

A. They are soluble in acidic solutions.

B. They appear as fine granules at 10× microscopic power.

C. They frequently develop after refrigeration of urine.

D. They commonly are present in the urine of healthy people.

14. **Triple phosphate crystals are composed of**

A. ammonium, calcium, phosphate

B. magnesium, calcium, phosphate

C. uric acid, ammonium, phosphate

D. ammonium, magnesium, phosphate

15. **All of the following statements regarding granular casts are true** *except*

A. Granular casts have a higher refractive index than hyaline casts.

B. They are found in equal ratio with hyaline casts.

C. Granules arise from intracellular lysosomal particles.

D. Granular casts may occur in normal healthy people.

16. **All of the following statements regarding cystinuria are true** *except*

A. Cystine crystals are flat, clear, colorless hexagons.

B. It demonstrates a negative birefringent pattern under polarized microscopy.

C. Cystine crystals are only soluble in ammonia.

D. It is an inherited autosomal recessive disorder that also is seen in Wilson disease.

17. **Which abnormal crystal is depicted in the figure below? (Figure 28.32)**

A. Cholesterol crystals

B. Tyrosine crystals

C. Uric acid crystals

D. Cystine crystals

18. **All of the following statements regarding red blood cell casts are true** *except*

A. Their presence indicates glomerular injury.

B. They basically are hyaline casts with red blood cells.

C. They may be mistaken for fatty casts.

D. Proteinuria is infrequently seen concurrently with red blood cell casts.

19. **Which urine sediment cast is represented in the following photomicrograph? (Figure 28.45)**

A. Granular cast

B. Red blood cell cast

C. Waxy cast

D. Renal tubular epithelial cell cast

20. **Which organism is seen in the following photomicrograph? (Figure 28.50)**

A. *Trichomonas vaginalis*

B. *Schistosoma hematobium*

C. *Enterobius vermicularis*

D. *Gardnerella vaginalis*

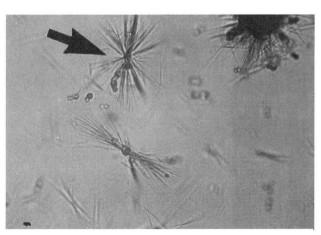

FIGURE 28.32.

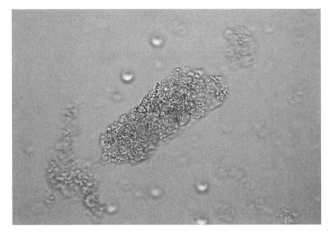
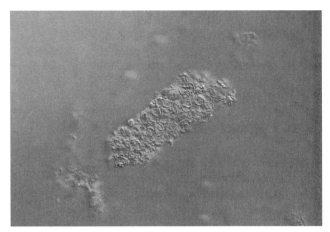

FIGURE 28.45.

Indicate whether each of the following statements is true (T) or false (F).

21. The point at which a solution is frozen or vaporized is proportional to the osmolality.

22. An adult human normally produces 1 to 2 L of urine a day.

23. Quality assurance (QA) is the most important concept in urinalysis because QA ensures consistency and accuracy of results.

24. Urine dipstick is a simple, rapid, inexpensive, and accurate method of urinalysis with narrow interobserver variation.

25. Urine dipstick is an effective screening method for galactosemia, an inborn error of galactose metabolism.

26. Patients with nephrotic syndrome commonly excrete >4 g of protein per day in the urine.

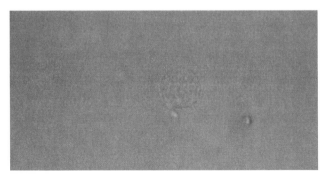

FIGURE 28.50.

27. Standard urine dipsticks fail to detect Bence Jones proteins, which are present in approximately one half patients with multiple myeloma.

28. A patient with rhabdomyolysis will have a positive urine dipstick reaction for hemoglobin in addition to microscopic evidence of hematuria.

29. Alkalization of urine may retard or inhibit the formation of uric acid stones.

30. β-Hydroxybutyric acid, a ketone body, is not detected by urine dipstick analysis.

31. The presence of yellow foam after vigorous shaking of the urine sample is a crude method of detecting increased amounts bilirubin.

32. A negative nitrite dipstick reaction excludes a bacterial infection.

33. Identification of small numbers of erythrocytes (red blood cells) and leukocytes (white blood cells) in urine sediment is abnormal.

34. Hyaline, granular, and cellular casts appear in the urinary sediment in normal, healthy individuals.

35. Hyaline casts typically are translucent and rarely observed in the urine.

36. "Glitter" cells are degenerating lymphocytes with large intracytoplasmic vacuoles.

37. **Inclusion bodies in renal tubule epithelial cells may be seen with lead toxicity, and with herpes, cytomegalovirus, and measles infection.**

38. **Neutral fat, the major component of oval fat bodies, accounts for the Maltese cross pattern seen under polarized light.**

39. **Detection of indinavir crystals in patients with acquired immunodeficiency syndrome is an unexpected complication of therapy.**

40. **Eggs of *E. vermicularis,* a nocturnal intestinal parasitic organism, may be present in the urine.**

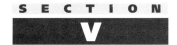

CYTOGENETICS

29 Basic Cytogenetics
30 Clinical Cytogenetics
31 Prenatal Cytogenetic Diagnosis
32 Cytogenetic Studies in Neoplastic Hematologic Disorders
33 Chromosome-Breakage Syndromes: Clinical Features, Cytogenetics, and Molecular Genetics
34 Solid Tumor Cytogenetics

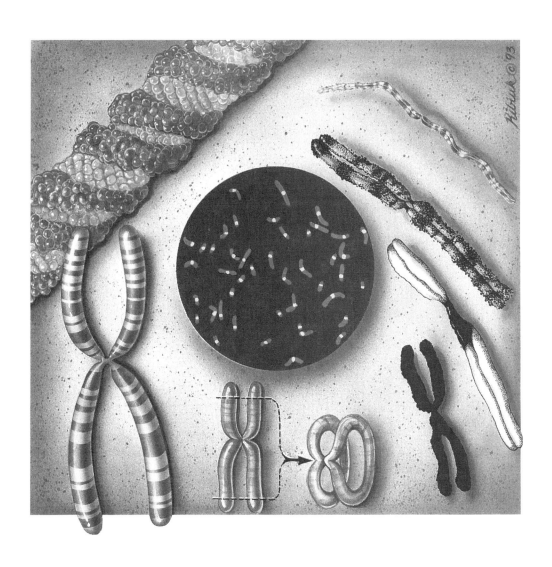

29

BASIC CYTOGENETICS

QUESTIONS

Select the one best answer of the choices offered.

1. **All of the following statements regarding chromosome staining and identification are true *except***

    A. Quinacrine mustard is a fluorescing dye that stains each chromosome in a specific banding pattern.
    B. Autoradiography is the method of choice for identification of 22 pairs of autosomes and X and Y chromosomes.
    C. Gains or losses of whole chromosomes can be detected by Giemsa stain, quinacrine mustard, and autoradiography.
    D. Giemsa stain is more sensitive than autoradiography in detecting deletions, duplications, and inversions of chromosomes.

2. **Which of the following statements regarding chromosome structure is true?**

    A. The 30-nm solenoid forms the " beads on a string" structure.
    B. The-145 bp DNA helix is coiled around a pentamer of histones.
    C. The 10-nm fiber nucleosome is the basic subunit of the chromosome.
    D. DNA linkers associated with H2b histone separate nucleosomes.

3. **All the following statements regarding telomeres are true *except***

    A. They allow complete replication of the chromosome end.
    B. Lack of telomeres will cause cell immortality and carcinoma.
    C. They enable cells to distinguish chromosome ends from breaks in the DNA.
    D. Telomeres may regulate gene expression, cell senescence, and neoplastic proliferation.

4. **The ends of the chromosome are called**

    A. solenoids
    B. nucleosomes
    C. telomeres
    D. histones

5. **All of the following statements regarding centromere are true *except***

    A. Its position is always on the chromosome center.
    B. It is essential for spindle apparatus attachment.
    C. It is required for proper chromosomal segregation during mitosis and meiosis.
    D. It serves as point of attachment for both sister chromatids.

6. **The centromere divides the chromosome into arms and is referred to as**

    A. nucleosome
    B. primary constriction
    C. kinetochore
    D. linker DNA

7. **All the following statements regarding heterochromatin are true *except***

    A. It consists of repetitive DNA.
    B. It remains condensed during telophase.
    C. Constitutive and facultative heterochromatin remains visible during interphase.
    D. constitutive heterochromatin contains transcribable DNA.

8. **A meiosis chiasma is the microscopic manifestation of**

    A. karyolysis
    B. satelliting
    C. crossing over
    D. α-satelliting

9. **Meiosis includes all of the following *except***
   A. pairing
   B. recombination
   C. reduction in chromosome number to haploid (1N)
   D. resting state

10. **The synaptonemal complex begins to appear during meiosis, but the chromosomes are held together by chiasmata at the**
   A. telomere
   B. diplotene
   C. leptotene
   D. pairing

11. **All of the following statements are true regarding gametogenesis *except***
   A. Transition from spermatogonia to mature sperm requires 60 to 65 days.
   B. In females, the first meiotic division occurs in puberty.
   C. The second meiotic division in females occurs in the fallopian tube after fertilization.
   D. Transition from oogonia to a mature ova requires years to complete.

12. **Staining reaction of Q banding**
   A. is reserved for visualization of polymorphism on the Y chromosome
   B. darkly stains chromosome bands
   C. requires Romanowsky dyes
   D. is better than the G banding method

13. **R bands are rich in**
   A. adenine-thymidine
   B. guanine-cytosine
   C. adenine-guanine
   D. thymidine-cytosine

14. **All of the following statements regarding the C banding method of chromosome staining are true *except***
   A. It is used to identify dicentric chromosomes.
   B. It is used to trace origin of specific abnormalities (e.g., Down syndrome).
   C. Base composition of DNA is mainly GC rich.
   D. It is useful in identification of chromosomal variants.

15. **The X chromatin body (Barr body)**
   A. is abnormally seen in females
   B. is absent in males with Klinefelter syndrome
   C. is seen in Turner syndrome
   D. is microscopically evident in cells with an inactivated X chromosome

16. **The single X hypothesis is the observation of**
   A. Barr
   B. Bertram
   C. Lyon
   D. Turner

17. **The XIST (X inactive specific transcripts) gene, which is close to and may represent the inactivating center, has been identified to be at**
   A. t (Y;12)
   B. Xq11
   C. Xq13
   D. t (Y;22)

18. **Genomic imprinting of chromosome 15 has been associated with**
   A. Angelman syndrome
   B. Beckwith-Wiedemann syndrome
   C. neonatal diabetes
   D. Turner syndrome

19. **The first use of deletions to map chromosomes was in**
   A. Duffy blood group
   B. family studies
   C. gonadal development studies
   D. *Drosophila*

20. **The most direct cytogenetic method of gene localization has been**
   A. mapping studies
   B. polyethylene glycol
   C. electron microscopy
   D. *in situ* hybridization

Indicate whether each of the following statements is true (T) or false (F).

21. **Phytohemagglutinin inhibits cell division at metaphase.**

22. **Chromosome 1 has the shortest length in the normal human autosomal karyotype.**

23. **The arms of chromosome 22 are equal in length and can be referred as a metacentric chromosome.**

24. **The greatest advances in the field of cytogenetics have been the utilization of fluorescence *in situ* hybridization (FISH).**

25. In humans, the telomeres in germ line cells are significantly longer than in the somatic tissue cells.

26. If the arms of the chromosome are equal, the chromosome is referred to as telocentric.

27. α-Satellite regions of human chromosomes are located at the nucleosome.

28. The kinetochore functions as the region of attachment of microtubules.

29. Patients with scleroderma have antibodies against centromere proteins (CENPs).

30. In meiosis, chromosomes are at their greatest length at leptotene.

31. Completion of meiotic and mitotic divisions typically requires 15 to 32 hours.

32. The centromere divides the chromosome into three arms designated p (short arm), q (long arm), and n (null or no arm).

33. R banding staining reaction is the reverse of G/Q banding and is useful in detecting abnormalities in chromosomal ends.

34. According to the Lyon hypothesis of X inactivation, preferential inactivation of the maternal or paternal X chromosome occurs, which is reversible in germ cells.

35. Loss of the paternal genes in 15q results in Prader-Willi syndrome (PWS).

30

CLINICAL CYTOGENETICS

QUESTIONS

Select the one best answer of the choices offered.

1. **About ____% of newborns have a chromosome abnormality.**
   A. 0.001
   B. 0.01
   C. 0.1
   D. 0.6

2. **About ____% of first-trimester miscarriages have a chromosome abnormality.**
   A. 10
   B. 25
   C. 35
   D. 50

3. **About ____% of first-trimester miscarriages are triploid.**
   A. 1
   B. 3
   C. 5
   D. 7

4. **Tetraploidy (4N) usually results from a failure of cell division after**
   A. translocations
   B. meiosis
   C. mitosis
   D. inversions

5. **When an individual chromosome is gained or lost, the karyotype is**
   A. euploid
   B. diploid
   C. aneuploid
   D. haploid

6. **Classic trisomy syndromes include all of the following *except***
   A. Down
   B. Edward
   C. Barr
   D. Patau

7. **Trisomy 8 is a common abnormality in**
   A. leukemia
   B. solid cancer
   C. Down syndrome
   D. Edward syndrome

8. **Trisomy 7 is a common abnormality in**
   A. leukemia
   B. solid cancer
   C. Down syndrome
   D. Edward syndrome

9. **In Down syndrome, it has been established that >90% of nondisjunctional events occur during ____ meiosis.**
   A. paternal
   B. maternal
   C. conception
   D. 10 weeks of gestation

10. **The average maternal age for trisomy 21 children is**
    A. 25
    B. 30
    C. 35
    D. 40

11. **Mosaics for all the following trisomies are well known *except***
    A. 6
    B. 13
    C. 18
    D. 21

12. The average gene is ____ kb in length.

    A. 10
    B. 20
    C. 30
    D. 40

13. Cri-du-chat syndrome is characterized by deletion of

    A. 4p–
    B. 5p–
    C. 18p–
    D. 18q–

14. Breakage in both arms of a chromosome and repair by fusion at the two breakpoints result in

    A. deletion syndrome
    B. mosaicism
    C. bonding
    D. circular chromosome

15. In an isochromosome, the arms are

    A. at odds
    B. complementary
    C. isometric
    D. mirror images

16. Balanced reciprocal translocations are found in 1 of ____ livebirths.

    A. 100 to 300
    B. 500 to 700
    C. 9,000 to 12,000
    D. 15,000 to 20,000

17. The reciprocal translocation ____ is seen in approximately 1 of 5,000 normal subjects.

    A. t (11;22) (q23;q11)
    B. t (6;9) (q23;q11)
    C. t (11;22) (q12;q11)
    D. t (11;22) (q23;q13)

18. An inversion is a two-break rearrangement in which a chromosome segment is turned

    A. 45°
    B. 90°
    C. 180°
    D. 270°

19. The frequency of balanced pericentric inversion in the general population is approximately 1 in

    A. 300
    B. 600
    C. 900
    D. 1,200

20. The frequency of balanced paracentric inversion in the general population is approximately 1 in

    A. 500
    B. 750
    C. 1,000
    D. 1,250

21. The feature found in almost all chromosome imbalances is

    A. hypertelorisms
    B. growth retardation
    C. low-set ears
    D. micrognathia

22. Wolf syndrome is characterized by deletion of a segment of

    A. long arm of chromosome 6
    B. short arm of chromosome 4
    C. short arm of chromosome 6
    D. long arm of chromosome 11

23. Cri-du-chat syndrome is characterized by rearrangement of chromosome

    A. 4
    B. 5
    C. 6
    D. 7

24. The incidence of trisomy 8 mosaicism is estimated to be 1 in ____ newborns.

    A. 1,000
    B. 5,000
    C. 10,000
    D. 18,000

25. The overall incidence of Beckwith-Wiedemann syndrome has been estimated as 1 in ____ live births.

    A. 5,000
    B. 10,000
    C. 14,000
    D. 18,000

26. Wilms tumor, aniridias, genitourinary malformation, and mental retardation (WAGR) syndrome is associated with loss of

    A. band 8p10
    B. band 10p11
    C. band 11p13
    D. band 13q14

27. **Patau syndrome is characterized by trisomy**
    A. 8
    B. 9
    C. 11
    D. 13

28. **The contiguous gene syndrome of retinoblastoma and birth defects is associated with an interstitial deletion of a small segment of chromosome**
    A. 6
    B. 8
    C. 11
    D. 13

29. **Prader-Willi syndrome patients have an interstitial deletion of 15q11.2–q12 or q13 that always includes loss of subband**
    A. 15q11.2
    B. 14q11
    C. 15q12
    D. 15q5

30. **Edward syndrome is associated with trisomy**
    A. 8
    B. 14
    C. 18
    D. 21

31. **One in _____ infants has Down syndrome.**
    A. 400 to 600
    B. 800 to 1,000
    C. 1,200 to 1,500
    D. 2,000 to 3,000

32. **Most translocations associated with Down syndrome are der (21;21) or**
    A. der (11;21)
    B. der (13;21)
    C. der (14;21)
    D. der (20;21)

33. **As many as _____% of trisomy 21 conceptions results in miscarriage.**
    A. 25
    B. 50
    C. 75
    D. 100

34. **The phenotype of cat's-eye syndrome includes all of the following *except***
    A. coloboma of the iris
    B. preauricular pit
    C. imperforate anus

    D. verruca plans

35. **Patients with DiGeorge syndrome have deletions involving band**
    A. 22q11
    B. 11p22
    C. 10q12
    D. 10p15

36. **The incidence of monosomy X is about 1 in _____ newborns.**
    A. 500
    B. 1,000
    C. 3,000
    D. 5,000

37. **Features that appear in approximately 75% of patients with Turner syndrome include all of the following *except***
    A. high arched palate
    B. short or webbed neck
    C. mulberry molars
    D. shield chest

38. **Triple X syndrome (47,XXX) appears in 1 of _____ liveborn females.**
    A. 1,000
    B. 4,000
    C. 7,000
    D. 15,000

39. **The incidence of Klinefelter syndrome (47,XXY) is approximately 1 in _____ male newborns.**
    A. 500
    B. 700
    C. 1,000
    D. 3,000

40. **The fragile X syndrome accounts for approximately _____% of mental retardation among males.**
    A. 5
    B. 10
    C. 15
    D. 20

Indicate whether each of the following statements is true (T) or false (F).

41. **Down syndrome is the most common single identified cause of mental retardation.**

42. **Robertsonian translocation arises from the fusion of two acrocentric chromosomes.**

43. Cat's-eye syndrome can be suspected in infants with a plaintive, meowing cry, low birth weight, and failure to thrive.

44. The key features of Williams syndrome include supravalvular aortic stenosis, small stature, long philtrum, and hoarse voice.

45. Gigantism and generalized organomegaly are features of Beckwith-Wiedemann syndrome.

46. Edward syndrome has a characteristic hyperkinetic behavior with a stiff ataxic gait.

47. Children with Klinefelter syndrome are attentive with above average IQ.

48. Women who have one or more miscarriages have an increased risk of miscarriage in future pregnancies compared with women who have no history of miscarriage.

49. Simple probability dictates that 2% of couples with two pregnancies will have two miscarriages.

50. Tissue biopsy samples are routine specimens for chromosome analysis.

PRENATAL CYTOGENETIC DIAGNOSIS

QUESTIONS

Select the one best answer of the choices offered.

1. **Indications for prenatal cytogenetic or α-fetoprotein (AFP) testing include all of the following** *except*

   A. advanced maternal age
   B. previous offspring with chromosome abnormality
   C. abnormal complete blood count (CBC)
   D. one parent carries a chromosome rearrangement

2. **Chorionic villus sampling (CVS) is routinely performed at ____ weeks of gestation.**

   A. 10 to 12
   B. 16 to 20
   C. 28 to 30
   D. 34 to 40

3. **X-linked conditions include all of the following** *except*

   A. Duchenne muscular dystrophy
   B. hemophilia A
   C. Hunter syndrome
   D. Cri-du-chat syndrome

4. **Amniocentesis carries approximately ____ risk of miscarriage or infection.**

   A. 1/125
   B. 1/300
   C. 1/500
   D. 1/1,000

5. **All of the following statements regarding amniocentesis are true** *except*

   A. Risk to fetus and mother are lower than CVS.
   B. It requires follow-up with CVS.
   C. It is cheaper to perform than CVS.
   D. There is a lower percentage of indeterminate cytogenetic results (mosaicism).

6. **All the following statements regarding spina bifida are true** *except*

   A. The disease is exclusively genetically inherited.
   B. 95% of patients with spina bifida are born to couples with no family history.
   C. Intrauterine exposure to isotretinoin is a known risk factor for developing the disease.
   D. Spina bifida may be associated with Roberts syndrome.

7. **____ is the major protein in fetal plasma in early pregnancy.**

   A. Albumin
   B. γ-Globulin
   C. AFP
   D. Fibrinogen

8. **Peak levels of AFP are attained in fetal plasma at ____ weeks of gestation.**

   A. 6 to 8
   B. 8 to 10
   C. 10 to 12
   D. 12 to 14

9. **After 22 weeks of gestation, the fetal liver gradually switches from production of AFP to primarily production of**

   A. albumin
   B. clotting factors
   C. transferrin
   D. γ-globulin

10. **Maternal serum AFP values tend to be ____% higher in patients of African-American descent.**

    A. 6 to 8
    B. 10 to 12
    C. 12 to 15
    D. 20 to 25

11. **Pregnant women with insulin-dependent diabetes have a ____% rate of birth defects compared with the general population incidence of 3% to 5%.**

    A. 10 to 15
    B. 15 to 20
    C. 20 to 25
    D. 25 to 30

12. **A maternal serum AFP (MSAFP) value of 4.5 MoM**

    A. is diagnostic of spina bifida
    B. within cutoff range for singleton pregnancy
    C. is diagnostic of yolk sac (endodermal sinus) tumor
    D. indicates twin pregnancy needs to be ruled out

13. **All of the following are causes of elevated levels of MSAFP *except***

    A. oligohydramnios
    B. polyhydramnios
    C. bilateral renal agenesis
    D. sacrococcygeal teratoma

14. **Down syndrome screening markers include**

    A. Acetylcholinesterase (AChE), human chorionic gonadotropin (HCG), progesterone, estriol
    B. MSAFP, AChE, progesterone, estriol
    C. MSAFP, estriol, HCG, inhibin A
    D. MSAFP, HCG, inhibin A, progesterone

15. **Amniotic fluid gives a characteristic microscopic feature known as (see Figure 31.4)**

    A. colonies
    B. rosettes
    C. ferning
    D. rouleaux

16. **The optimal size for a CVS sample for laboratory examination is ____ mg.**

    A. 1 to 2
    B. 2 to 4
    C. 3
    D. 5 to 15

17. **All of the following are sources of growth failure of amniotic fluid samples *except***

    A. blood contaminant
    B. hygroma fluid
    C. urine sample
    D. cold damage during transport

18. **The risk of mental retardation (with or without birth defects) is ____% with an unbalanced chromosome rearrangement.**

    A. 25
    B. 50
    C. 75
    D. About 100

19. **All of the following statements regarding trisomy 20 mosaicism are true *except***

    A. A trisomy 20 syndrome has not been described.

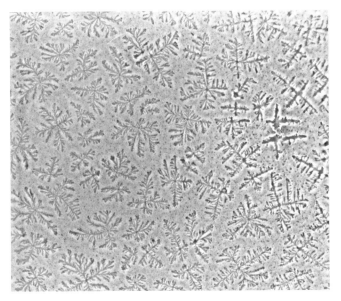
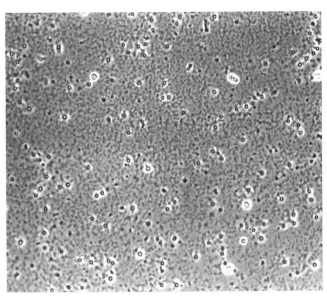

FIGURE 31.4.

B. 1 in 1,000 fluid cell cultures reveals a true trisomy 20 mosaicism.

C. Most newborns have a normal phenotype at birth.

D. 6% of cases have abnormalities.

20. About _____% of prenatal genetic studies reveals fetal mosaicism.

    A. 0.3
    B. 0.6
    C. 1.8
    D. 2.4

Indicate whether each of the following statements is true (T) or false (F).

21. Amniocentesis for prenatal genetic diagnosis typically is performed at 16 to 20 weeks of gestation.

22. Direct preparation of uncultured cytotrophoblast from CVS has a lower false-negative rate than the short-term culture method.

23. In the United States, a maternal age of 25 years is the accepted age at which physicians routinely offer prenatal chromosome analysis.

24. Prenatal diagnosis with amniocentesis or CVS is 99.9% sensitive in detecting birth defects and/or metal retardation.

25. The second most common reason for amniocentesis is for the prenatal diagnosis of spina bifida.

26. Most laboratories set a cutoff range of 2.0 to 2.5 MoM for MSAFP.

27. AFP is a predictable marker for spina bifida throughout pregnancy.

28. Chromosomal analysis requires the treatment with a hypotonic solution to disperse chromosomes with the cell membrane.

29. The College of American Pathologists (CAP) recommends analysis of at least 15 metaphase cells taken from 15 different colonies and representing at least two independent cultures.

30. Tetraploidy is a common artifact of harvest procedure in monolayer cultures.

31. Identification of a chromosomal abnormality in some but not all cells is diagnostic of a true fetal mosaicism.

32. Chorionic villus cell karyotype studies exhibit true mosaicism in approximately 2% of studies.

33. True mosaicism is likely only when abnormal colonies are detected in independent preparations.

34. Most amniotic fluid cell colonies represent multiple clones, and most CVS colonies represent single clones.

35. If mosaicism involves a chromosome that is imprinted, uniparental disomy studies may be indicated.

32

CYTOGENETIC STUDIES IN NEOPLASTIC HEMATOLOGIC DISORDERS

QUESTIONS

Select the one best answer of the choices offered.

1. **All of the following statements regarding the different types of chromosomal abnormalities are true** *except*
   A. Polyploidy refers to chromosome complements that are multiple of 23.
   B. Aneuploidy results from endoreduplication.
   C. Inversions are either pericentric or paracentric.
   D. Isochromosomes arise from a break and fusion of sister chromatids.

2. **All of the following statements regarding chromosome evolution and tumor progression are true** *except*
   A. Additional chromosome abnormalities appear in sporadic malignant cells by "chromosome evolution."
   B. The observation of t(9;22)(q34;q11.2) and trisomy 8 in a subset of cells in chronic myeloid leukemia is evidence of a subclone.
   C. Patients with *de novo* acute myeloid leukemia show similar prognosis to patients with acute myeloid leukemia evolving from the myelodysplastic syndrome.
   D. t(8;22)(q24;q11) translocation is an example of oncogene activation.

3. **All of the following statements regarding cytogenetic analysis are true** *except*
   A. Chromosome analysis of peripheral blood is informative in some coetaneous T-cell lymphomas.
   B. >95% of blood specimens produce adequate metaphases.
   C. Successful chromosome studies are possible 2 to 3 weeks after chemotherapeutic agent administration.

   D. Cytogenetic analysis sometimes is successful, even on low-volume body fluid specimens that appear to lack cells by cytopathologic evaluation.

4. **All of the following statements regarding collection and transportation of cytogenetic specimens are true** *except*
   A. Chromosome analysis requires 7.0 to 10.0 mL of peripheral blood.
   B. Chromosome analysis requires 0.25 to 0.5 mL of bone marrow.
   C. Transportation time and environmental conditions do not affect the laboratories' success in obtaining analyzable metaphases.
   D. The anticoagulant of choice is sodium citrate.

5. **All of the following statements regarding processing specimens for chromosome analysis are true** *except*
   A. The 24-hour unstimulated culture is superior to the direct preparation technique in processing hematologic specimens for cytogenetic studies.
   B. The 24-hour unstimulated culture is successful in >90% of bone marrow specimens.
   C. The direct *in situ* method is successful in specimens with a low mitotic index.
   D. Mitogens such as phytohemagglutinin and pokeweed, used to stimulate division of neoplastic cells, can stimulate normal B and T cells.

6. **All of the following statements regarding the advantages of the fluorescence in situ hybridization (FISH) technique are true** *except*
   A. Accrediting agents for FISH are well established.
   B. FISH is less expensive than conventional cytogenetics.
   C. FISH can be performed on both metaphase and interphase cells.
   D. FISH probes can easily be made as "home-brew" products.

Match each of the following types of FISH probes with the corresponding chromosomal abnormality.

7. **Telomere-specific probe**

8. **Locus-specific probe**

9. **Chromosome-specific probe**

10. **Centromere-specific probe**
    A. Abnormalities involving the ends of chromosomes
    B. Numerical abnormalities
    C. Cryptic translocations
    D. Structural abnormalities

Match each of the following with the appropriate FISH strategy.

11. **Moderately sensitive strategy for detection of t(9;22)(q34;q11.2)**

12. **Most sensitive strategy for detection of t(9;22)(q34;q11.2)**

13. **Strategy used for detection of breakpoints within the ALK gene on chromosome 2p23**

14. **Least sensitive strategy for detection of t(9;22)(q34;q11.2)**
    A. Break-apart FISH strategy
    B. Single-fusion FISH (S-FISH) strategy
    C. Extra signal FISH (ES-FISH) strategy
    D. Double-fusion FISH (D-FISH) strategy

15. **All of the following statements regarding chromosomal abnormalities in hematologic disorders are true *except***
    A. Translocations are the most common chromosomal abnormalities.
    B. −7 is the most common monosomy.
    C. +8 is the most common trisomy.
    D. 5q− is the most common deletion.

16. **All of the following statements regarding the incidence of acute leukemia are true *except***
    A. The yearly incidence of acute lymphoblastic leukemia (ALL) is higher in children compared with adults.
    B. Among adults with acute leukemia, 20% have ALL and 80% have acute myelogenous leukemia (AML).
    C. AML in adults older than 55 years often have chromosomal abnormalities associated with progression of myelodysplastic syndromes.

D. The yearly incidence of AML in adults of age 70 is 15 in 100,000.

17. **All of the following statements regarding t(1;14)(p32;q11) are true *except***
    A. Defined gene breakpoints are amenable to Southern blot or reverse transcriptase polymerase chain reaction (RT-PCR).
    B. Specific for T-cell acute lymphoblastic leukemia (T-ALL) in 10% to 30% of patients.
    C. Translocation involves the TAL1 gene on chromosome 1 and the IgH gene on chromosome 14.
    D. Positive cerebrospinal fluid and high white count are common.

18. **All of the following statements regarding t(8;21)(q22;q22) are true *except***
    A. It occurs in 10% to 30% of AML-M2 and 7% of AML-M4.
    B. 60% of females have associated loss of the X chromosome.
    C. Generally it has a poor prognostic significance.
    D. Involves the ETO gene on chromosome 8 and the AML1 gene on chromosome 21.

Match each of the following chromosomal translocations with the corresponding hematologic malignancy.

19. **t(8;14)(p11;p13)**

20. **t(1;19)(q23;p13)**

21. **t(8;21)(q22;q22)**

22. **t(10;14)(q24;q11)**
    A. AML-M2
    B. Pre–B-cell ALL
    C. T-cell ALL
    D. ALL-L3

23. **All of the following statements regarding t(12;21)(p13;q22) are true *except***
    A. It has a good prognostic significance.
    B. Involves the TEL gene on chromosome 12 and the AML1 gene on chromosome 21.
    C. It is present in 25% of children with ALL.
    D. It is easy to detect by conventional cytogenetic studies.

24. **All of the following statements regarding t(15;17)(q22;q21) are true *except***
    A. Patients are resistant to all-*trans* retinoic acid therapy.

B. It involves the PML gene on chromosome 15 and the RARα gene on chromosome 17.

C. Median age of onset is 38 years.

D. Patients frequently present with disseminated intravascular coagulation.

25. **All of the following statements regarding inv(16) (p13;q22) are true** *except*

A. Most common cytogenetic variant is t(16;16) (p13;q22).

B. It is present in 100% of patients with AML-M4.

C. It is clinically associated with lymphadenopathy and hepatomegaly.

D. It involves the MYH11 gene on chromosome 16p13 and the CBFβ gene on chromosome 16q22.

26. **All of the following statements regarding the myelodysplastic syndromes are true** *except*

A. "5q– syndrome" is not recognized as an FAB subgroup.

B. Chromosomally abnormal clones are found in 31% of patients with refractory anemia and 29% of patients with refractory anemia with ringed sideroblasts.

C. Overall, 80% of patients with myelodysplastic syndromes have a chromosomal anomaly.

D. Many patients with myelodysplastic syndromes progress to acute leukemia.

27. **All of the following statements regarding t(9;22) (q34;q11.2) and chronic myeloid leukemia (CML) are true** *except*

A. Other cytogenetic abnormalities, including multiple copies of Ph chromosome, +8, and i(17q), can be detected during the chronic phase of CML.

B. Lymphoid blast crisis can occur in CML.

C. "Ph-negative CML" does not exist.

D. >90% of patients with CML have t(9;22) in all metaphases.

28. **All of the following hematologic neoplasms may be associated with t(11;14)(q13;q32)** *except*

A. B-cell prolymphocytic leukemia

B. Mantle cell lymphoma

C. B-cell chronic lymphocytic leukemia

D. Multiple myeloma

Match each of the following chromosomal translocations with the corresponding lymphoproliferative disorder.

29. **t(14;18)(q32;q21)**

30. **t(14;19)(q32;q13)**

31. **t(9;14)(p13;q32)**

32. **t(8;14)(q24;q32)**

33. **t(2;5)(p23;q35)**

A. Burkitt lymphoma

B. Follicular lymphoma

C. Small lymphocytic lymphoma

D. Lymphoplasmacytic lymphoma

E. Anaplastic large cell lymphoma

34. **All of the following statements regarding t(14;19) (q32;q13) are true** *except*

A. It occurs in B-cell chronic lymphocytic leukemia and small lymphocytic lymphoma.

B. It involves the IgH gene on chromosome 14 and the *Bcl*-2 gene on chromosome 19.

C. It is associated with trisomy 12 in 50% of the patients.

D. It has a poor prognostic significance.

CHROMOSOME-BREAKAGE SYNDROMES: CLINICAL FEATURES, CYTOGENETICS, AND MOLECULAR GENETICS

QUESTIONS

Select the one best answer of the choices offered.

1. **Chromosome instability syndromes that demonstrate an autosomal recessive mode of inheritance include all of the following** *except*

    A. ataxia-telangiectasia
    B. Bloom syndrome
    C. Fanconi anemia
    D. Xeroderma pigmentosum

2. **Clinical features of Bloom syndrome include all of the following** *except*

    A. tall stature
    B. beaked nose
    C. sun sensitivity
    D. immunologic impairment

3. **Typical dermatologic lesions in Bloom syndrome include all of the following** *except*

    A. photosensitivity
    B. hyperpigmentation
    C. pustules
    D. café-au-lait spots

4. **The most characteristic cytogenetic abnormality in Bloom syndrome is**

    A. symmetrical homologous Qr chromosome configuration
    B. nonhomologous Qr chromosome configuration
    C. trisomy 15
    D. monosomy 8

5. **Clinical features of Fanconi anemia include all of the following** *except*

    A. short stature
    B. renal anomalies
    C. skeletal anomalies
    D. decreased skin pigmentation

6. **What is the therapy of choice for Fanconi anemia?**

    A. Blood transfusions
    B. Bone marrow transplant
    C. Radiation
    D. Chemotherapy

7. **Which malignancy is predominately associated with Fanconi anemia?**

    A. Basal cell carcinoma
    B. Osteosarcoma
    C. Neuroblastoma
    D. Acute myelogenous leukemia

8. **Clinical features of ataxia-telangiectasia include all of the following** *except*

    A. cerebellar ataxia
    B. ocular apraxia
    C. hypoplasia of radii and thumbs
    D. immunodeficiency

9. **Which serum immunoglobulin is characteristically decreased in ataxia-telangiectasia?**

    A. IgA
    B. IgM
    C. IgG1
    D. IgG3

10. **What type of malignancy are patients with ataxia-telangiectasia at increased risk of developing?**

    A. Skin cancer

B. Sarcomas

C. Neural tumors

D. Lymphoid malignancies

11. On what chromosome is the ATM gene for ataxia-telangiectasia located?

A. 15

B. 11

C. 6

D. X

12. Clinical features of Nijmegen breakage syndrome include all of the following *except*

A. immunodeficiency

B. short stature

C. scleral telangiectasia

D. cerebellar ataxia

13. The truncated nibrin protein in Nijmegen breakage syndrome normally functions in

A. cell cycle regulator

B. DNA double-strand break repair

C. apoptosis

D. protein transport

14. The clinical features of xeroderma pigmentosum include all of the following *except*

A. sun sensitivity

B. numerous freckles

C. keratoconjunctivitis sicca

D. microcephaly

15. What type of malignancy are patients with xeroderma pigmentosum at increased risk of developing?

A. Skin cancer

B. Sarcomas

C. Neural tumors

D. Lymphoid malignancies

16. The clinical features of Werner syndrome include all of the following *except*

A. scleroderma-like skin changes

B. tall stature

C. premature graying of hair

D. high-pitched or hoarse voice

Indicate whether each of the following statements is true (T) or false (F).

17. In xeroderma pigmentosum, excessive chromatid breakage occurs after exposure to magnetic radiation.

18. Bloom syndrome is more common in patients of Irish decent than in Ashkenazi Jews.

19. Failure to unwind G4 DNA may be a possible explanation of the genomic instability in Bloom syndrome.

20. Ataxia-telangiectasia cells demonstrates decreased telomere shortening.

21. Ataxia-telangiectasia cells are strikingly hyperresponsive to the chromosome breaking action of x-rays.

22. Cataracts develop during the third decade in Werner syndrome.

23. Hyperkeratosis and calluses of the feet and ankles are seen frequently in Werner syndrome.

24. Thyroid carcinomas are the most common malignancies in Werner syndrome.

25. The function of the WRN protein is DNA double-strand repair.

SOLID TUMOR CYTOGENETICS

QUESTIONS

Select the one best answer of the choices offered.

1. _____ is associated with a poor prognostic outlook in acute lymphocytic leukemia and acute undifferentiated leukemia.
   A. t(5;12)(q21;q23)
   B. t(4;11)(q21;q23)
   C. t(17;19)(q17;q21)
   D. t(18;19)(q19;q21)

2. HITES medium contains all of the following *except*
   A. hydrocortisone
   B. insulin
   C. testosterone
   D. estradiol

3. In molecular allotyping, DNA is harvested from tumor cells and normal cells and assessed for
   A. diploid cell lines
   B. loss of restriction fragment length polymorphisms
   C. clonal abnormalities
   D. leukemias

4. The majority of meningiomas have a simple monosomy
   A. 17
   B. 21
   C. 22
   D. 13

5. The important gene locus associated with retinoblastoma was detected as deletions of the long arm of chromosome
   A. 5
   B. 7
   C. 11
   D. 13

6. N-myc amplification and deletion are associated with a poor prognosis in neuroblastoma.
   A. 1p
   B. 3p
   C. 5q
   D. 7q

7. The consistent change in pleomorphic adenomas is
   A. t (3;4)(p11;q11)
   B. t (4;6)(p11;q12)
   C. t (5;7)(p7;q11)
   D. t (3;8)(p12;q12)

8. Small cell carcinoma of the lung demonstrates a consistent deletion of the short arm of chromosome
   A. 3
   B. 5
   C. 11
   D. 17

9. Familial adenomatous polyposis is often associated with a loss of alleles on chromosome
   A. 3q
   B. 4p
   C. 5q
   D. 7q

10. The primary site for chromosome change in renal cell carcinoma is found on chromosome
   A. 1
   B. 3
   C. 4
   D. 6

11. Wilms tumor has been associated with constitutional deletion of
   A. 3p
   B. 5p
   C. 7q
   D. 11p

12. Isochromosome has been observed in >90% of teratomas and seminomas.

    A. 3p
    B. 5p
    C. 10p
    D. 12p

13. Melanoma candidate tumor suppressor gene has been associated with chromosome deletion

    A. 3p
    B. 5q
    C. 6q
    D. 9p

14. Ninety percent of Ewing sarcomas characteristically demonstrate translocation

    A. t(11;22)
    B. t(11;14)
    C. t(1;13)
    D. t(X; 18)

15. A highly specific chromosome change in synovial sarcoma is

    A. t(X;17)(p11;q10)
    B. t(X;18)(p11;q11)
    C. t(X;18)(p10;q10)
    D. t(X;15)(p11;q12)

16. In general, low-grade noninvasive bladder tumors have

    A. diploid karyotypes
    B. polyploid karyotypes
    C. aneuploid karyotypes
    D. normal karyotypes

Indicate whether each of the following statements is true (T) or false (F).

17. Allelotyping uses primer sets that flank individual polymorphic sequence repeat polymorphisms (SSRPs) that have already been mapped to each chromosome arm.

18. Comparative genomic hybridization (CGH) combines fluorescence hybridization techniques with a conventional metaphase spread.

19. The t (9;22) translocation in chronic myelogenous leukemia (CML) results in the active production of both message and a protein called p210 bcr/abl.

20. Amplification of N-myc protooncogenes have been implicated as prognostically important in neuroblastoma.

21. Individuals with von Recklinghausen disease (NF-1) characteristically develop acoustic neuromas.

22. Neurofibromatosis type 1 (NF-1) has been mapped to chromosome 17q11.2.

23. Patients with squamous cell carcinoma with 11q13 rearrangements generally demonstrate a good clinical outcome.

24. Adenocarcinomas and acinic cell carcinomas often show deletions of 6q and trisomies for chromosome 7.

25. Parathyroid adenoma gene 1 (PRAD 1) was identified as cyclin D, which is overexpressed in parathyroid tumors with inversion of chromosome 11.

26. Familial polyposis coli (FPC), also known as Lynch syndrome, is an inherited predisposition to colorectal cancer that is characterized by microsatellite instability as a result of DNA replication errors.

27. FPC is an autosomal dominant condition, with nearly all affected patients developing colon cancer by or in their 50s.

28. Mesoblastic nephroma cytogenetically are characterized by simple numerical changes, the most consistent being +11.

29. Patients with low copy number of N-myc amplification have a much better likelihood of survival.

30. HER-2/neu oncogene has been correlated with a shortened disease-free interval and decreased overall survival in breast cancer.

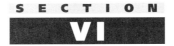

HLA TYPING

35 HLA: Structure, Function, and Methodologies
36 Molecular HLA Typing
37 HLA: The Major Histocompatability Complex: Applications
38 Bone Marrow Transplantation

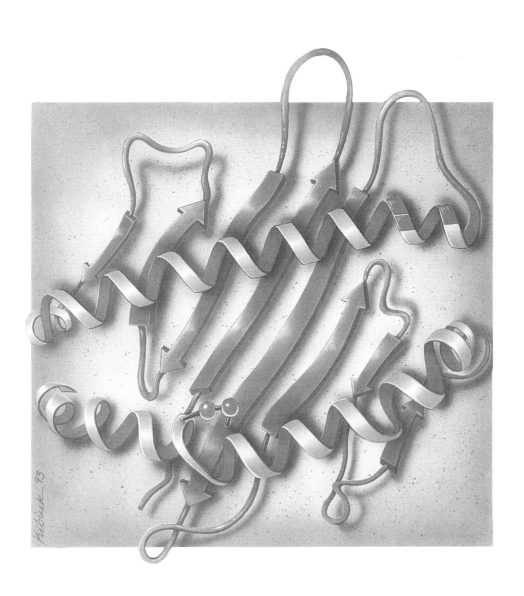

HLA: STRUCTURE, FUNCTION, AND METHODOLOGIES

QUESTIONS

Select the one best answer of the choices offered.

1. **Histocompatibility antigens serve as self-recognition molecules, thus triggering the T-cell–dependent immune response.**

   A. True   B. False

2. **The genetic complex controlling the production of histocompatibility antigens in man is located on**

   A. distal one third of the short arm of chromosome 6
   B. proximal one third of the short arm of chromosome 8
   C. distal two thirds of the short arm of chromosome 8
   D. proximal one third of the short arm of chromosome 6

3. **The genetic complex or HLA haplotype can be divided into ____ major regions.**

   A. 2
   B. 3
   C. 4
   D. 5

4. **Public antigens are specific epitopes that are found associated with each of the different specifications of an entire family of HLA molecules.**

   A. True   B. False

5. **Soluble HLA antigens are shed from**

   A. anuclear mature red cells
   B. nucleated cells
   C. erythroblasts
   D. A and C
   E. A, B, and C

6. **The class II antigens are constitutive products of nucleated cells.**

   A. True   B. False

7. **Most regularly, the class II antigens are found on**

   A. monocytes
   B. endothelial cells
   C. macrophages
   D. A and C
   E. A, B, and C

8. **Class II antigens can act in the capacity of controlling the immune response.**

   A. True   B. False

9. **There is a strong association of the HLA-B53 allele with recovery from a potentially lethal form of malaria.**

   A. True   B. False

10. **DNA-based methods are particularly useful in identifying HLA class II antigens in patients with**

    A. leukemia
    B. aplastic anemia
    C. immunosuppressive therapy
    D. A and C
    E. A, B, and C

36

MOLECULAR HLA TYPING

QUESTIONS

Select the one best answer of the choices offered.

1. **The most common methodologies used to detect nucleotide sequence polymorphism of HLA alleles include**

   A. sequence-specific primers
   B. sequence-specific oligonucleotide probing
   C. polymerase chain reaction (PCR) followed by sequencing
   D. none of the above

2. **The dot-blot procedure may replace serologic typing of volunteers of bone marrow donor registries.**

   A. True   B. False

37

HLA: THE MAJOR HISTOCOMPATABILITY COMPLEX: APPLICATIONS

QUESTIONS

Select the one best answer of the choices offered.

1. **The antigens of the ABO blood group system are fully expressed in all tissues of the human body with the exception of tissues from the central nervous system.**

   A. True   B. False

2. **Survival of cadaveric kidney grafts at 5 years with an HLA mismatch of 2 is _____ %.**

   A. 68
   B. 72
   C. 82
   D. 94

3. **HLA-DR matching alone does not improve long-term graft survival.**

   A. True   B. False

4. **Accelerated solid-organ graft rejection occurs**

   A. 2 to 5 posttransplant days
   B. while the patient is on the operating table
   C. within 3 months of transplant
   D. within 3 weeks of transplant

5. **If a heart transplant candidate has preformed panel-reactive anti-HLA antibodies, a T-cell cross-match should be performed.**

   A. True   B. False

6. **In liver transplantation, HLA matching for DR has a reverse effect. That is, patients with grafts poorly matched for class II antigens appear to do better than those with well-matched grafts.**

   A. True   B. False

7. **It has been noted in lung transplantation that antibodies to class II major histocompatibility complex antigens can be particularly dangerous.**

   A. True   B. False

8. **Antibody screening by cytotoxicity methods includes**

   A. panels of purified T cells to detect class I antigens
   B. B cells for the detection of class II antigens
   C. patient's own cells to detect autoantibodies
   D. A and B
   E. A, B, and C

9. **Positive B-cell cross-matches have been implicated in early rejection of both cardiac and lung transplants.**

   A. True   B. False

10. **Flow cytometric techniques are sensitive methods in solid allograft recipient workups because it is not dependent on complement binding.**

    A. True   B. False

11. **Flow cytometric cross-matches offer advantages over complement-dependent cytotoxicity testing, including**

    A. IgG antibodies can be identified without additional treatment of the patient's serum.
    B. Cell viability is not critical.
    C. It is unnecessary to prepare separate suspensions of T cells and B cells.
    D. A and C
    E. A, B, and C

12. **Immunophilin-binding drugs include cyclosporine.**

    A. True   B. False

13. Tacrolimus is a macrolide antibiotic.

    A. True   B. False

14. Both rheumatoid arthritis and insulin-dependent diabetes mellitus are strongly associated with

    A. DR2

    B. DR3

C. DR8

D. DR4

15. The HLA system is the only polymorphic alloantigenic system in humans whose function is known.

    A. True   B. False

38

BONE MARROW TRANSPLANTATION

QUESTIONS

Select the one best answer of the choices offered.

1. **Indications for bone marrow transplantation include**

    A. rescue from high-dose chemoradiotherapy
    B. therapy for defective genes
    C. delivery of anticancer immunotherapy
    D. A and C
    E. A, B, and C

2. **The most visible manifestation(s) of graft versus host disease is (are)**

    A. liver
    B. skin
    C. gut
    D. all of the above
    E. none of the above

3. **"Linkage disequilibrium" is the theory that HLA antigens are evolutionarily selected as incomplete haplotypes.**

    A. True   B. False

4. **African-Americans are far more polymorphic for HLA than other racial groups.**

    A. True   B. False

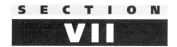
HEMATOLOGY

39 Hematopoiesis and Hematopoietic Growth Factors
40 Peripheral Blood and Bone Marrow: Morphology, Counts and Differentials, and Reactive Disorders
41 Red Blood Cell Disorders
42 Thalassemia and Hemoglobinopathy Syndromes
43 Acute Leukemia and Myelodysplastic Syndromes
44 Chronic Lymphoproliferative Disorders, Immunoproliferative Disorders, and Malignant Lymphoma
45 Chronic Myeloproliferative Disorders

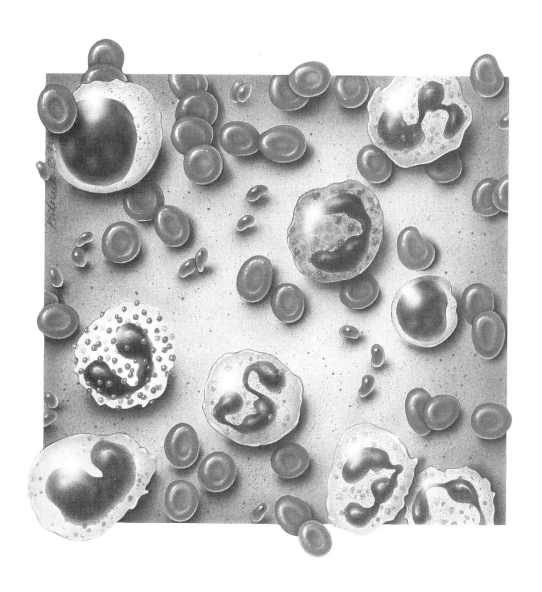

HEMATOPOIESIS AND HEMATOPOIETIC GROWTH FACTORS

QUESTIONS

Select the one best answer of the choices offered.

1. **Which of the following stages of human development marks the replacement of the embryonic liver by the bone marrow as the dominant site of hematopoiesis?**

   A. 15 to 20 mm
   B. 20 to 25 mm
   C. 25 to 30 mm
   D. 30 to 35 mm

2. **All of the following regarding hematopoiesis in the spleen of the embryo and fetus are true** *except*

   A. The spleen is a center of myelopoiesis until the time of birth.
   B. Wandering mesenchymal cells invade the spleen around the 70-mm stage of human development.
   C. The white pulp forms by the differentiation of mesenchymal cells that have grouped around the splenic arterioles.
   D. The white pulp forms around the fifth month of gestation.

3. **The cell divisions that give rise to erythropoietin-sensitive erythroid progenitor cells are largely erythropoietin independent.**

   A. True   B. False

4. **All of the following mediators participate in regulating early divisions of granulocytes** *except*

   A. interleukin-3 (IL-3)

   B. IL-1
   C. stem cell factor (SCF)
   D. granulocyte-macrophage colony-stimulating factor (GM-CSF)

5. **All of the following cytokines play an inductive role in the production of eosinophils** *except*

   A. IL-3
   B. IL-5
   C. tumor necrosis factor (TNF)
   D. GM-CSF

6. **Which of the following mediators appears to play a major role in the later stages of megakaryopoiesis?**

   A. IL-3
   B. IL-6
   C. SCF
   D. GM-CSF

Match each of the following with the corresponding lymphocyte subset (each answer might be used more than once).

7. **Direct stimulation of TCR/CD3**

8. **IL-7**

9. **IL-2**

10. **IL-4**

   A. CD8 T lymphocytes
   B. CD4 T lymphocytes
   C. B lymphocytes

PERIPHERAL BLOOD AND BONE MARROW: MORPHOLOGY, COUNTS AND DIFFERENTIALS, AND REACTIVE DISORDERS

QUESTIONS

Select the one best answer of the choices offered.

1. **The cytoplasmic granulation of the bands is different compared with segmented neutrophils.**

   A. True B. False

2. **All of the following morphologic criteria of the lymphocytes are true *except***

   A. inconspicuous nucleoli
   B. prominent parachromatin
   C. basophilic cytoplasm
   D. azurophilic granules may be identified

3. **All of the following statements regarding the morphologic criteria of the granulocytes are true *except***

   A. Promyelocytes are medium-sized cells (12 to 16 µm).
   B. Myeloblasts are the youngest identifiable cells in the granulocytic series.
   C. Chromatin of the metamyelocytes is dense, with no nucleolus evident.
   D. The Golgi hof may be quite prominent in myelocytes.

4. **All of the following statements regarding the morphologic criteria of the erythroid precursors are true *except***

   A. Hemoglobinization is evident in the orthochromatic normoblasts.
   B. Reticulocytes lack a nucleus.
   C. Pronormoblasts are the largest erythroid precursors (15 to 22 µm).
   D. Basophilic normoblasts exhibit prominent nucleoli.

5. **All of the following statements regarding the lymphopoiesis are true *except***

   A. Further differentiation and maturation of T-lymphocyte precursors occur in the thymus.
   B. B lymphocytes differentiate to maturity within the bone marrow.
   C. B lymphocytes migrate from the bone marrow to the paracortical regions of the lymph nodes.
   D. Morphology offers a limited perspective of lymphopoiesis.

6. **All of the following statements regarding the anticoagulants used for hematologic studies are true *except***

   A. Citrate is the most commonly used anticoagulant for coagulation and special platelet studies.
   B. Citrate should not be used for routine hematologic studies.
   C. Heparin may cause clumping of platelets or leukocytes.
   D. EDTA produces significant morphologic artifacts on blood film if allowed to stand for more than 2 to 3 hours.

7. **All of the following statements regarding hematocrit are true *except***

   A. Hematocrit is the ratio of the volume of red blood cells to the volume of plasma.
   B. Spun hematocrits may give spurious high results.
   C. Most hematocrits are now calculated directly from red blood cells (RBC) and mean corpuscular volume (MCV).
   D. Hematocrit is a less accurate measure of anemia than direct determination of hemoglobin concentration.

8. **All of the following statements regarding the red blood cell indices are true *except***

    A. Mean corpuscular hemoglobin (MCH) is calculated from hemoglobin and RBC.
    B. MCV is determined by the distribution of the red blood cell histogram.
    C. MCH is the most useful of the red blood cell indices.
    D. MCH concentration is of minimal diagnostic use.

9. **All of the following conditions might be associated with increased red cell distribution width (RDW) *except***

    A. iron deficiency anemia
    B. thalassemia trait
    C. S-β-thalassemia
    D. hemoglobin H

10. **All of the following statements regarding the differential white blood cell count (WBC) are true *except***

    A. Traditional manual differential count has poor sensitivity, specificity, and predictive values.
    B. Traditional manual differential count is the gold standard of differential WBCs.
    C. Categorization of immature granulocytes can be accurately identified only on a manual smear.
    D. The digital image analysis system is the standard in automated differential counts.

11. **All of the following conditions are associated with high mean platelet volume (MPV) *except***

    A. May-Hegglin anomaly
    B. myelodysplastic syndrome
    C. megaloblastic anemia
    D. Bernard-Soulier syndrome

12. **Döhle bodies represent endoplasmic reticulum and are a very reliable sign of an infectious process.**

    A. True   B. False

13. **All of the following findings are considered among the features of the leukemoid reaction *except***

    A. absence of basophilia
    B. leukocyte alkaline phosphatase (LAP) score <10
    C. total WBC of 10.0 to 100.0×10^9/L
    D. myeloid:erythroid (M:E) ratio of 5 to 10:1

14. **All of the following clinical conditions are associated with neutropenia *except***

    A. Fanconi anemia
    B. storage disorders
    C. myelofibrosis
    D. hyperthyroidism

15. **All of the following clinical conditions are associated with eosinophilia *except***

    A. graft versus host disease
    B. rheumatoid arthritis
    C. acute infections
    D. systemic mastocytosis

16. **All of the following clinical conditions are associated with lymphopenia *except***

    A. Whipple disease
    B. DiGeorge syndrome
    C. dilantin administration
    D. ataxia telangiectasia

17. **All of the following statements regarding May-Hegglin anomaly are true *except***

    A. It is an autosomal recessive disorder.
    B. Large abnormal Döhle bodies are identified in neutrophils and monocytes.
    C. Döhle bodies consist of rough endoplasmic reticulum.
    D. Giant platelets are identified, but platelet function studies are within normal.

Match each of the following morphologic findings with the corresponding leukocyte disorder.

18. **Giant, cytoplasmic lysosomal inclusions**

19. **Neutrophils with dumbbell-shaped nucleus**

20. **Promyelocytes and myelocytes with nuclear indentation and segmentation**

21. **Morphologically unremarkable neutrophils**

    A. Hereditary hypersegmentation in neutrophils
    B. Chronic granulomatous disease
    C. Chediak-Higashi syndrome
    D. Pelger-Huet anomaly

41

RED BLOOD CELL DISORDERS

QUESTIONS

Select the one best answer of the choices offered.

1. The concentration of red cell 2,3-diphosphoglycerate increases shortly after the onset of anemic hypoxia.

    A. True   B. False`

2. All of the following diseases might be associated with a microcytic hypochromic anemia *except*

    A. anemia of chronic disease
    B. iron deficiency anemia
    C. sideroblastic anemia
    D. aplastic anemia

3. All of the following diseases might be associated with a macrocytic anemia *except*

    A. aplastic anemia
    B. myelodysplastic syndrome
    C. thalassemia
    D. liver disease

4. All of the following statements regarding heme synthesis are true *except*

    A. Increased free erythrocyte protoporphyrin is the most sensitive laboratory indicator for iron-deficient erythropoiesis
    B. The final step of heme synthesis occurs in the mitochondria.
    C. The major rate-limiting step is the combination of succinyl CoA and glycine to form δ-aminolevulinic (ALA) acid under the influence of ALA synthetase.
    D. The action of heme synthetase is specific for iron.

5. All of the following statements regarding iron deficiency anemia are true *except*

    A. An elevated serum ferritin should indicate the presence of adequate iron stores.
    B. Atransferrinemia results in hemosiderosis.
    C. Nonheme iron must be in the ferrous state to facilitate absorption.
    D. Iron is absorbed primarily in the duodenum or upper jejunum.

6. All of the following serum chemistry findings are consistent with iron deficiency anemia *except*

    A. increased transferrin
    B. decreased transferrin saturation
    C. decreased soluble fragment of transferrin receptor (sTfR) in serum
    D. decreased serum ferritin early during the course of the disease

7. All of the following peripheral blood and bone marrow findings are consistent with iron deficiency anemia *except*

    A. poikilocytosis
    B. thrombocytopenia
    C. mean corpuscular volume (MCV), mean corpuscular hemoglobin (MCH), and mean corpuscular hemoglobin concentration (MCHC) proportionally reduced
    D. decreased sideroblasts in bone marrow

8. All of the following statements regarding hereditary sideroblastic anemia are true *except*

    A. The disease is due to impaired utilization of iron, resulting in diminished heme synthesis.
    B. Pyridoxine can be an effective therapy.
    C. Hereditary forms of sideroblastic anemia are significantly less common than the acquired forms.
    D. Most hereditary forms have been traced to an autosomal recessive pattern of inheritance.

9. All of the following statements regarding hereditary hemochromatosis are true *except*

    A. The juvenile hemochromatosis locus is present on chromosome 1q.
    B. Genotypic testing should be limited to the more common C282Y *HEF* gene mutation.
    C. The hemochromatosis gene *HFE* gene encodes for a nonclassic MHC class I molecule.
    D. Genotypic analysis is recommended for patients with excess iron staining on liver biopsy.

10. **All of the following findings are consistent with anemia of chronic disease** *except*
   A. diminished iron stores
   B. sustained release of interleukin-1 (IL-1)
   C. decreased erythrocyte survival time
   D. decreased serum transferrin

11. **In anemia of chronic disease, lactoferrin competes with transferrin for binding of iron.**
   A. True
   B. False

12. **All of the following laboratory findings are found in anemia of chronic disease** *except*
   A. decreased sideroblasts in the bone marrow
   B. minimal anisopoikilocytosis
   C. decreased ferritin
   D. normal transferrin

13. **Megaloblastic anemias are a group of disorders characterized by reduced rates of DNA and RNA synthesis.**
   A. True
   B. False

14. **Megaloblastic anemia results from failure of conversion of deoxyuridine monophosphate (dUMP) to deoxythymidine monophosphate (dTMP), with subsequent formation of deoxyuridine triphosphate (dUTP).**
   A. True
   B. False

15. **All of the following statements regarding vitamin B_{12} are true** *except*
   A. >50% of the vitamin B_{12} entering the intestine arrives via the enterohepatic circulation.
   B. Free vitamin B_{12} is bound to R proteins.
   C. Transcobalamin II binds only 10% to 25% of vitamin B_{12} in the plasma.
   D. Transcobalamin II is a less significant carrier of vitamin B_{12}.

16. **All of the following statements regarding pernicious anemia are true** *except*
   A. Anti-intrinsic factor antibodies are of two types: blocking and binding.
   B. Antibodies to parietal cell cytoplasm are present in 90% of the patients.
   C. Pernicious anemia results from decreased secretions of the intrinsic factor.
   D. Anti-intrinsic factor antibodies are the primary etiologic agents in pernicious anemia.

17. **All of the following statements regarding the laboratory evaluation of vitamin B_{12} deficiency are true** *except*
   A. Detection of anti-intrinsic factor antibodies is helpful to confirm the diagnosis.
   B. Renal dysfunction may significantly alter results of the Schilling test.
   C. Urinary excretion of methylmalonic acid is essential to establish the diagnosis.
   D. Vitamin B_{12} deficiency due to poor intestinal malfunction can be established using the Schilling test.

18. **All of the following statements regarding the folic acid and folates are true** *except*
   A. Green leafy vegetables, fruits, and dairy products provide the greatest sources.
   B. They are thermostable.
   C. Body stores are limited.
   D. Tetrahydrofolate is a precursor to DNA synthesis.

19. **All of the following statements regarding laboratory evaluation of folic acid deficiency are true** *except*
   A. In vitamin B_{12} deficiency, serum folate is decreased.
   B. Serum folate levels are sensitive to short-term variation in vitamin intake.
   C. Serum folate concentrations are <3 ng/mL.
   D. Red cell folate levels better reflect tissue folate levels.

20. **The following clinical features are among the diagnostic triad of vitamin B_{12} deficiency anemia** *except*
   A. weakness
   B. paresthesias
   C. sore tongue
   D. lemon yellow skin

21. **Neurologic manifestations are absent in folic acid deficiency.**
   A. True
   B. False

22. **All of the following peripheral blood and bone marrow findings are consistent with megaloblastic anemia** *except*
   A. pseudo Pelger-Huët neutrophils
   B. complex hypersegmentation of megakaryocytes
   C. giant bands
   D. increased erythroblasts in bone marrow

23. **All of the following statements regarding drug-related bone marrow injury are true** *except*
   A. The idiosyncratic drug reaction of chloramphenicol cannot be related to drug dose or mode of administration.

B. Hematopoietic suppression associated with heavy alcohol intake is self-limited.
C. In benzene exposure, the dysplastic changes noted in the marrow may evolve to erythroleukemia.
D. Drug-related bone marrow injury always has some uniform effects on the three hematopoietic cell lines.

24. **All of the following peripheral blood and bone marrow findings are consistent with aplastic anemia** *except*
    A. foci of erythroblasts in the bone marrow
    B. no significant dysplasia in peripheral blood smear
    C. predominance of erythroid precursors on bone marrow aspirate smears
    D. increased number of iron-laden histiocytes in the bone marrow

Match each of the following findings with the corresponding type of congenital dyserythropoietic anemia (CDA) (each answer may be used more than once).

25. **Positive acidified serum test**

26. **Autosomal dominance mode of inheritance**

27. **The most common form of CDA**

28. **Giant erythroblasts with up to 12 nuclei**

29. **Spongy nuclear configuration**
    A. Type I CDA
    B. Type II CDA
    C. Type III CDA

30. **All of the following are considered inherited hemolytic disorders** *except*
    A. aldolase deficiency
    B. thalassemias
    C. stomatocytosis
    D. paroxysmal nocturnal hemoglobinuria (PNH)

31. **All of the following statements regarding hereditary spherocytosis are true** *except*
    A. defective ankyrin
    B. In approximately 10% of cases, anemia is severe.
    C. autosomal dominance mode of inheritance
    D. defective interaction of spectrin with protein 4.1

32. **The most frequent structural abnormality in hereditary elliptocytosis is quantitative deficiency of protein 4.1.**
    A. True   B. False

33. **All of the following statements regarding hereditary stomatocytosis are true** *except*
    A. Patients present with mild anemia.
    B. Structural abnormality in hereditary stomatocytosis is defective spectrin dimer-dimer interaction.
    C. There is increased permeability to both sodium and potassium ions.
    D. Splenectomy sometimes is indicated.

34. **All of the following statements regarding glucose-6-phosphate dehydrogenase (G6PD) deficiency are true** *except*
    A. G6PD Mediterranean has a half-life of few hours compared with 60 days for G6PD.
    B. G6PD A is found in approximately 20% of American black males.
    C. Deficiency in G6PD accounts for 99% of cases of hemolytic anemia attributable to enzyme deficiencies in the Embden-Meyerhof pathway.
    D. G6PD A− is deficient in aging red blood cells.

35. **All of the following statements regarding pyruvate kinase deficiency are true** *except*
    A. The dysfunctional abnormality is attributed to altered kinetic rate of the enzyme.
    B. Red blood morphology is unremarkable.
    C. Single copy of a defective gene causes no significant alteration of enzyme activity.
    D. Acquired form of pyruvate kinase deficiency sometimes is seen with the myelodysplastic syndrome.

36. **IgM-coated red cells are readily found in the circulation.**
    A. True   B. False

37. **Spherocytes are frequent in ABO-related hemolysis, but are a minor feature of Rh incompatibility.**
    A. True   B. False

38. **Up to 30% of chronic lymphocytic leukemia cases are associated with warm autoimmune hemolytic anemia.**
    A. True   B. False

39. **Approximately 95% of cold-reacting antibodies show anti-I specificity.**
    A. True   B. False

40. **Cold agglutinins associating mycoplasma pneumonia are directed against the I antigen.**
    A. True   B. False

41. **All of the following statements regarding paroxysmal cold hemoglobinuria (PCH) are true *except***

    A. The disease usually is self-limited.
    B. Hemolysis occurs after the blood has been chilled then warmed to 37°C.
    C. PCH is the result of an anti-P antibody.
    D. PCH has an autosomal dominant pattern of inheritance.

Match each of the following drugs with the appropriated hemolytic mechanism.

42. **Penicillin**

43. **Methyldopa**

44. **Quinidine**

45. **Cephalothin**

    A. Innocent bystander mechanism
    B. Nonimmune absorption of proteins
    C. Hapten mechanism
    D. True autoimmune hemolytic anemia

46. **PNH is an acquired, clonal hematopoietic stem cell disorder.**

    A. True   B. False

47. **All of the following statements regarding PNH are true *except***

    A. Flow cytometric analysis of red blood cells incubated with monoclonal antibodies is a sensitive and specific test for diagnosis of PNH.
    B. The membrane inhibitor of reactive lysis (CD59) is lacking on the red blood cell membrane.
    C. The disease is limited to the red blood cells.
    D. The sucrose hemolysis test is less specific than the acidified serum lysis test (Ham test) for diagnosis of PNH.

THALASSEMIA AND HEMOGLOBINOPATHY SYNDROMES

QUESTIONS

Match each of the following globin chains with the corresponding type of hemoglobin (Hb).

1. α_2/δ_2

2. $\alpha_2/^G\gamma_2$

3. α_2/ε_2

4. ζ_2/ε_2
   A. Hb F
   B. Gower 1
   C. Hb A_2
   D. Gower 2

5. **All of the following statements regarding the oxygen dissociation curve are true *except***
   A. Increase in pH leads to shift to the left of the oxygen dissociation curve.
   B. 2,3-diphosphoglycerate (2,3-DPG) increases the oxygen affinity of Hb.
   C. P_{50} for normal men is close to 27 mm Hg.
   D. Increase in temperature reduces the oxygen affinity of Hb.

6. **All of the following statements regarding the genetic control of Hb are true *except***
   A. $^A\gamma$-chains have alanine and $^G\gamma$-chains have phenylalanine as the 136th amino acid residue.
   B. The α-gene is present on chromosome 16.
   C. Production of the δ-chain is approximately 0.5% of the total globin chain production at birth.
   D. The α1-gene is responsible for approximately two thirds of the α-chains.

Match each of the following Hb abnormalities with the corresponding common finding (each answer may be used more than once).

7. **Hb H**

8. **Hb C**

9. **Glucose-6-phosphate dehydrogenase deficiency**

10. **Thalassemia minor**
    A. Crystals
    B. Microcytic hypochromic red cells without significant anemia
    C. Heinz bodies

11. **The following could give false-positive results in the solubility test for detection of Hb S *except***
    A. presence of many nucleated red blood cells in the peripheral blood
    B. large amounts of proteins in patient's plasma
    C. incomplete lysis of red blood cells
    D. severe anemia

Match each of the following with the corresponding Hb electrophoresis method.

12. **Run both on alkaline and acidic pH**

13. **Utilizes agar and citrate-citric buffer**

14. **Hb C, Hb E, and Hb O_{Arab} migrate together**

15. **Glycosylated Hb, methemoglobin, and glycerated Hb are seen.**
    A. Acid electrophoresis
    B. Isoelectric focusing
    C. Globin-chain electrophoresis
    D. Cellulose acetate electrophoresis

16. **All of the following statements regarding α-thalassemia are true *except***

    A. Hb$_{Barts}$ is seen in adults.
    B. Deletion of both α-globin genes from the same chromosome is called α-thalassemia 1.
    C. Some of the deletions involving the α-globin genes are the most common single gene disorder in the world.
    D. Brilliant cresyl blue stain causes Hb H to precipitate in red blood cells.

17. **All of the following statements regarding Hb H disease are true *except***

    A. Heinz bodies are present in the red blood cells.
    B. Morphology of the red blood cells is within normal range.
    C. It is a form of thalassemia intermedia.
    D. Hb H is a tetramer of β-globin chains.

18. **All of the following statements regarding β-thalassemia minor are true *except***

    A. S/β$^+$-thalassemia compound heterozygotes have Hb A levels between 5% and 30%.
    B. It requires no therapy.
    C. Doubling level of Hb F is the hallmark of β^0-thalassemia and β$^+$-thalassemia minor.
    D. It is not possible to distinguish between β^0-thalassemia minor and β$^+$-thalassemia minor on a hematologic basis.

19. **All of the following statements regarding β-thalassemia major are true *except***

    A. There is marked erythroid hypoplasia.
    B. The excess α-globin chains do not form a soluble tetramer.
    C. Periodic acid-Schiff (PAS)–positive inclusions are present in the erythroid precursors in the bone marrow.
    D. The disease is masked at birth by the production of γ-globin chains.

20. **All of the following statements regarding αβ-thalassemia are true *except***

    A. Hb F is increased to 5% to 20% in αβ-thalassemia minor.
    B. αβ-thalassemia minor is less severe than β-thalassemia.
    C. Homozygous αβ-thalassemia is a severe form of thalassemia.
    D. Hb electrophoresis shows the presence of 100% Hb F in homozygous αβ-thalassemia.

21. **All of the following statements regarding Hb Lepore are true *except***

    A. The Hb consists of 75% Hb F and 25% Hb Lepore in homozygotes.
    B. Three different types of anti-Lepore Hb have been reported .
    C. Hb Lepore migrates with Hb S on cellulose acetate in alkaline buffer.
    D. Homozygous Hb Lepore presents clinically as thalassemia minor.

22. **All of the following statements regarding Hb S are true *except***

    A. Hb S is common in endemic areas of falciparum malaria.
    B. It results from a point mutation in the sixth codon of the β-chain.
    C. Hb S molecules tend to form tactoids under conditions of reduced oxygen tension.
    D. The prevalence of sickle cell trait is 2.0% in American blacks.

Match each of the following disorders with the expected Hb A and Hb S findings.

23. **Hb SC**

24. **Hb S/β$^+$ thalassemia**

25. **Sickle cell anemia (Hb SS)**

26. **Hb S/α thalassemia 1**

    A. Hb A 75%, Hb S 25%
    B. Hb A 0%, Hb S 50%
    C. Hb A 0%, Hb S 95%
    D. Hb A 5% to 30%, Hb S 60% to 90%

27. **The following findings may occur in sickle cell trait *except***

    A. painless hematuria
    B. isosthenuria
    C. markedly increased Hb A$_2$
    D. sudden death

28. **All of the following findings are consistent with sickle cell anemia *except***

    A. increased susceptibility to infection by *Pneumococcus*
    B. normal Hb F levels
    C. hand-foot syndrome
    D. splenomegaly in childhood

29. All of the following statements regarding Hb SC disease are true *except*

A. Frequency of renal papillary necrosis is less than sickle cell anemia.

B. Frequency of cerebrovascular accidents is equal to that of sickle cell anemia.

C. Life expectancy is slightly shortened.

D. There is a higher rate of spontaneous early abortions.

30. All of the following laboratory findings are consistent with Hb SC disease *except*

A. rare sickle cells

B. crystals

C. boat-shaped cells

D. Hb A_2 will be contained within Hb S by Hb electrophoresis at alkaline pH.

31. Hb S in combination with hereditary persistence of fetal Hb is a benign disorder.

A. True   B. False

32. All of the following statements regarding Hb C disorders are true *except*

A. The red cells show reduced mean corpuscular volume (MCV), but increased mean corpuscular hemoglobin concentration (MCHC) in Hb C heterozygotes (Hb AC).

B. High-performance liquid chromatography is necessary for quantitation of Hb A_2 in the presence of Hb C.

C. Hb C is found exclusively in blacks.

D. Extracellular crystals are identified in Hb C disease.

33. All of the following statements regarding Hb E are true *except*

A. Homozygous Hb E disease is a benign disorder.

B. It occurs mainly in Africa.

C. It is the second most common Hb variant.

D. Hb E migrates with Hb C, Hb O_{Arab}, and Hb A_2 on cellulose acetate.

34. All of the following statements regarding unstable Hbs are true *except*

A. The Carrell test is a screening test for the presence of unstable Hbs.

B. Bites cells are identified in the peripheral blood smears.

C. Hb Köln is a low oxygen affinity variant.

D. Several unstable Hbs migrate with Hb A.

35. All of the following statements regarding M Hbs are true *except*

A. Cyanosis is due to methemoglobin.

B. Hb $M_{Saskatoon}$ and Hb $M_{Hyde\ Park}$ have been associated with significant hemolysis.

C. Cyanosis is due to hypoxia.

D. Most of the M Hbs separate from Hb A on alkaline electrophoresis.

43

ACUTE LEUKEMIA AND MYELODYSPLASTIC SYNDROMES

QUESTIONS

Select the one best answer of the choices offered.

1. **Acute leukemias are hyperproliferative disorders that result in the production of new cells at a rapid pace.**
   A. True   B. False

Match each of the following major types of leukemia with its corresponding relative incidence.

2. **B-cell chronic lymphocytic leukemia**

3. **Acute myelogenous leukemia (AML)**

4. **Acute lymphoblastic leukemia (ALL)**

5. **Chronic myelogenous leukemia**
   A. 15%
   B. 45%
   C. 10%
   D. 30%

6. **All of the following statements regarding ALL are true *except***
   A. Only 1% to 3% of ALL cases in adults and children are of the FAB-L3 subtype.
   B. ALL is slightly more common in boys than girls.
   C. Approximately 50% of ALL patients will have a peripheral white blood cell count (WBC) above 50.0×10^9/L.
   D. ALL is the most common cancer in children younger than 15 years.

7. **The present protocols for treatment of high-risk patients mandates application of the FAB morphologic classification of ALL into L1, L2, or L3.**
   A. True   B. False

Match each of the following morphologic criteria with the corresponding FAB type of ALL (each answer might be used more than once).

8. **Irregular nuclear shape**

9. **Small inconspicuous nucleoli**

10. **Deeply basophilic cytoplasm**

11. **Predominant small cells**

12. **Sharply punched vacuoles**

13. **Heterogeneous, intermediate to large cells**
    A. FAB-L1
    B. FAB-L2
    C. FAB-L3

14. **All of the following statements regarding the cytochemistry of ALL are true *except***
    A. Terminal deoxynucleotidyl transferase (TdT) is a nuclear staining.
    B. Periodic acid-Schiff (PAS) is positive in 40% to 60% of ALL cases.
    C. TdT is positive in B-precursor, but not in T-cell ALL.
    D. Oil red O is an excellent marker for ALL-L3.

15. **All of the following statements regarding immunophenotypic classification of ALL are true *except***
    A. Lack of CD10 expression appears to be associated with a poorer prognosis.
    B. CD19 is present in >95% of ALL cases.
    C. Pre–B-cell ALL is characterized by expression of cytoplasmic μ.
    D. CD34 is consistently identified in ALL.

16. **All of the following statements regarding ALL are true *except***

    A. ALL with t(4;11) has a relatively good prognosis.
    B. Pre–B-cell ALL is commonly associated with t i(1;19).
    C. CD10 expression is found in one third to one half of B-cell ALL (Burkitt leukemia) cases.
    D. The earliest stage of B-cell development has been associated with ALL with t i(4;11).

17. **All of the following statements regarding T-cell ALL are true *except***

    A. Patients have a higher incidence of CNS relapse compared with B-cell ALL.
    B. The most sensitive markers are CD3, CD4, and CD8.
    C. A mediastinal mass is found in >50% of cases.
    D. CD10 can be detected in T-cell ALL.

18. **All of the following statements regarding lymphoblastic lymphoma are true *except***

    A. A mediastinal mass often is found.
    B. Most lymphoblastic lymphomas are B cell in origin.
    C. It can be distinguished from other types of lymphomas based on TdT reactivity.
    D. Males are affected more frequently.

19. **All of the following chromosomal translocations are associated with poor prognosis in ALL *except***

    A. t i(8;14)
    B. t i(9;22)
    C. t i(12;21)
    D. t i(4;11)

Match each of the following chromosomal abnormalities encountered in ALL with the corresponding type of ALL.

20. **t i(9;22)**

21. **t i(4;11)**

22. **t i(8;22)**

23. **t i(12;21)**

    A. Identified in 25% of childhood ALL
    B. Most commonly identified in infant ALL (<2 years)
    C. Identified in 20% of adult ALL
    D. Identified in surface immunoglobulin-positive ALL

24. **All of the following statements regarding ALL with t i(4;11) are true *except***

    A. Splenomegaly is commonly identified.

B. Immunophenotypic analysis shows HLA-DR$^+$, CD34$^+$, CD19$^+$, CD10$^-$, and CD20$^-$.
    C. It typically has FAB-L2 morphology.
    D. Median survival is about 5 years.

25. **AML is not a disorder of rapidly proliferating cells but rather an accumulation of incompetent, long-surviving cells.**

    A. True   B. False

Match each of the following FAB subtypes of AML with the corresponding relative incidence.

26. **M0**

27. **M1**

28. **M2**

29. **M3**

    A. 28%
    B. 8%
    C. 1%
    D. 18%

30. **All of the following statements regarding FAB classification of AML are true *except***

    A. The ability to reproduce the various FAB groups is well proven.
    B. FAB classification of AML does not provide important prognostic information to the patient.
    C. FAB classification distinguishes AML into eight major subtypes: FAB-M0 to FAB-M7.
    D. FAB classification of AML relies on the degree of granulocytic, monocytic, erythroid, and megakaryocytic differentiation.

Match each of the following diagnostic criteria with the corresponding FAB subtype of AML.

31. **≥90% blasts in bone marrow**

32. **≥50% nucleated red blood cells in marrow**

33. **≤80% myeloblasts and granulocytic precursors and >20% monocytes in marrow**

34. **Negative staining with myeloperoxidase, sulanblack b, and nonspecific esterase is noted in which FAB subtype of acute myelogenous leukemia**

    A. M4
    B. M0
    C. M6
    D. M1

Match each of the following types of AML with the corresponding FAB subtype.

35. Acute erythroleukemia

36. AML with maturation

37. Acute monocytic leukemia

38. Acute promyelocytic leukemia

39. Acute megakaryoblastic leukemia

  A. M3
  B. M7
  C. M6
  D. M2
  E. M5

40. All of the following statements regarding FAB-M1 are true *except*

  A. <10% of the marrow cells show evidence of granulocytic differentiation at or beyond the promyelocytic stage.
  B. <3% of the leukemic blasts demonstrate MPO and/or SBB positivity.
  C. The blasts show a minimal number of Auer rods.
  D. Differential diagnosis includes ALL-L2, AML-M5a, and AML-M7.

41. All of the following statements regarding FAB-M2 are true *except*

  A. Patients with t (8;21) have poor prognosis.
  B. Blasts from patients with t (8;21) exhibit the "crushed" orange granularity in the cytoplasm.
  C. Blasts are >20%, but <90% of the marrow cellularity.
  D. Approximately 5% to 30% of FAB-M2 patients demonstrate t (8;21).

42. All of the following statements regarding FAB-M3 are true *except*

  A. Median age at diagnosis is 35 to 40 years.
  B. t (11;17) is seen in FAB-M3.
  C. Hypogranular (FAB-M3v) has less incidence of disseminated intravascular coagulation compared with classic FAB-M3.
  D. Typical FAB-M3 cases are CD13⁺, CD33⁺, CD34⁻, and HLA-DR⁻.

43. All of the following statements regarding FAB-M4e are true *except*

  A. The sum of myeloblasts and granulocytic precursor cells are <80% of the marrow cells.
  B. Abnormalities of chromosome 16 are consistently identified.
  C. Peripheral blood eosinophilia is frequently identified.
  D. FAB-M4e has a good prognosis.

44. All of the following statements regarding FAB-M5 are true *except*

  A. FAB-M5b shows more differentiation than FAB-M5a.
  B. Both FAB-M5a and FAB-M5b are associated with a high incidence of extramedullary infiltration.
  C. FAB-M5a is more commonly diagnosed in the pediatric age group.
  D. Together, FAB-M2 and FAB-M5 account for approximately two thirds of all AML cases.

45. All of the following criteria for diagnosis of FAB-M7 are true *except*

  A. platelet peroxidase by ultracytochemistry with electron microscopy
  B. immunophenotypic positivity for CD14 and CD64
  C. strong reactivity with the acetate substrate of nonspecific esterase
  D. absence reactivity with α-naphthyl butyrate esterase

46. All of the following are included in the FAB classification of myelodysplastic syndromes *except*

  A. refractory cytopenia with multilineage dysplasia
  B. idiopathic refractory sideroblastic anemia
  C. chronic myelomonocytic leukemia
  D. refractory anemia with excess blasts in transformation

47. All of the following are included in the proposed World Health Organization (WHO) classification of myelodysplastic syndromes *except*

  A. refractory anemia with ringed sideroblasts
  B. 5q– syndrome
  C. refractory anemia with excess blasts in transformation
  D. refractory cytopenia with multilineage dysplasia

48. All of the following are considered low-risk prognostic factors in myelodysplastic syndromes *except*

  A. absence of chromosomal abnormalities
  B. numerous ringed sideroblasts
  C. low colony-forming unit (CFU) capacity
  D. refractory anemia with normal platelet and WBC

44

CHRONIC LYMPHOPROLIFERATIVE DISORDERS, IMMUNOPROLIFERATIVE DISORDERS, AND MALIGNANT LYMPHOMA

QUESTIONS

Select the one best answer of the choices offered.

1. **All of the following characteristics are consistent with chronic lymphocytic leukemia *except***

   A. most cases are of B-cell type
   B. positive CD5 and negative CD23
   C. peripheral blood lymphocytes >5,000/mm³
   D. mixed and focal interstitial pattern of bone marrow involvement

2. **All of the following findings are consistent with chronic lymphocytic leukemia *except***

   A. trisomy 12
   B. free light chain in urine
   C. T-cell antigen receptor rearrangement
   D. increased DNA content

3. **Richter syndrome is an acute lymphoblastic transformation of chronic lymphocytic leukemia.**

   A. True   B. False

4. **All of the following findings are associated with worse prognosis in chronic lymphocytic leukemia *except***

   A. trisomy 12
   B. prolymphocytes >15,000/mm³
   C. interstitial marrow infiltrate
   D. thrombocytopenia (<100 × 10⁹/L)

5. **All of the following statements regarding prolymphocytic leukemia are true *except***

   A. There is positive FMC7 and CD23.
   B. Prolymphocytes comprise >55% of the peripheral blood lymphocytes.
   C. There is strongly reacting sIg.
   D. Most of the cases are of the B-cell type.

6. **Tartrate-resistant acid phosphatase (TRAP) stain is useful to distinguish prolymphocytic leukemia from hairy cell leukemia.**

   A. True   B. False

7. **All of the following features are consistent with hairy cell leukemia *except***

   A. splenomegaly
   B. leukocytosis
   C. male predominance
   D. dry tap

8. **All of the following markers are positive in hairy cell leukemia *except***

   A. FMC7
   B. TRAP
   C. CD25
   D. CD79b

9. **The following findings favor T-cell lymphoproliferative disorder more than B-cell process *except***

   A. cytopenia
   B. skin lesions
   C. clefting of the nucleus
   D. cytoplasmic granules

10. **Most of the T-cell prolymphocytic leukemia cases are of the cytotoxic/suppressor (CD8) phenotype.**

    A. True   B. False

11. **All of the following statements regarding large granular lymphocyte leukemia are true *except***

    A. Lymphocytes of the T-cell phenotype are +/− for CD57.

B. Lymphocytes of the natural killer (NK)-cell pheno-type are +/− for CD57.

C. Lymphocytes of the NK-cell phenotype are +/− for CD3.

D. Bone marrow usually is not involved.

12. **All of the following statements regarding Sézary syndrome/mycosis fungoides (SS/MF) are true *except***

A. Presence of a small percentage of convoluted cells in the peripheral blood is diagnostic of SS.

B. Cells of SS/MF are CD4⁺/CD7⁻.

C. SS is primarily a disorder of the skin with secondary blood involvement.

D. Late in the course of MF, dissemination occurs and convoluted lymphoid cells may be seen in the peripheral blood.

13. **All of the following features are consistent with adult T-cell leukemia/lymphoma *except***

A. indolent T-cell disorder

B. CD4 phenotype

C. lytic bone lesions

D. relative marrow sparing

14. **The following findings are consistent with plasma cell myeloma *except***

A. monoclonal gammopathy in urine

B. large sheets of atypical plasma cells on bone marrow sections

C. bone marrow aspirate smears with ≥10% atypical plasma cells

D. binucleated plasma cells

15. **The following are major clinical/pathologic criteria for diagnosis of plasma cell myeloma *except***

A. plasmacytoma

B. >1 g per day α-chains or β-chains in urine without other significant proteinuria

C. lytic bone lesions

D. >30% marrow plasmacytosis

16. **All of the following are consistent with plasma cell leukemia *except***

A. poor prognosis

B. >30% plasma cells in peripheral blood

C. less involvement of the bone marrow

D. >5,000 plasma cells per cubic millimeter in peripheral blood

17. **The best procedure to detect a monoclonal gammopathy is immunofixation.**

A. True   B. False

18. **All of the following statements regarding Waldenström macroglobulinemia are true *except***

A. Waldenström macroglobulinemia is the bone marrow counterpart of lymphoplasmacytoid lymphoma.

B. Prognosis is intermediate between chronic lymphocytic leukemia and plasma cell myeloma.

C. The disease is characterized by an immunoglobulin M monoclonal gammopathy and lytic bone lesions.

D. The infiltrate in the bone marrow consists of small lymphocytes, plasmacytoid lymphocytes, and plasma cells.

19. **All of the following statements regarding heavy-chain disease are true *except***

A. γ-chain disease is the most common form of heavy-chain disease.

B. 70% of the patients with γ heavy-chain disease have a neoplastic disease.

C. Chronic lymphocytic leukemia/small lymphocytic lymphoma is the most common morphologic entity associated with production of μ heavy chains.

D. Patients with α-chain disease usually present with gastrointestinal symptoms.

Match each of the following leukemic/marrow counterparts with its corresponding lymphomatous counterpart.

20. **L3 acute lymphoblastic leukemia**

21. **Plasma cell myeloma**

22. **Chronic lymphocytic leukemia**

23. **Waldenström macroglobulinemia**

24. **L1 and L2 acute lymphoblastic leukemia**

A. Small lymphocytic lymphoma

B. Lymphoplasmacytoid lymphoma

C. Lymphoblastic lymphoma

D. Plasmacytoma

E. Burkitt lymphoma

Match each of the following morphologic features with corresponding type of lymphoid aggregates (each answer may be used more than once).

25. **Poorly circumscribed spreading border**

26. **Distinctly atypical cell type**

27. **Mild nuclear contour irregularity**

28. Well-circumscribed border

A. Benign
B. Malignant
C. Both

Match the following immunologic findings with the corresponding type of lymphoma.

CD5⁻, CD23⁻, CD43⁻, CD10⁺

CD10⁺, CD19⁺, TdT⁺

CD5⁺, CD23⁻, cyclin D1⁺

29. CD5⁺, CD23⁺, CD43⁺

A. Mantle cell lymphoma
B. Follicle center cell lymphoma

C. Lymphoblastic lymphoma
D. Small lymphocytic lymphoma

30. The requirement to diagnose bone marrow involvement by Hodgkin disease is seeing a cellular infiltrated consistent with Hodgkin disease and at least one mononuclear variant of Reed-Sternberg cells.

A. True   B. False

31. All of the following statements regarding posttransplant lymphoproliferative disorders (PTLD) are true *except*

A. PTLD is highly associated with Epstein-Barr virus.
B. The lymphoma usually is of B-cell phenotype.
C. The lymphoma frequently presents as widespread nodal involvement.
D. Patients with polymorphic lymphoproliferative disease are most likely to respond to antiviral therapy.

CHRONIC MYELOPROLIFERATIVE DISORDERS

Select the one best answer of the choices offered.

1. **According to the World Health Organization (WHO) classification of myeloid neoplasms, each of the following diseases is considered a chronic myeloproliferative disorder** *except*

   A. essential thrombocythemia
   B. polycythemia vera (PV)
   C. chronic myelomonocytic leukemia
   D. chronic idiopathic myelofibrosis

2. **According to the WHO classification of myeloid neoplasms, each of the following entities is considered a myelodysplastic/myeloproliferative disorder** *except*

   A. chronic neutrophilic leukemia
   B. chronic myelomonocytic leukemia
   C. juvenile myelomonocytic leukemia
   D. atypical chronic myeloid leukemia

3. **All of the following statements regarding the BCR-ABL hybrid protein are true** *except*

   A. The BCR-ABL oncoprotein confers protection of the chronic myeloid leukemia cells from apoptosis.
   B. The BCR-ABL hybrid protein is a constitutively active cytoplasmic protein kinase C isoform.
   C. The BCR-ABL protein is produced as a result of the translocation of chromosome 9 and 22 [t (9;22)(q34;q11)].
   D. The BCR-ABL protein transforms the hematopoietic cells to become independent of cytokine and growth factors.

4. **Bone marrow morphologic findings in chronic myeloid leukemia do not add significant information for diagnostic purposes.**

   A. True   B. False

5. **All of the following are peripheral blood findings in chronic myelogenous leukemia (CML)** *except*

   A. Auer rods
   B. eosinophilia
   C. monocytosis
   D. occasional blasts

6. **The morphologic features of the bone marrow in chronic myeloid leukemia include all of the following** *except*

   A. pseudo-Gaucher cells
   B. decreased megakaryocytes
   C. small hypolobated megakaryocytes
   D. myeloid to erythroid ratio of 10:1 or greater

7. **All of the following statements regarding genetic studies in CML are true** *except*

   A. The Philadelphia chromosome is the abnormal short chromosome 22.
   B. Up to 10% of CML cases are negative for t (9;22) by standard cytogenetics.
   C. Old peripheral blood may be used for detection of t(9;22) by fluorescence *in situ* hybridization (FISH) analysis.
   D. Polymerase chain reaction (PCR) analysis of the BCR-ABL fusion gene is a viable alternative to karyotyping.

8. **All of the following statements regarding t (9;22) are true** *except*

   A. It involves the major breakpoint cluster region (M-bcr) on chromosome 22 in CML.
   B. It may involve the major breakpoint cluster region (M-bcr) on chromosome 22 in acute lymphoblastic leukemia.
   C. It may involve the minor breakpoint cluster region (m-bcr) on chromosome 22 in acute lymphoblastic leukemia.
   D. Acute lymphoblastic leukemia patients with t (9;22) usually are more responsive to chemotherapy.

9. **Flow cytometric analysis is a useful diagnostic tool in the chronic phase of CML.**

    A. True   B. False

10. **All of the following statements regarding the leukocyte alkaline phosphatase (LAP) score test are true *except***

    A. The LAP score test is performed on fresh, heparinized peripheral blood.
    B. The LAP score is decreased in CML.
    C. The LAP score is decreased in leukemoid reactions.
    D. The LAP score is decreased in paroxysmal nocturnal hemoglobinuria.

11. **The following findings are consistent with leukemoid reactions *except***

    A. total leukocytic count >50 × 10⁹/L
    B. normal cytogenetic analysis
    C. basophilia
    D. neutrophilia

12. **The following findings are consistent with chronic myelomonocytic leukemia *except***

    A. erythroid precursors >15%
    B. basophils <2%
    C. monocytes >1 × 10⁹/L
    D. metamyelocytes, myelocytes, and promyelocytes >10%

13. **The following criteria are consistent with atypical CML *except***

    A. basophilia
    B. trilineage dysplasia
    C. median survival <2 years
    D. immature granulocytes between 10% and 20%

14. **The following laboratory findings are consistent with juvenile CML *except***

    A. Philadelphia chromosome, usually by molecular studies
    B. absolute peripheral monocytosis, usually >5 × 10⁹/L
    C. elevated hemoglobin F >10%
    D. monosomy 7 in approximately 25% of patients

15. **The following clinical features are consistent with juvenile CML *except***

    A. café-au-lait spots
    B. better prognosis in patients >2 years old at presentation
    C. xanthomas
    D. lymphadenopathy

16. **The following findings are consistent with the accelerated phase of CML *except***

    A. basophils >20%
    B. blasts <30%
    C. platelets >600 × 10⁹/L
    D. isochromosome 17q

17. **Any of the following findings is considered diagnostic of blastic transformation in CML *except***

    A. >30% blasts in peripheral blood or bone marrow
    B. development of lymphoblastic lymphoma
    C. development of extramedullary myeloid tumor
    D. emergence of a second Philadelphia chromosome

18. **In CML, the lymphoid blast crisis is associated with longer median survival and better response to therapy when compared with the myeloid blast crisis.**

    A. True   B. False

19. **The following findings are characteristic of the lymphoid blast crisis in CML *except***

    A. less frequent organomegaly
    B. lower blast percentage
    C. abrupt transformation without preceding accelerated phase
    D. less extensive involvement of the bone marrow by blasts

20. **The overwhelming majority of the lymphoid blast crises in CML show a B-lineage with a relatively common aberrant expression of myeloid antigens.**

    A. True   B. False

21. **All of the following markers are useful in differentiating the lymphoid from the myeloid blast crisis in CML *except***

    A. CD79a
    B. CD3
    C. CD34
    D. TdT

22. **All of the following statements regarding PV are true *except***

    A. There are low levels of serum erythropoietin.
    B. Definitive diagnosis is made based on increased red blood cells (>6 × 10¹²/L), increased hemoglobin concentration, and elevated hematocrit.
    C. Erythromelalgia and transient ocular defects are detected in PV patients.
    D. Platelets uncommonly are >1,000 × 10⁹/L

23. All of the following bone marrow findings may be identified in PV *except*

A. normal reticulin stain
B. increased iron stores
C. absence of dysplasia in the erythroid precursors
D. large, hyperlobulated megakaryocytes

24. All of the following are among the major criteria established by the Polycythemia Vera Study Group for diagnosis of PV *except*

A. splenomegaly
B. red cell mass >32 mL/kg (female)
C. evidence of clonality
D. normal arterial oxygen saturation (≥92%)

25. All of the following are among the proposed minor revised criteria for diagnosis of PV *except*

A. splenomegaly by isotope/ultrasound scan
B. thrombocytosis (>400 × 10^9/L)
C. spontaneous burst-forming unit erythroid (BFU-E) growth
D. increased vitamin B$_{12}$ (≥900 mg/L) or increased unsaturated vitamin B$_{12}$ binding capacity (>2200 mg/L)

26. All of the following statements regarding the progression of PV are true *except*

A. Acute leukemia develops in 10% to 20% of untreated patients.
B. Approximately 10% of the patients will develop postpolycythemic myeloid metaplasia (spent phase).
C. Blastic progression in PV is predominantly myeloid.
D. Blastic progression usually is without a previous myelodysplastic stage.

27. The following clinical findings are consistent with essential thrombocythemia (ET) *except*

A. <5% of patients with platelet count >1,000 × 10^9/L have ET.
B. Both arterial and venous thrombosis occur with equal frequency.
C. Arterial thrombosis involves mainly the cerebral vasculature.
D. Hemorrhage occurs with excessively high platelet counts.

28. All of the following are among the criteria established by the Polycythemia Vera Study Group for diagnosis of ET *except*

A. decreased iron stores in bone marrow
B. hemoglobin ≤13 g/dL

C. absent collagen fibrosis of bone marrow
D. absent Philadelphia chromosome

29. All of the following are among the B criteria in the proposed revised diagnostic criteria for ET *except*

A. normal erythrocyte sedimentation rate
B. spontaneous growth of BFU-E
C. no increase in red cell mass
D. splenomegaly on isotopic scan

30. All of the following statements regarding pathogenesis of chronic idiopathic myelofibrosis are true *except*

A. Marked myelofibrosis is secondary to stimulation of fibroblasts by cytokines produced by megakaryocytes.
B. Monoclonality of fibroblasts is detected by molecular studies.
C. Transforming growth factor-β promotes angiogenesis.
D. Transforming growth factor-β up-regulates collagen synthesis.

31. The following clinical features are characteristic of chronic idiopathic myelofibrosis *except*

A. osteosclerosis
B. mildly to moderately enlarged spleen
C. hepatomegaly
D. elderly patients

32. All of the following peripheral blood smear findings are indicative of leukoerythroblastosis *except*

A. metamyelocytes
B. nucleated red blood cells
C. teardrop red blood cells
D. myelocytes

33. All of the following bone marrow findings are characteristic of chronic idiopathic myelofibrosis *except*

A. cellular hypoplasia
B. cellular hyperplasia
C. collagen deposition
D. normal megakaryocytes

Match each of the following megakaryocytic morphologies with the most likely diagnosis.

34. Relatively within normal

35. Large, pleomorphic

36. Small, hypolobulated

37. Large, hyperlobulated

A. Chronic idiopathic myelofibrosis
B. CML
C. Essential thrombocythemia
D. PV

38. The following are among the Optional Criteria proposed by the Italian cooperative study group for diagnosis of myelofibrosis with myeloid metaplasia *except*

A. no Philadelphia chromosome
B. erythroblasts in peripheral blood
C. splenomegaly
D. abnormal megakaryocytes in bone marrow

39. All of the following criteria regarding the hypereosinophilic syndrome (HES) are true *except*

A. The heart is the most commonly involved organ.
B. Eosinophils are $>1.5 \times 10^9$/L.

C. Eosinophils are consistently polyclonal.
D. Evidence of organ/tissue damage is a prerequisite for diagnosis of HES.

40. All of the following are proposed diagnostic criteria for chronic eosinophilic leukemia *except*

A. Eosinophils are positive for chloracetate esterase.
B. Myeloblasts comprise >5%, but <30%.
C. Absent Philadelphia chromosome
D. Presence of CBFβ-MYH11 rearrangement

41. The following chromosomal aberrations may be detected in chronic eosinophilic leukemia *except*

A. isochromosome 17
B. loss of the Y chromosome
C. trisomy 8
D. t (16;16)

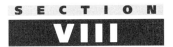

SECTION VIII

COAGULATION

46 Overview of Hemostasis
47 Laboratory Evaluation of Platelet Disorders
48 Coagulation Abnormalities
49 Thrombophilia

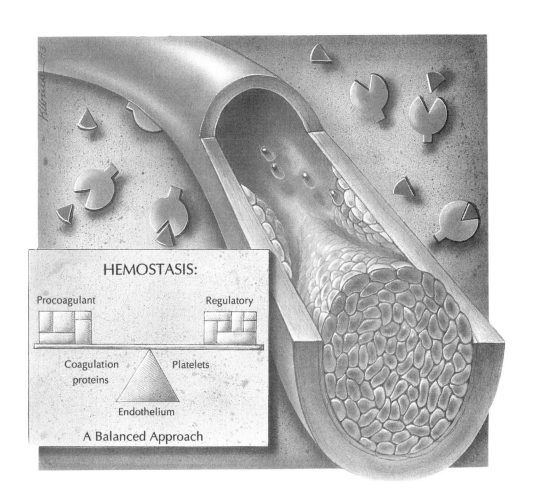

46

OVERVIEW OF HEMOSTASIS

QUESTIONS

Select the one best answer of the choices offered.

1. **All of the following statements regarding thrombo-poietin (TPO) are true** *except*
   A. The effect of TPO is mediated by interaction with cMpl receptor.
   B. TPO affects the burst-forming unit megakary-ocyte, but not the colony-forming unit megakary-ocyte.
   C. Erythropoietin modulates the effect of TPO on megakaryocyte development.
   D. Severe thrombocytopenia occurs in experimental animals in which the gene for cMpl is inactivated.

Match each of the following platelet proteins/receptors with the corresponding biologic function.

2. **Apolipoprotein E**

3. **P-selectin (CD62P)**

4. **GpIIb/IIIa (CD41/CD61)**

5. **PECAM-1 (CD31)**

6. **GpIb/IX/V (CD42b/CD42c/CD42a/CD42d)**
   A. Adhesion molecule
   B. von Willebrand factor receptor
   C. Fibrinogen receptor
   D. Stimulation of nitric oxide (NO) synthetase
   E. Mediates interaction with leukocytes

7. **All of the following are platelet α-granule proteins** *except*
   A. serotonin
   B. protein S
   C. fibrinogen
   D. vitronectin

8. **The adhesion of platelets to subendothelial structures is mediated primarily by the interaction between von Willebrand factor and GpIIb/IIIa.**
   A. True   B. False

9. **All of the following substances are promoters of platelet activation** *except*
   A. thromboxane A_2
   B. NO
   C. phosphatidylinositol-bis-phosphate
   D. inositol triphosphate

10. **Fibronectin is the major protein involved in cross-linking platelets** *in vivo.*
    A. True   B. False

11. **All of the following are characteristics of the contact system serine proteases** *except*
    A. They are not dependent on ionic calcium for activation.
    B. Molecular weight for each monomeric unit is 80 to 85 kDa.
    C. They are not absorbed by $BaSO_4$ or $Al(OH)_3$.
    D. They require vitamin K for complete synthesis.

12. **The following proteins comprise the contact system serine proteases** *except*
    A. factor XII
    B. factor XI
    C. factor X
    D. prekallikrein

13. **All of the following vitamin-K–dependent coagulation proteins possess enzymatic activity** *except*
    A. protein C
    B. prothrombin
    C. protein S
    D. factor IX

14. **Thrombin activates all of the following coagulation proteins** *except*

A. high-molecular-weight kininogen
B. fibrinogen
C. factor XIII
D. factor VIII

15. **All of the following are components of the "pro-thrombinase complex"** *except*

    A. factor Va
    B. factor Xa
    C. factor VIIIa
    D. phospholipid

16. **In the presence of tissue factor and calcium, factor VIIa activates factor IX.**

    A. True   B. False

17. **Each of the following proteins functions as a cofactor in the coagulation cascade** *except*

    A. high-molecular-weight kininogen
    B. factor XIa
    C. factor VIIIa
    D. factor Va

18. **All of the following statements regarding fibrin formation are true** *except*

    A. The fibrin gel is stabilized by factor XIIIa.
    B. The fibrin monomers polymerize in a staggered overlap.
    C. The A and B subunits of factor XIII are under separate genetic control.
    D. Thrombin activation of factor XIII is inhibited by noncross-linked fibrin.

19. **All of the following are inhibitors of platelet aggregation** *except*

    A. NO
    B. endothelial glycocalyx
    C. prostaglandin I$_2$ (prostacyclin)
    D. ADPase

20. **NO is a potent vasodilator that causes an increase in platelet cytoplasmic cyclic GMP levels.**

    A. True   B. False

21. **All of the following statements regarding NO synthetase are true** *except*

    A. The activity of constitutive NO synthetase is regulated by calcium concentration.
    B. A number of inflammatory mediators can stimulate the production of inducible NO synthetase.
    C. The constitutive NO synthetase provides a more persistent supply of NO.
    D. Platelets contain a constitutive NO synthetase that can generate low levels of NO.

Match each of the following regulators of fibrin clot formation with its specific action.

22. **Fibrinolytic system**

23. **Tissue factor pathway inhibitor**

24. **Protein C system**

25. **Serine protease inhibitors**

    A. Inhibition of factor tissue factor/factor VIIa
    B. Degradation of factors Va and VIIIa
    C. Neutralization of thrombin and factor Xa
    D. Degradation of fibrin

Match each of the following components of the protein C system with its biologic function.

26. **Factor V**

27. **Thrombomodulin**

28. **Thrombin**

29. **Protein S**

    A. Cofactor for thrombin activation of protein C
    B. Cofactor for degradation of factor VIIIa by activated protein C
    C. Cofactor for protein C
    D. Activates protein C

Match each of the components of the fibrinolytic system with its biologic function.

30. **Kallikrein**

31. **Plasminogen activator inhibitor-1**

32. **Annexin II**

33. **Fibrin**

    A. Cell surface receptor for plasminogen and tissue plasminogen activator (tPA)
    B. Inhibition of tPA, urokinase, and activate protein C
    C. Cofactor for activation of plasminogen by tPA
    D. Conversion of prourokinase to urokinase

34. **All of the following statements regarding bleeding disorders are true** *except*

    A. Mucocutaneous bleeding is suggestive of a platelet disorder.
    B. Routine coagulation screening tests include platelet count, bleeding time, prothrombin time (PT), and activated partial thromboplastin time (APTT).
    C. Screening tests usually are normal in bleeding disorders due to fibrinolytic abnormalities.
    D. Hemophilia A is the most common congenital bleeding disorder.

47

LABORATORY EVALUATION OF PLATELET DISORDERS

QUESTIONS

Select the one best answer of the choices offered.

1. **All of the following statements regarding the bleeding time (BT) are true except**

   A. BT may be normal in patients with significant mucocutaneous bleeding.
   B. The template BT is the most commonly performed method.
   C. BT is a useful, routine preoperative screening procedure.
   D. BT usually is prolonged in thrombocytopenia.

2. **All of the following statements regarding platelet aggregation studies are true *except***

   A. Normal platelets tend to aggregate to ristocetin (1.0 mg/mL) in a monophasic pattern.
   B. Adenosine diphosphate and epinephrine induce a biphasic wave of platelet aggregation.
   C. Platelets from patients with platelet-type von Willebrand disease (vWD) and type 2B vWD aggregate to ristocetin at a higher concentration >1.0 mg/mL.
   D. Thrombin is not commonly used as a platelet agonist in the clinical laboratory.

3. **vWD is the most common congenital bleeding disorder known.**

   A. True   B. False

4. **All of the following statements regarding vWD are true *except***

   A. The clinical manifestations of type 3 vWD may mimic those of hemophilia A.
   B. vWD typically is inherited as an autosomal dominant trait.
   C. von Willebrand factor (vWF) is an obligate carrier of factor VIII in plasma.
   D. vWF is a mediator of platelet aggregation.

Match each of the following defects with the corresponding vWD disease subtype.

5. **Absence of high-molecular-weight multimers of vWF**

6. **Moderate quantitative deficiency of vWF**

7. **Abnormal GpIb/IX/V**

8. **Mild deficiency of high-molecular-weight multimers of vWF**

   A. Type 2A vWD
   B. Platelet-type vWD
   C. Type 1 vWD
   D. Type 2B vWD

9. **All of the following are consistent with Bernard-Soulier syndrome *except***

   A. giant platelets
   B. functional abnormality of the GpIb/IX/V complex
   C. autosomal recessive mode of inheritance
   D. decreased concentration of the high-molecular-weight multimers of vWF

10. **All of the following statements regarding disorders of platelet activation are true *except***

    A. Platelet aggregation with ADP and epinephrine shows a primary wave defect.
    B. Storage pool disorders result from abnormalities of platelet α-granules and dense granules.
    C. Normal platelet response to ristocetin is detected.
    D. Response to arachidonic acid may be delayed.

11. **All of the following findings are consistent with Glanzmann thrombasthenia *except***

    A. diminished clot retraction
    B. abnormal GpIIb/IIIa complex
    C. increased fibrinogen in platelets α-granules
    D. lack of platelet aggregation with normal fibrinogen levels

12. **Platelet aggregation studies have a major role in evaluating patients with acquired platelet dysfunction.**

    A. True   B. False

13. **All of the following are possible therapeutic options for managing clinical bleeding in patients with uremia *except***

    A. cryoprecipitate
    B. correction of anemia
    C. factor VIII
    D. conjugated estrogens

14. **Measurement of platelet-associated IgG is a useful tool in the routine evaluation of adult patients with idiopathic thrombocytopenic purpura (ITP).**

    A. True   B. False

Match each of the following parameters with the corresponding type of autoimmune thrombocytopenia (each answer may be used more than once).

15. **Other autoimmune disorders often are present.**

16. **F = M**

17. **Most frequent in childhood**

18. **Frequent clinical remissions**

19. **F > M**

    A. Acute ITP
    B. Chronic ITP

20. **Changes in BT are not diagnostic for ITP nor predictive of the clinical manifestations of the disorder.**

    A. True   B. False

21. **Alloimmune thrombocytopenia usually occurs in patients with PLA2 (HPA-1b) phenotype who receive blood products from PLA1 (HPA-1a)-positive donors.**

    A. True   B. False

Match each of the following drugs with the corresponding mechanism for immunologic destruction of platelets.

22. **Quinidine**

23. **Penicillin**

24. **Heparin**

    A. Immune–complex interaction with the Fc receptor on the platelet surface
    B. Drug binds to and alters platelet surface glycoproteins (GpIb/IX/V)
    C. Drug serves as a hapten that binds to the platelet surface (FcγRIIa)

Match each of the following with the corresponding disease (each answer may be used more than once).

25. **Congenital or acquired loss of protease function**

26. ***Escherichia coli* (O157:H7)**

27. **Presence of abnormally large vWF multimers**

28. **Neurologic symptoms**

29. **Microvascular endothelial cell injury**

30. **Giant platelets**

    A. Thrombotic thrombocytopenic purpura
    B. Hemolytic uremic syndrome
    C. Both

48

COAGULATION ABNORMALITIES

QUESTIONS

Select the one best answer of the choices offered.

1. **All of the following statements regarding hemophilia A are true *except***

   A. Factor VIII gene comprises approximately 0.1% of the X chromosome.
   B. Both deletions and point mutations have been detected in patients with hemophilia A.
   C. A significant number of cases of hemophilia A occur due to *de novo* mutations.
   D. Patients with severe hemophilia A have factor VIIIc levels between 2% to 15%.

2. **All of the following statements regarding hemophilia A are true *except***

   A. The treatment of choice in mild/moderate hemophilia A is 1-deamino-8-D-arginine vasopressin (DDAVP).
   B. One unit of recombinant factor VIII per kilogram of body weight will raise factor VIII levels approximately 0.2%.
   C. Porcine factor VIII has been used successfully to treat patients with factor VIIIc inhibitors.
   D. Prothrombin complex concentrates (factors II, VII, IX, and X) have been used successfully to treat acute hemorrhage in patients with factor VIIIc inhibitors.

3. **Prothrombin complex concentrates (II, VII, IX, and X) are considered the treatment of choice for patients with hemophilia B (Christmas disease).**

   A. True   B. False

4. **All of the following statements regarding hemophilia C are true *except***

   A. The gene for factor XI is located on the distal end of the long arm of chromosome 4.
   B. Homozygous patients have factor XI activity <20%.

   C. The major physiologic substrate for factor XIa is factor X.
   D. Heterozygous patients typically have a negative bleeding history.

5. **All of the following statements regarding factor VII deficiency are true *except***

   A. Heterozygous patients present with a spectrum of clinical bleeding.
   B. Thromboembolic episodes have been reported in patients with factor VII deficiency.
   C. Factor VII deficiency is inherited in an autosomal recessive manner.
   D. Factor VII can be activated by thrombin and factors IXa, Xa, and XIIa.

6. **All of the following statements regarding factor X deficiency are true *except***

   A. Systemic amyloidosis is an important differential diagnostic consideration.
   B. The Russell viper venom time is normal in factor X deficiency.
   C. Hereditary factor X deficiency is an autosomal recessive disorder.
   D. Fresh frozen plasma is an effective therapeutic regimen.

7. **Deficiencies of the following coagulation factors may be associated with clinical bleeding *except***

   A. factor XIII
   B. factor V
   C. factor II
   D. factor XII

8. **All of the following statements regarding heparin are true *except***

   A. Heparin requires antithrombin in order to express its anticoagulant activities.
   B. Unfractionated heparin is a much powerful platelet aggregator compared with low-molecular-weight heparin.

C. Subcutaneous administration is the preferred mode of heparin administration.

D. >95% of the laboratories use activated partial thromboplastin time (APTT) as a means of monitoring heparin.

9. **All of the following statements regarding heparin-associated thrombocytopenia (HAT) are true *except***

A. Type I HAT is associated with antibodies directed against a complex of heparin and platelet factor 4 (H-PF4).

B. Type II HAT can be seen in situations where the patient is only minimally exposed to heparin.

C. In type I HAT, platelet count usually returns to the original baseline value prior to the initiation of heparin therapy.

D. Low-molecular-weight heparin might induce HAT.

10. **All of the following statements regarding laboratory monitoring of oral anticoagulant therapy are true *except***

A. The majority of patients are satisfactorily anticoagulated with international normalized ratios (INRs) of 2.0 to 3.0.

B. Oral anticoagulants block the reductase enzyme in the vitamin K pathway, which increases the level of protein induced by vitamin K antagonist (PIVKA).

C. The introduction of INR had emphasized the need for higher doses of oral anticoagulants.

D. The INR expresses the ratio of the patient's prothrombin time (PT) to the mean of the normal range raised to the power of international sensitivity index

11. **All of the following statements regarding the lupus anticoagulant (LA) are true *except***

A. LA interferes with one or more of the *in vitro* phospholipid-dependent tests of coagulation.

B. LA often is associated with an increased risk of thrombosis.

C. The presence or absence of time dependency is not a useful differential diagnostic point to separate factor VIIIc inhibitors from LA.

D. In the platelet neutralization procudure (PNP) test, a significant prolongation of the APTT baseline value is positive for the presence of LA.

Match each of the following findings with the corresponding type of disseminated intravascular coagulation (DIC) (each answer may be used more than once).

12. **Prolonged APTT, PT, and thrombin time (TT)**

13. **Bleeding**

14. **Increased fibrin/fibrinogen degradation products**

15. **Decreased antithrombin**

16. **Thrombosis**

A. Acute DIC
B. Chronic DIC
C. Both

17. **The presence of any of the following will lead to an increase in TT *except***

A. paraproteins
B. heparin
C. warfarin (Coumadin)
D. dysfibrinogenemia

49

THROMBOPHILIA

QUESTIONS

Select the one best answer of the choices offered.

1. **All of the following statements regarding anti-thrombin (AT) deficiency are true** *except*

   A. Type II AT deficiency results in reduced synthesis of a biologically normal protein.
   B. AT deficiency is inherited as an autosomal dominant abnormality.
   C. Most thromboembolic events are venous.
   D. AT-deficient patients have levels of 40% to 50% of normal.

2. **All of the following statements regarding protein C are true** *except*

   A. Protein S is a cofactor for activated protein C.
   B. Activated protein C, in the presence of protein S, inactivates factors Va and Xa.
   C. The gene for protein C is found on chromosome 2.
   D. Activated protein C is inhibited by protein C inhibitor and α_1-antitrypsin.

3. **All of the following statements regarding protein C deficiency are true** *except*

   A. Most thromboembolic events are venous.
   B. Heterozygous protein C deficiency is associated with purpura fulminans.
   C. In type II protein C deficiency, the antigenic level of protein C deficiency is within normal limits.
   D. Patients with heterozygous protein C deficiency typically have a protein C level of 40% to 50% of normal.

4. **All of the following statements regarding protein S deficiency are true** *except*

   A. Acquired deficiencies of protein S have been described in patients with lupus anticoagulant.
   B. Type II protein S-deficient patients have decreased amounts of both free and bound protein S.
   C. Plasma levels of protein S decrease in patients with vitamin K deficiency.
   D. Bound protein C comprises approximately 40% of the plasma compartment.

Match each of the following anticoagulation proteins with the corresponding target (each answer may be used more than once).

5. **Protein S**

6. **Antithrombin**

7. **Heparin cofactor II**

8. **Protein C**

   A. Factor X
   B. Factor VIIIa
   C. None of the above

9. **All of the following statements regarding activated protein C resistance/factor V Leiden are true** *except*

   A. Factor V Leiden is found in approximately 5% of patients who present with an initial deep vein thrombosis.
   B. The Invader Technology is quicker and costs less than polymerase chain reaction (PCR) for molecular identification of factor V Leiden.
   C. Carriers of factor V Leiden without a history of thrombosis have an absolute risk of thrombosis of approximately 0.45% per year.
   D. There is a decreased ability to down-regulate factor Va by activated protein C.

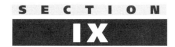

SECTION IX

MICROBIOLOGY

50 Specimen Collection and Processing for Microbiology

51 Bacteriology

52 Fungi and Fungal Infections

53 *Chlamydia*, *Mycoplasma*, and *Rickettsia*

54 Aerobic Actinomycetes

55 Antimicrobial Susceptibility Testing

56 Molecular Techniques for Diagnosis of Infectious Diseases

57 Role of the Clinical Microbiology Laboratory in Hospital Epidemiology and Infection Control

58 Autopsy Microbiology

59 Diagnostic Virology

60 Parasitology

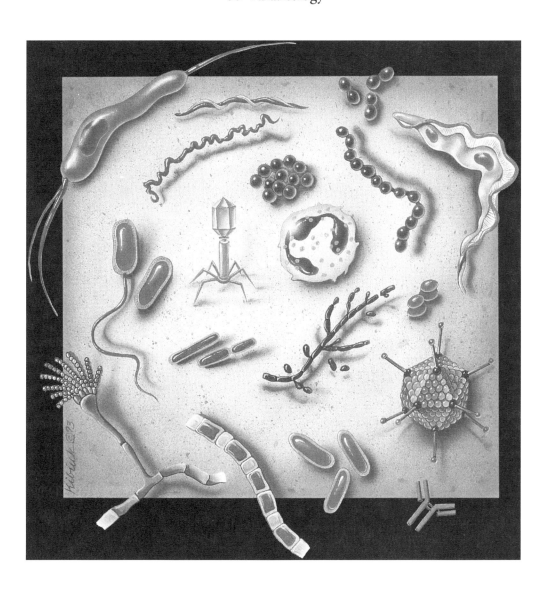

SPECIMEN COLLECTION AND PROCESSING FOR MICROBIOLOGY

QUESTIONS

Select the one best answer of the choices offered.

1. **For delays in transport, most microbiologic specimens should be refrigerated** *except*

   A. blood
   B. cerebrospinal fluid
   C. anaerobic specimens
   D. all of the above
   E. none of the above

2. **Specimens not routinely accepted for anaerobic culture are**

   A. sputa
   B. catheterized urine
   C. bowel contents
   D. A, B, and C
   E. A and C

3. **The temperature of incubation usually is 35°C for bacteria and viruses and 30°C for fungi.**

   A. True   B.   False

4. **No more than four blood culture sets should be submitted in a 24-hour period.**

   A. True   B. False

5. **The optimal time to collect a blood sample for *Loa loa* extremities is**

   A. any time
   B. noon
   C. midnight

6. **With a duration of symptoms of <25 hours, the probable infection causing meningitis is**

   A. *Brucella* sp
   B. *Candida* sp
   C. pyogenic bacteria
   D. *Coccidioides immitis*

7. **Anaerobic culture is not routinely performed on cerebrospinal fluid specimens.**

   A. True   B. False

8. **The VDRL (Venereal Disease Research Laboratory test) is the only useful test for detecting syphilis antibodies in CSF.**

   A. True   B. False

9. **Otitis media most often is caused by organisms derived from the respiratory flora.**

   A. True   B. False

10. **Feces optimally should be examined within 2 hours of collection.**

    A. True   B. False

11. **The reference method for detection of cytotoxin, such as the one produced by *Clostridium difficile*, is cell culture assay.**

    A. True   B. False

12. **Fungal culture of stool is not recommended.**

    A. True   B. False

13. **Organisms such as are always pathogenic in genital tract specimens.**

    A. *Chlamydia trachomatis*
    B. Group B streptococci
    C. *Haemophilus ducreyi*
    D. A and C
    E. A, B, and C

14. **Cultures for *Actinomyces* sp should be incubated anaerobically for 14 days.**

    A. True   B. False

15. *Trichomonas vaginalis* most often is detected by examination of a wet mount examination of vaginal or urethral discharge, prostatic secretions, or urine sediment.

    A. True   B. False

16. >10 squamous epithelial cells in a respiratory specimen is contaminated with saliva.

    A. True   B. False

17. **Legionellosis can be diagnosed by**

    A. culture
    B. detection of antigens in the urine
    C. serologic testing
    D. A and C
    E. A, B, and C

18. *Burkholderia cepacia* is an important respiratory pathogen in persons with cystic fibrosis.

    A. True   B. False

19. **No culture methods are available for** *Pneumocystis carinii*.

    A. True   B. False

20. **Vincent angina is an acute necrotizing ulcerative tonsillitis.**

    A. True   B. False

21. **Acceptable methods of urine collection include**

    A. midstream clean catch
    B. catheterization
    C. Foley catheter tip
    D. A and B
    E. A, B, and C

22. **Most commonly isolated viruses from urine are**

    A. cytomegalovirus (CMV)
    B. herpes simplex virus (HSV)
    C. adenovirus
    D. A and B
    E. A, B, and C

51

BACTERIOLOGY

QUESTIONS

Select the one best answer of the choices offered.

1. **The most frequently isolated species of staphylococci are**

    A. *Staphylococcus aureus*
    B. *Staphylococcus epidermidis*
    C. *Staphylococcus saprophyticus*
    D. A and B
    E. A, B, and C

2. **The most common toxin-induced disease associated with *S. aureus* is**

    A. scalded skin syndrome
    B. gastroenteritis
    C. toxic shock syndrome
    D. pustule

3. ***S. aureus, S. epidermidis,* and *S. saprophyticus* are associated with the majority of staphylococcal infections.**

    A. True   B. False

4. ***S. epidermidis* causes nosocomial infections, especially in patients with indwelling foreign bodies.**

    A. True   B. False

5. ***S. saprophyticus* causes urinary tract infections in young women.**

    A. True   B. False

6. **The genus *Abiotrophia* includes**

    A. Streptococcus mitis
    B. Streptococcus crista
    C. Streptococcus sanguis
    D. A and C
    E. A, B, and C

7. **Streptococci and enterococci are facultative anaerobes. (Figure 51.2)**

    A. True   B. False

8. **β-Hemolytic streptococci do not require routine susceptibility testing because they remain routinely susceptible to**

    A. erythromycin
    B. penicillin
    C. vancomycin
    D. B and C
    E. A, B, and C

9. **Pelvic inflammatory disease caused by preexisting gonococcal cervicitis occurs in up to ____% of women with gonorrhea. (Figure 51.4)**

    A. 5
    B. 10
    C. 20
    D. 30
    E. 40

10. **Humans are the only natural host for *Neisseria meningitidis*.**

    A. True   B. False

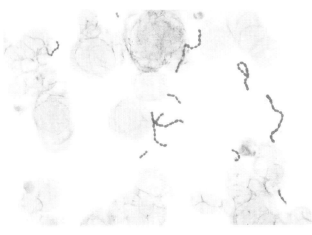

FIGURE 51.2.

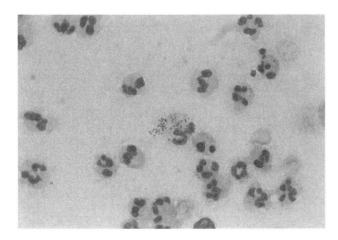

FIGURE 51.4.

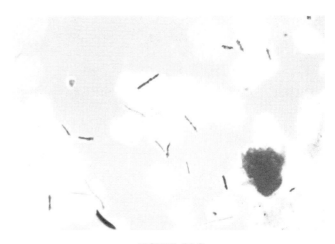

FIGURE 51.6.

11. The sensitivity of the Gram stain relative to culture for the detection of gonococci in urethral cultures from symptomatic men is
    A. 20% to 40%
    B. 30% to 50%
    C. 50% to 70%
    D. 70% to 90%
    E. 95% to 100%

12. *Neisseria gonorrhoeae* grows on selective media and produces acid from glucose and maltose.
    A. True   B. False

13. Approximately ____% of strains of *Branhamelllla catarrhalis* produce β-lactamase.
    A. 20
    B. 40
    C. 65
    D. 85
    E. 95

14. The most important pathogen(s) in the genus *Bacillus* are (Figure 51.6)
    A. *B. virgi*
    B. *B. cereus*
    C. *B. anthracis*
    D. B and C
    E. A and C

15. The genus *Erysipelothrix* contains the species
    A. rhusiopathiae
    B. haemolyticum
    C. tonsillarum
    D. A and C
    E. A, B, and C

16. Anthrax occurs worldwide and is primarily a disease of herbivores.
    A. True   B. False

17. *Yersinia pestis* may have a "safety pin" appearance on Gram stain.
    A. True   B. False

18. The Widal test is used to help diagnose *Salmonella typhi*.
    A. True   B. False

19. *Aeromonas* causes infections in humans, including
    A. diarrhea
    B. bacteremia
    C. cellulitis
    D. A and B
    E. A, B, and C

20. *Vibrio* species have characteristics such as
    A. Gram positive
    B. curved rod
    C. oxidase position
    D. B and C
    E. A, B, and C

21. The primary treatment for epidemic cholera is fluid replacement.
    A. True   B. False

22. *Helicobacter pylori* has not been recovered from the environment.
    A. True   B. False

23. Categories of *Legionella* infections include
A. nonpneumonic
B. extrapulmonary
C. subclinical
D. A and B
E. A, B, and C

24. The drug of choice for treatment of *Legionella* infections is
A. penicillin
B. tetracycline
C. fluoroquinolone
D. ampicillin

25. *Haemophilus* species are
A. facilitative anaerobic
B. nonmotile
C. pleomorphic
D. A and B
E. A, B, and C

26. Most Gram-negative nonfermentative bacilli are strict anaerobes.
A. True   B. False

27. Nonfermentative bacilli comprise approximately ____% of all Gram-negative rods isolated in the clinical laboratory.
A. 1 to 3
B. 5 to 10
C. 15 to 20
D. 30 to 40

28. Melioidosis, a rare infection in North America, is caused by *Acinetobacter*.
A. True   B. False

29. *Pseudomonas aeruginosa* is characterized in the laboratory by
A. a grape-like order
B. β-hemolysis
C. a variety of pigments
D. A and B
E. A, B, and C

30. *Moraxella* is part of the normal flora of the mucous membranes in humans.
A. True   B. False

31. Facultative anaerobic Gram-negative bacilli include
A. *Gardnerella*
B. *Pseudomonas*
C. *Pasteurella*
D. A and C
E. A, B, and C

32. *Pasteurella multocida* can cause
A. localized infection after an animal bite
B. chronic pulmonary disease
C. gingivitis
D. A and B
E. A, B, and C

33. Organism(s) that upon isolation can be highly suspicious of endocarditis is(are)
A. *Haemophilus*
B. *Actinobacillus*
C. *Eikenella*
D. A and B
E. A, B, and C

34. *Actinobacillus* is generally susceptible to
A. streptomycin
B. choramphenicol
C. erythromycin
D. A and B
E. A, B, and C

35. Brucellosis is primarily a genitourinary tract infection in animals.
A. True   B. False

36. Humans are the only known reservoir for *Bordetella pertussis*.
A. True   B. False

37. Medically important Gram-negative cocci include
A. *Prevotella*
B. *Veillonella*
C. *Peptostreptococcus*
D. A and C
E. A, B, and C (see Table 51.27)

38. *Clostridium perfringens* is a Gram-positive rod with square ends and usually does not contain a spore. (Figure 51.17)
A. True   B. False

39. The family Leptospiraceae contains the genera
A. *Leptospira*
B. *Borrelia*
C. *Leptonema*
D. A and C
E. B and C

40. Relapsing fever is transmitted to humans by infected soft-shelled ticks of the genus *Ixodes*.
A. True   B. False

TABLE 51.27. RECENT TAXONOMIC CHANGES OF ANAEROBIC BACTERIA

Current Nomenclature	Previous Nomenclature
Bacteroides distasonis	*Porphyromonas*
Bacteroides furcosus	*Porphyromonas*
Bacteroides putredinis	*Rikenella*
Campylobacter gracilis	*Bacteroides gracilis*
Campylobacter showae	*New species*
Campylobacter cuvus	*Wolinella cuvus*
Campylobacter rectus	*Wolinella rectus*
Dialister pneumosintes	*Bacteroides pneumosintes*
Johnsonella ignava	*Clostridium*
Porphyromonas catoniae	*Oribaculum catoniae*
Prevotella dentalis	*Mitsuokella dentalis*
Prevotella enoeca	New species
Prevotella pallens	New species
Prevotella tonnerae	New species
Sutterella wadsworthensis	New genus and species

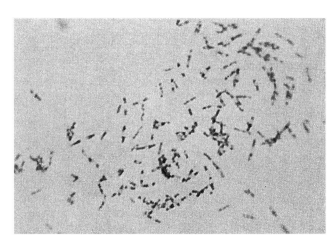

FIGURE 51.17.

41. The nontreponemal test becomes nonreactive in primary syphilis _____ years after therapy.

    A. 0.25
    B. 0.50
    C. 0.75
    D. 1.0

42. Pathogenic spirochetes belong to the genera

    A. *Treponema*
    B. *Borrelia*
    C. *Leptospira*
    D. A and B
    E. A, B, and C

52

FUNGI AND FUNGAL INFECTIONS

QUESTIONS

Select the one best answer of the choices offered.

1. **Fungi are eukaryotic organisms.**

   A. True   B. False

2. **Fungi have cell walls containing complex**

   A. glucans
   B. mannans
   C. decans
   D. A and B
   E. A, B, and C

3. **The main growth forms of fungi include**

   A. yeast
   B. mold
   C. trichophyte
   D. A and B
   E. A, B, and C

4. **Systemic mycoses include**

   A. *Histoplasma capsulatum*
   B. *Microsporum*
   C. *Penicillium marneffei*
   D. A and C
   E. A, B, and C

5. ***Coccidiodes immitis* is endemic only to**

   A. Ohio river valley
   B. Mississippi river valley
   C. southeastern United States
   D. lower Sonoran life zone regions

6. ***Tinea cruris* is an infection of the**

   A. scalp
   B. trunk
   C. feet
   D. groin

7. ***Microsporium* is identified by observation if its microconidia.**

   A. True   B. False

8. **The most common subcutaneous mycosis(es) is(are)**

   A. lymphocutaneous sporotrichosis
   B. chromoblastomycosis
   C. eumycotic mycetoma
   D. A and B
   E. A, B, and C

9. **Medlar bodies are associated with (see Figure 52.7)**

   A. sporotrichosis
   B. chromoblastomycosis
   C. mycetoma
   D. tenia

10. **Dimorphic endemic fungal pathogens include**

    A. *H. capsulatum*
    B. *C. immitis*
    C. *Penicillium marneffei*
    D. A and B
    E. A, B, and C

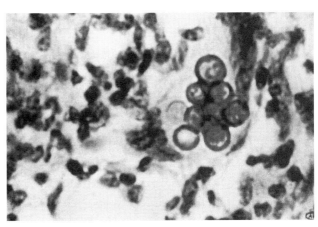

FIGURE 52.7.

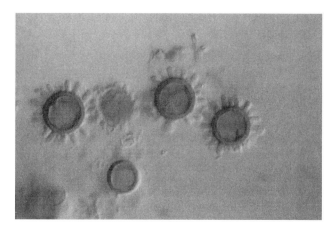

FIGURE 52.9.

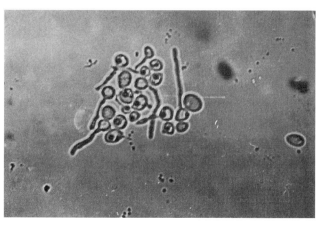

FIGURE 52.15.

11. The tissue phase of *H. capsulatum* is a small budding yeast cell ____ mm in diameter. (See Figure 52.9.)

   A. 1 to 2
   B. 3 to 4
   C. 2 to 5
   D. 5 to 7
   E. 7 to 9

12. Coccidioidomycosis also is called

   A. valley bumps
   B. desert rheumatism
   C. Posadas disease
   D. A and B
   E. A, B, and C

13. The budding yeast cells in the form of a "mariner's wheel" is typical of

   A. histoplasmosis
   B. coccidioidomycosis
   C. paracoccidioidomycosis
   D. A and B
   E. A, B, and C

14. The most well-known cause(s) of opportunistic mycosis(es) is(are)

   A. *Candida*
   B. *Cryptococcus neoformans*
   C. *Aspergillus* sp
   D. A and B
   E. A, B, and C

15. *Candida parapsilosis* has become an important cause of nosocomial infections.

   A. True   B. False

16. Germ tube production is noted with (see Figure 52.15)

   A. *Candida albicans*
   B. *Candida dubliniensis*
   C. *Candida stellatoidea*
   D. A and B
   E. A, B, and C

17. Tinea versicolor is caused by *Malassezia furfur*.

   A. True   B. False

18. Rhinocerebral zygomycosis is caused primarily by *Rhizopus arrhizus*. (See Figure 52.19.)

   A. True   B. False

19. *Alternaria* species are important causes of paranasal sinusitis.

   A. True   B. False

20. *Pneumocystis carinii* now is considered to be a fungus based on molecular/genetic evidence.

   A. True   B. False

21. The hallmark of *P. carinii* infection is

   A. lobar pneumonia
   B. interstitial pneumonia
   C. lobular pneumonia
   D. A and C
   E. A, B, and C

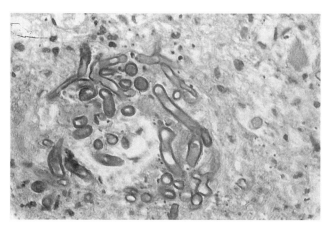

FIGURE 52.19.

53

CHLAMYDIA, MYCOPLASMA, AND RICKETTSIA

QUESTIONS

Select the one best answer of the choices offered.

1. *Chlamydia trachomatis* is reportedly the most common sexually transmitted disease in developed countries.
   A. True   B. False

2. **Trachoma represents the single greatest cause of blindness in the world.**
   A. True   B. False

3. **In women, *C. trachomatis* causes**
   A. mucopurulent cervicitis
   B. proctitis
   C. vaginitis
   D. A and B
   E. A, B, and C

4. **Horder spots, a maculopapular rash, is associated with *Chlamydia psittaci*. (See Figure 53.1.)**
   A. True   B. False

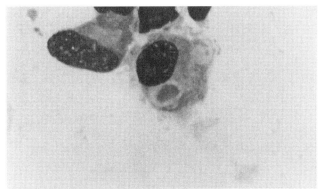

FIGURE 53.1.

5. **The tetracyclines are extremely effective agents for treatment of psittacosis.**
   A. True   B. False

6. **Mycoplasmas are members of the class Mollicutes.**
   A. True   B. False

7. **The most common clinical syndrome resulting from *Mycoplasma pneumonia* is**
   A. tracheobronchitis
   B. interstitial pneumonia
   C. pleuritis
   D. laryngitis

8. **Illness caused by *M. pneumonia* may be complicated by**
   A. urticaria
   B. erythema nodosum
   C. erythema multiforme
   D. A and B
   E. A, B, and C

9. **During the summer months, *M. pneumonia* may cause up to ____% of all pneumonias.**
   A. 10
   B. 20
   C. 30
   D. 50
   E. 70

10. **M. pneumonia* is the most common cause of pneumonia in children 5 to 15 years of age.**
    A. True   B. False

11. **Mycoplasma hominis* is recovered more often from the**
    A. cervix
    B. vagina
    C. endometrium
    D. anus

12. **Genera now considered to include human pathogens in the family Rickettsiaceae are**
    A. *Orientia*
    B. *Ehrlichia*
    C. *Bartonellaceae*
    D. A and B
    E. A, B, and C

13. **Rickettsiae are transmitted among mammalian reservoirs by arthropod vectors. (See Figure 53.4.)**
    A. True   B. False

14. ***Rickettsia typhi* is transmitted by fleas.**
    A. True   B. False

15. **Epidemic typhus is caused by**
    A. *Rickettsia felis*
    B. *Rickettsia prowazekii*
    C. *Rickettsia typhi*
    D. *Rickettsia rickettsiae*

16. ***Orientia tsutsugamushi* causes scrub typhus.**
    A. True   B. False

17. **Q fever is caused by**
    A. *Ehrlichia chaffeensis*
    B. *Ehrlichia morulae*
    C. *Coxiella burnetii*
    D. *Ehrlichia phagocytophila*

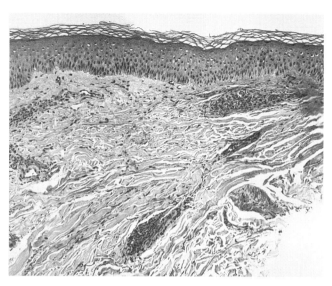

FIGURE 53.4.

18. **The genus *Bartonella* contains the species**
    A. *quintana*
    B. *henselae*
    C. *verruga*
    D. A and B
    E. A, B, and C

19. **Cat scratch disease results from infection with**
    A. *Bartonella henselae*
    B. *Bartonella bacilliformis*
    C. *Bartonella quintana*
    D. *Bartonella verruga*

54

AEROBIC ACTINOMYCETES

QUESTIONS

Select the one best answer of the choices offered.

1. **Mycolic acids are present in the cell walls of all of the following genera** *except*

   A. *Myocobacterium*
   B. *Oerskovia*
   C. *Corynebacterium*
   D. *Nocardia*

2. **All of the following genera may exhibit some acid fastness** *except*

   A. *Myocobacterium*
   B. *Rhodococcus*
   C. *Nocardia*
   D. *Streptomyces*

3. **The characteristics of *Mycobacterium* include all of the following** *except*

   A. acid fastness
   B. long mycolic acid chains
   C. inability to grow on laboratory media
   D. variable growth rate between species

4. **Yellow to orange pigment development after exposure of the organism to light is seen with which Runyon group?**

   A. Group I (photochromogen)
   B. Group II (scotochromogen)
   C. Group III (nonphotochromogen)
   D. Group IV (rapid grower)

5. **Which *Mycobacterium* produces visible colonies on solid agar within 7 days?**

   A. *M. tuberculosis*
   B. *M. xenopi*
   C. *M. bovis*
   D. *M. chelonae*

6. **An individual was cleaning her aquarium when she accidentally received an abrasion. A granulomatous lesion developed at the site of injury; it ulcerated and eventually healed. The most likely causative agent of the lesion is**

   A. *M. tuberculosis*
   B. *M. avium*
   C. *M. ulcerans*
   D. *M. marinum*

7. **Which *Mycobacterium* has an association with prosthetic valve endocarditis?**

   A. *M. ulcerans*
   B. *M. gordonae*
   C. *M. fortuitum*
   D. *M. kansasii*

8. **The best respiratory tract specimen for culture from a patient with strong clinical indication of tuberculosis infection is**

   A. early morning
   B. afternoon
   C. evening
   D. before bedtime

9. **Genetic probes are specific for the identification of all of the following *Mycobacterium except***

   A. *M. avium*
   B. *M. gordonae*
   C. *M. bovis*
   D. *M. kansasii*

10. **Mycobacteria have a high ____ content that is responsible for "acid fast" characteristics.**

   A. chitin
   B. lipid
   C. amino acid
   D. polysaccharide

11. **All of the following stains are used to visualize mycobacteria** *except*

    A. Ziehl-Neelsen
    B. Gram
    C. Kinyoun
    D. auramine O fluorochrome

12. **A long delicate, branched beaded Gram-positive filamentous organism was isolated from an immunocompromised patient. The organism is most characteristic of**

    A. *Nocardia*
    B. *Mycobacterium*
    C. *Staphylococcus aureus*
    D. *Pseudomonas aeruginosa*

13. **Which *Rhodococcus* species has been associated with clinical opportunistic infections?**

    A. *R. equi*
    B. *R. ruber*
    C. *R. fascians*
    D. *R. rhodnii*

14. **Which actinomycetes characteristically are mucoid, clear white, and turns salmon-pink, red within 2 to 5 days?**

    A. *M. tuberculosis*
    B. *Nocardia*
    C. *M. gordonae*
    D. *Rhodococcus*

15. **Which of the following organisms listed below demonstrates orange, tiny, pitting colonies and cause a self-limited pustular desquamatous keratitis of the hands and forearms?**

    A. *Actinomadura*
    B. *Nocardiopsis*
    C. *Streptomyces*
    D. *Dermatophilus*

Indicate whether each of the following statements is true (T) or false (F).

16. **All personnel working in the laboratory with a low risk of exposure to *M. tuberculosis* should be given a tuberculin skin test annually.**

17. **A 24-hour pooled respiratory tract collection is acceptable because of the increase amount of organisms obtained.**

18. **Kinyoun acid-fast stain does not require constant heating and is easier to perform compared to Ziehl-Neelsen acid-fast stain.**

19. **Acid-fast stained smears with carbolfuchsin requires scanning at least 30 fields at high magnification.**

20. ***Streptomyces annulatus* and *Streptomyces somaliensis* are the only common species associated with human disease.**

55

ANTIMICROBIAL SUSCEPTIBILITY TESTING

QUESTIONS

Select the one best answer of the choices offered.

1. **All of the following are responsibilities of laboratories performing antimicrobial susceptibility testing** *except*
   A. select the isolate to be tested
   B. use standardized procedures whenever possible
   C. prescribe which antimicrobials to use
   D. accurately report results

2. **All of the following are frequently used** *in vitro* **susceptibility tests** *except*
   A. disk diffusion
   B. broth microdeletion
   C. broth macrodeletion
   D. agar dilution

3. **Minimum inhibitory concentration (MIC) is defined as**
   A. the lowest concentration of antimicrobial agent (in μg/mL) that inhibits the growth of a bacterium
   B. the lowest concentration of antimicrobial agent (in μg/mL) that kills a bacterium
   C. the lowest therapeutic concentration of antimicrobial agent that inhibits a bacterium
   D. the lowest concentration of antibiotic that produces a zone of inhibition

4. **The concentration of calcium and magnesium ions contained in Mueller-Hinton medium is important when testing the activity of aminoglycosides against**
   A. *Escherchia coli*
   B. *Pseudomonas aeruginosa*
   C. *Staphylococcus aureus*
   D. *Serratia marcescens*

5. **To enhance the expression of resistance to oxacillin in staphylococci, the cation-adjusted Mueller-Hinton broth must contain**
   A. 0.1% serum
   B. 10 to 12 mg/L Zn
   C. 2.0% NaCl
   D. hemin

6. **All of the following statements regarding susceptibility testing are true** *except*
   A. Portions of four to five similar colonies are used to prepare the inoculum.
   B. Tests for oxacillin resistance in staphylococci should be incubated 24 hours.
   C. Inoculated tests are incubated 18 to 24 hours in room air incubator.
   D. Turbidity of the inoculum should be adjusted to a 1.0 McFarland standard.

7. **The disk diffusion method is approved only for**
   A. anaerobes
   B. all microorganisms
   C. rapidly growing organisms
   D. slowly and rapidly growing organisms

8. **All of the following statements regarding the disk diffusion test are true** *except*
   A. The depth of agar should be 4 mm.
   B. The zone of inhibition produced measures the bactericidal activity of the antimicrobic.
   C. Blood-supplemented plates may be used to test fastidious bacteria.
   D. The zone of inhibition diameter is inversely proportional to MIC.

9. **All of the following statements regarding the E-test are true** *except*
   A. It is an agar diffusion test that provides an MIC result.
   B. It compares favorably with the broth dilution test.
   C. It uses a plastic strip that has a continuous gradient of antimicrobic immobilized on one side.
   D. It can be used only for testing fastidious organisms.

10. **All of the following methods are used to detect the presence of β-lactamase** *except*
    A. iodometric
    B. chromogenic cephalosporin
    C. acetyltransferase
    D. acidimetric

11. Which of the following organisms usually is tested for β-lactamase production?

A. *S. aureus*
B. *Haemophilus influenzae*
C. *Neisseria gonorrhoeae*
D. *Moraxella* catarrhalis

12. Minimum bactericidal concentration (MBC) is defined as the lowest concentration of antimicrobic that kills at least _____ of the original inoculum.

A. 90%
B. 95%
C. 99.9%
D. 100%

13. The serum bactericidal test (SBT) measures

A. a trailing endpoint in the MIC test
B. absence of killing by an antimicrobic

C. MBC to MIC ratio of ≥32:1
D. presence of ≥6 colonies in the zone of inhibition

14. The SBT is used in all of the following situations *except*

A. cases of urinary tract infections
B. cases of endocarditis
C. cases of osteomyelitis treated with combination therapy
D. patients switched from parenteral or oral therapy

15. Vancomycin, gentamicin, and tobramycin are added alone or in combination to cultures of *Enterococcus faecium*. The results shown in the figure illustrate (see Figure 55.9)

A. antagonism between vancomycin and tobramycin
B. indifference between all drugs

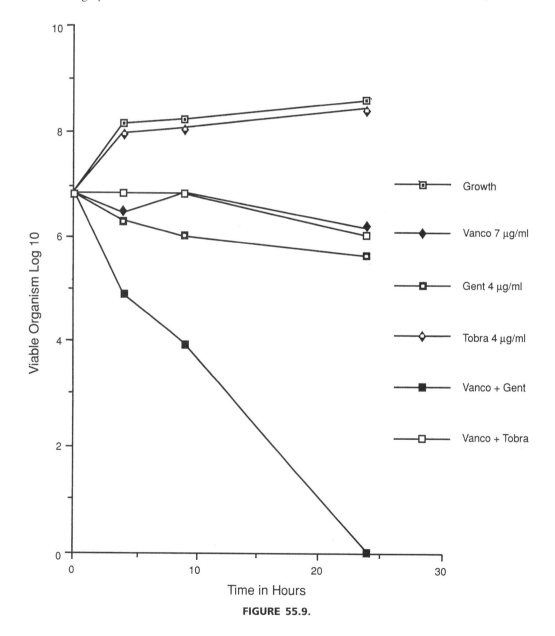

FIGURE 55.9.

C. synergism between vancomycin and gentamicin

D. organism resistant to vancomycin and gentamicin

Indicate whether each of the following statements is true (T) or false (F).

16. No quantitative antimicrobial susceptibility testing results can be given with the disk diffusion method.

17. Extended spectrum β-lactamase (ESBL) producing strains of *E. coli* and *Klebsiella* carry mutated TEM and SHV plasmids that code this enzyme.

18. Strains of *H. influenzae* capable of producing chloramphenicol acetyltransferase that renders them resistant to chloramphenicol have been isolated in the community.

19. The time-kill kinetic assay currently is thought to be the best method to study *in vitro* drug synergy.

20. "Checkerboard" microdeletion is an alternative method of performing drug synergy studies.

56

MOLECULAR TECHNIQUES FOR DIAGNOSIS OF INFECTIOUS DISEASES

QUESTIONS

Select the one best answer of the choices offered.

1. **Which of the following is the most commonly used method for probe hybridization?**
   A. Solid phase
   B. Liquid phase
   C. *In situ* hybridization
   D. DNA gene arrays

2. **Compared to routine polymerase chain reaction (PCR), nested PCR**
   A. only decreases the sensitivity
   B. only increases the specificity
   C. increases both sensitivity and specificity
   D. decreases both sensitivity and specificity

3. **All of the following are reasons for quantitation of amplified product *except***
   A. type of cells used for DNA extraction
   B. minor differences in amplification efficiency
   C. sample preparation
   D. thermal cycler performances

4. **All of the following statements regarding transcription-based amplification systems are true *except***
   A. It is a rapid detection method.
   B. It requires a thermal cycler.
   C. Denaturation of RNA is not necessary.
   D. It uses single-tube assays.

5. **Real-time PCR is**
   A. a post-PCR detection method
   B. an isothermal RNA amplification method
   C. a signal amplification system
   D. a method in which target amplification and detection occur simultaneously

6. **DNA microarray**
   A. is an alternative method of DNA amplification
   B. combines PCR and solid-phase hybridization techniques
   C. is a signal detection method for quantitation of DNA
   D. is a DNA antibody assay

7. **Which of the following human diseases was identified by molecular methods to be associated with human herpes virus 8 (HHV-8)?**
   A. Bacillary angiomatosis
   B. Whipple disease
   C. Kaposi sarcoma
   D. Hepatitis C infection

8. **Which human papilloma virus (HPV) subtype determined by molecular methods is associated with a high risk of cervical cancer?**
   A. 6
   B. 11
   C. 16
   D. 42

9. **Resistance to all of the following antimicrobials was detected molecular methods *except***
   A. methicillin
   B. vancomycin
   C. pentavalent antimonials
   D. rifampin

10. **Molecular laboratory tests [which proficiency testing (PT) is extremely important] are under which category of testing according to Clinical Laboratory Improvement Amendments of 1988 (CLIA 88)?**
    A. waived test
    B. point-of-care test (POCT)
    C. high complexity test
    D. provider-performed microscopy

Indicate whether each of the following statements is true (T) or false (F).

11. Nonamplified probe technique has poor analytical sensitivity and is limited in clinical situations where the number of pathogens is the greatest (i.e., group A streptococcal pharyngitis).

12. Multiplex PCR is more sensitive than single primer set PCR reactions.

13. Ligase chain reaction (LGR) is a convenient and easily automated molecular technique.

14. Direct sequencing of PCR by capillary electrophoresis techniques has streamlined the sequencing processes.

15. Plasma human immunodeficiency virus (HIV) viral load is a better predictor of disease progression than CD4+ lymphocyte count.

57

ROLE OF THE CLINICAL MICROBIOLOGY LABORATORY IN HOSPITAL EPIDEMIOLOGY AND INFECTION CONTROL

QUESTIONS

Select the one best answer of the choices offered.

1. **An onset of symptoms >48 hours after admission is evidence of nosocomial acquisition.**

   A. True   B. False

2. **All of the following statements regarding nosocomial infections are true *except***

   A. Coagulase-negative staphylococcus is the most commonly encountered nosocomial pathogen.
   B. Surgical wound infections comprises 35% to 40% of all nosocomial infections.
   C. The most common cause of nosocomial urinary tract infections is *Escherichia coli*.
   D. Emergence of *Candida* sp has been seen over the last two decades.

3. **All of the following microorganisms are relatively easy to identify *except***

   A. *Candida* sp

B. *Aspergillus* sp
C. Enterobacteriaceae
D. *Enterococcus* sp

Match each of the following sources of cross-infection in nosocomial infection outbreak with the appropriate culture method.

4. **Respiratory therapy equipment**

5. **Environmental surfaces**

6. **Blood products**

7. **Intravenous devices**

   A. swab rinse or impression plate
   B. roth or membrane filter method
   C. roth rinse or swab rinse
   D. roth culture

58

AUTOPSY MICROBIOLOGY

QUESTIONS

Select the one best answer of the choices offered.

1. **All of the following statements regarding microbiology of autopsy tissue are true *except***
   A. Bowel manipulation increases the number of positive blood cultures.
   B. >10⁵ organisms per milliliter in lung tissue correlates well with clinical and pathologic pneumonia.
   C. Agonal and postmortem bacterial systemic invasion will occur regardless of the precautions undertaken during performing nonsterile autopsy techniques.
   D. Potential sites of bacterial dissemination include the normal flora of the oropharynx ad gastrointestinal tract.

2. **All of the following statements regarding postmortem culturing are true *except***
   A. Use of cultures should not be conducted because of antemortem antimicrobial therapy.
   B. If only one area is to be cultured, the spleen and heart blood are favored as reliable sites.
   C. Cultures from the lungs and kidneys will more accurately reflect the spectrum of bacteria affecting the patient.
   D. Special viral, fungal, or mycobacterial cultures, in addition to routine microbiology, should be considered in autopsies of immunocompromised patients.

3. **All of the following recommendations should be followed in postmortem culturing *except***
   A. Urine should be aspirated directly from the urinary bladder.
   B. Consider using a resin culture bottle if the patient has been on antibiotics.
   C. Dry the area to be cultured by searing with a hot steel spatula.
   D. Culture of abscesses should only be obtained from the peripheral wall of the lesion.

4. **Tissue from autopsy may be automatically plated for bacteriology, anaerobes, and fungi.**
   A. True   B. False

5. **Tissue specimens for viral cultures may be kept for up to 72 hours at 4°C, if any delay in transport to the laboratory is anticipated.**
   A. True   B. False

6. **Touch preparation can permit rapid identification of microorganisms in the morgue.**
   A. True   B. False

Match each of the following microorganisms with the corresponding host tissue reaction.

7. *Histoplasma*

8. *Aspergillus*

9. *Pneumocystis*

10. **Routine bacteria**
    A. Thrombosis
    B. Acute inflammation
    C. Chronic inflammation
    D. Caseous necrosis

Match each of the following microorganisms with the proper histologic stain for detection.

11. *Pneumocystis*

12. *Nocardia*

13. *Cryptococcus*

14. *Toxoplasma*

15. *Blastomyces*
    A. Acid fast
    B. Gomori methenamine silver nitrate (GMS)
    C. Hematoxylin and eosin
    D. Periodic acid-Schiff (PAS)
    E. Mucicarmine

59

DIAGNOSTIC VIROLOGY

QUESTIONS

Select the one best answer of the choices offered.

1. **The optimal temperature for storage and transport of specimens for viral culture and antigen detection is °C.**

   A. 2   C. 8
   B. 4   D. 16

2. **Advantages to viral antigen detection can include**

   A. Antigen detection test results are available sooner.
   B. Antigen detection tests do not require cell culture laboratory equipment.
   C. Specimen collection and transport conditions are less critical than for viral isolation.
   D. A and B
   E. A, B, and C

3. **Example(s) of nucleic acid amplification techniques is(are)**

   A. target amplification
   B. signal amplification
   C. probe amplification
   D. A and B
   E. A, B, and C

4. **In general, serologic tests for viruses are used when isolation/antigen detection tests are not available.**

   A. True   B. False

5. **The most common cause of acute sporadic encephalitis in the United States is**

   A. arbovirus

B. Parvovirus A
C. hantavirus
D. herpesvirus

6. **Cytomegalovirus (CMV) may be isolated in the absence of disease in one third of patients.**

   A. True   B. False

7. **Human herpesvirus types 6 and 7 are considered to be emerging pathogens.**

   A. True   B. False

8. **Human herpesvirus type 8 is the etiologic agent of**

   A. roseola
   B. mononucleosis syndrome
   C. Kaposi sarcoma
   D. A and B
   E. A, B, and C

9. **The hepatitis viruses that cause disease in the United States are**

   A. A, B, C, and D
   B. C and D
   C. A and B
   D. A, B, C, and D

10. **For human immunodeficiency virus (HIV), all positive screening enzyme-linked immunosorbent assays (ELISAs) are confirmed by Western blot or immunofluorescent assay (IFA).**

    A. True   B. False

60

PARASITOLOGY

QUESTIONS

Select the one best answer of the choices offered.

1. **Hemoflagellates include**
   A. *Plasmodium*
   B. *Leishmania*
   C. *Trypanosoma*
   D. A and B
   E. B and C

2. **The most common species of *Plasmodium* found worldwide is**
   A. *P. ovale*
   B. *P. malariae*
   C. *P. vivax*
   D. *P. falciparum*

3. **Complete cycles of the malaria parasite occur in a quartan pattern in *P. vivax*.**
   A. True   B. False

4. **Cestodes include**
   A. *Taenia solium*
   B. *Hymenolepsis diminuta*
   C. *Schistosoma mansoni*
   D. A and B
   E. B and C

5. **Malaria is transmitted by the *Anopheles* mosquito.**
   A. True   B. False

6. **In the thick-film preparation for diagnosis of malaria, blood is spread over the entire slide.**
   A. True   B. False

7. **The most common mixed malaria infection is attributable to a combination of (Figure 60.4)**
   A. *P. vivax* and *P. malariae*
   B. *P. malariae* and *P. falciparum*
   C. *P. ovale* and *P. vivax*
   D. *P. falciparum* and *P. vivax*

8. **Babesiosis is transmitted in nature by**
   A. soft-bodied tick
   B. hard-bodied tick
   C. flea
   D. mosquito

9. **Leishmaniasis is transmitted by**
   A. flea
   B. mosquito
   C. sand fly
   D. soft-bodied tick

10. **Chiclero ulcer is caused by**
    A. sand fly
    B. hard-bodied ticks
    C. *Leishmania mexicana*
    D. *P. ovale*

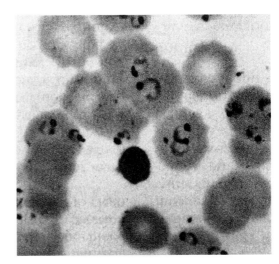

FIGURE 60.4. *Plasmodium falciparum.* Ring forms in film of peripheral blood. (From Garcia LS, Salzer AJ, Healy GR, et al. Blood and tissue protozoa. In: Murray PR, Baron EJ, Pfaller MA, et al., eds. *Manual of clinical microbiology,* 6th ed. Washington, DC: American Society for Microbiology, 1995:1171–1195, with permission.)

11. **Chagas disease is caused by**
    A. *Trypanosoma cruzi*
    B. *P. ovale*
    C. *Leishmania braziliensis*
    D. *Trypanosoma brucei gambiense*

12. ***Toxoplasma gondii* is a coccidian parasite.**
    A. True   B. False

13. **The life cycle (asexual and sexual reproduction) of *Toxoplasma gondii* occurs only in the cat.**
    A. True   B. False

14. **Of the free-living amebic infections, only ____ is able to exist temporarily in a flagellate as well as an ameboid form.**
    A. *Naegleria*
    B. *Acanthamoeba*
    C. *Balamuth*
    D. *Plasmodia*

15. **The cyst stage of *Entamoeba histolytica* contains ____ nuclei in the mature form.**
    A. 2
    B. 4
    C. 6
    D. 8

16. ***E. histolytica* has a worldwide distribution.**
    A. True   B. False

17. **Flagellate(s) found in humans is(are)**
    A. *Dientamoeba fragilis*
    B. *Chilomastix mesnili*
    C. *Enteromonas hominis*
    D. A and B
    E. A, B, and C

18. ***Giardia lamblia* causes an infection of the large intestine.**
    A. True   B. False

19. ***Balantidium coli* is a large nonciliated protozoan.**
    A. True   B. False

20. **Cryptosporidiosis is a zoonosis that can spread from animal reservoirs to humans.**
    A. True   B. False

21. **Helminths include**
    A. roundworms
    B. microsporidia
    C. flatworms
    D. A and C
    E. A, B, and C

22. **Whipworm infection is caused by**
    A. *Taenia*
    B. *Trichuris trichiura*
    C. *Clonorchis sinensis*
    D. *Enterobius vermicularis*

23. **The most common and widely distributed of the soil transmitted helminths is**
    A. *T. trichiura*
    B. *Ascaris lumbricoides*
    C. *E. vermicularis*
    D. *Necator americanus*

24. **The eggs of *Ancylostoma duodenale* and *N. americanus* are indistinguishable.**
    A. True   B. False

25. ***Strongyloides stercoralis* is the smallest intestinal nematode infecting humans.**
    A. True   B. False

26. **Trichinosis occurs throughout most of the world, except Australia and the Pacific Islands.**
    A. True   B. False

27. **Cutaneous larva migrans is an infection of the skin caused by the dog and cat hookworm *Ancylostoma braziliense*.**
    A. True   B. False

28. ***Loa loa* is transmitted by biting flies of the genus *Chrysops*.**
    A. True   B. False

29. **Trematodes or flukes are members of the Platyhelminthes.**
    A. True   B. False

30. **The blood flukes are members of the genus *Schistosoma*.**
    A. True   B. False

31. **The largest liver fluke is *Fasciola hepatica*.**
    A. True   B. False

32. **The principal lung fluke of humans is *Paragonimus westermani*.**
    A. True   B. False

33. **Obligate intravascular parasites inhabiting the venules of the intestine are**

A. *S. mansoni*
B. *Schistosoma japonicum*
C. *Schistosoma haematobium*
D. A and B
E. A, B and C

34. The pork tapeworm is *T. solium.* (Figure 60.55)

A. True   B. False

35. The fish tapeworm, *Diphyllobothrium latum*, inhabits the large intestine.

A. True   B. False

36. *Echinococcus granulosus* is a cause of hydatid disease.

A. True   B. False

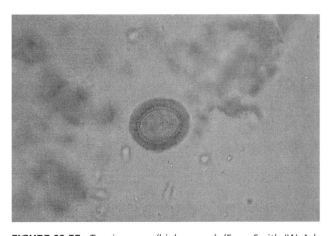

FIGURE 60.55. *Taenia* sp egg (high power). (From Smith JW, Ash LR, Thompson JH, et al. *Diagnostic medical parasitology: intestinal helminths.* Chicago: American Society of Clinical Pathologists, 1976, with permission.)

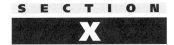

SECTION
X

IMMUNOPATHOLOGY

61 Basic Principles of Immunodiagnosis
62 Flow Cytometry
63 Cellular and Humoral Mediators of Inflammation
64 Monoclonal Gammopathies
65 Primary Immunodeficiency Diseases
66 Allergic Conditions
67 Receptor Assays of the Clinical Laboratory

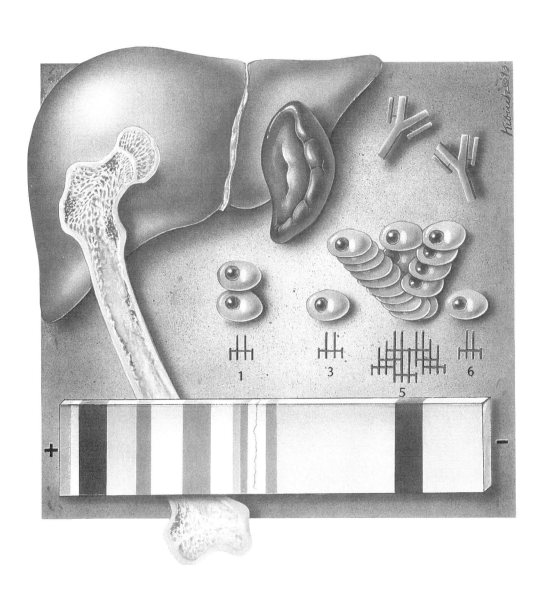

61

BASIC PRINCIPLES OF IMMUNODIAGNOSIS

QUESTIONS

Select the one best answer of the choices offered.

1. **Cytokines is a group of peptides such as**
   A. interleukins
   B. interferons
   C. tumor necrosis factors
   D. A and B
   E. A, B, and C

2. **A clone of plasma cells derived from a single B lymphocyte produces immunoglobulin molecules.**
   A. True   B. False

3. **Antibodies are protein molecules.**
   A. True   B. False

4. **The specific biologic function of each immunoglobulin class is determined by the tertiary structure of the constant domains. (Figure 61.3.)**
   A. True   B. False

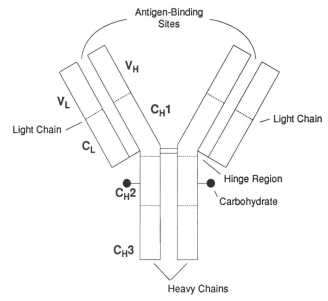

FIGURE 61.3.

5. **Variations of the passive agglutination technique include**
   A. Rose-Waaler test
   B. VDRL (Venereal Disease Research Laboratory test)
   C. Paul-Bunnell test
   D. A and C
   E. A, B, and C

6. **Cell lysis forms the base for the complement-fixation test.**
   A. True   B. False

7. **The molecular weight of the antigen is the major determinant of the time required for performance of a radial immunodiffusion assay.**
   A. True   B. False

8. **Electroimmunoassay is a technique in which an electric force is used to drive an antigen into a gel containing an antibody.**
   A. True   B. False

9. **A ligand is a substance that will not bind to or complex with another substance.**
   A. True   B. False

10. **Probe(s) used for labeling monoclonal antibodies is(are)**
    A. Texas red
    B. phycoerythrin
    C. rhodamine
    D. A and C
    E. A, B, and C

11. **An original method used in the differentiation of T and B lymphocytes is**
    A. immunodiffusion
    B. rocket electrophoresis
    C. resetting
    D. centrifugation

12. The mixed lymphocyte culture phenomenon is determined by the D locus of the HLA system.

A. True   B. False

13. Substance on the surface of a foreign body that enhances phagocytosis is called

A. antigen
B. complement
C. opsonin
D. precipitin

14. Functional complement assays include

A. hemolytic tube technique
B. immunoelectrophoresis
C. radial immunodiffusion
D. A and B
E. A and C

15. Indirect immunofluorescent staining is used to detect the presence of antigen in tissue.

A. True   B. False

FLOW CYTOMETRY

QUESTIONS

Match each of the following antigens with the corresponding cellular distribution.

1. **CD38**

2. **CD41**

3. **CD56**

4. **CD10**

5. **CD64**
   A. Common acute lymphoblastic leukemia
   B. Natural killer cells
   C. Monocytes
   D. Plasma cells
   E. Megakaryocytes

6. **All of the following antigens are expressed in precursor B acute lymphoblastic leukemia** *except*
   A. Tdt
   B. CD19
   C. CD20
   D. CD34

7. **All of the following antigens are expressed in pre-B acute lymphoblastic leukemia** *except*
   A. Tdt
   B. CD19
   C. CD10
   D. CD34

8. **All of the following antigens are characteristic of acute myelogenous leukemia M3** *except*
   A. HLA-DR
   B. CD13
   C. CD15
   D. CD33

9. **Which of the following markers distinguish chronic lymphocytic leukemia from mantle cell lymphoma?**
   A. CD5
   B. CD23
   C. CD19
   D. CD34

10. **All of the following antigens are expressed in B-cell prolymphocytic leukemia except**
    A. HLA-DR
    B. CD45 (bright)
    C. CD23
    D. Light chain (strong)

11. **Which of the following markers is expressed in plasma cell dyscrasia?**
    A. CD45 (bright)
    B. CD19
    C. CD11c
    D. CD38

12. **All of the following antigens are expressed in natural killer–large granular lymphocytic disorder** *except*
    A. CD3
    B. CD11c
    C. CD7
    D. CD16

Match each of the following types of lymphoma with the corresponding phenotype (each answer may be used more than once).

13. **Burkitt lymphoma**

14. **Follicular lymphoma**

15. **Mucosa-associated lymphoid tissue lymphoma (MALT)**

16. **Mantle cell lymphoma**
    A. CD19$^+$, CD5$^+$, CD10$^-$, CD23$^-$, cyclin D1$^+$
    B. CD19$^+$, CD 5$^-$, CD10$^+$
    C. CD19$^+$, CD5$^-$, CD10$^-$

17. **All of the following regarding paroxysmal nocturnal hemoglobinuria (PNH) are true except**
    A. Expression of CD55 and CD59 is diminished on erythrocytes.
    B. Expression of CD55 and CD59 is diminished on the granulocytes.
    C. Classic laboratory tests include the sucrose hemolysis test and the acid hemolysis test (Ham test).
    D. Flow cytometric analysis is not sensitive in the diagnosis of PNH II, when partial loss of CD55 and CD59 occurs.

18. **Analysis of cellular DNA by flow cytometry is limited by the fact that translocations escape detection.**
    A. True   B. False

19. **In most recent flow instruments, alignment is optimized by service engineers and, therefore, does not need to be checked on a daily basis.**
    A. True   B. False

Match each of the following patterns of light scatter in flow cytometric analysis with the corresponding population of blood cells.

20. **Very low side scatter/very low forward scatter**

21. **Very low side scatter/low forward scatter**

22. **High side scatter/high forward scatter**

23. **Intermediate side scatter/high forward scatter**
    A. Monocytes
    B. Cellular debris
    C. Granulocytes
    D. Lymphocytes

24. **In flow cytometric analysis, staining of the cells with multiple antibodies is best accomplished using an indirect immunofluorescence technique.**
    A. True   B. False

25. **It often is recommended for analysis of platelet activation by flow cytometry to fix the specimen with paraformaldehyde prior to staining.**
    A. True   B. False

26. **All of the following are intracellular antigens *except***
    A. CD3
    B. Myeloperoxidase
    C. CD20
    D. Tdt

27. **Histogram storage of data allows regating of flow cytometric data.**
    A. True   B. False

CELLULAR AND HUMORAL MEDIATORS
OF INFLAMMATION

QUESTIONS

Match each of the following with the corresponding family of cell adhesion molecules (CAMs).

1. **Leukocyte trafficking to peripheral lymph nodes**

2. **Cell recognition events during morphogenesis and inflammation**

3. **Cell differentiation and proliferation**

4. **Tight gap junctions and intercellular spacing**
   A. Immunoglobulin supergene family
   B. Cadherins
   C. Selectins
   D. Proteoglycans

Match each of the following substances with the corresponding type of granulocyte granules (each answer may be used more than once).

5. **Human neutrophil lipocalin**

6. **Lysozyme**

7. **Myeloperoxidase**

8. **Lactoferrin**

9. **Cathepsin G**
   A. Primary granules
   B. Secondary granules
   C. Both

Match each of the following substances with its corresponding biologic function.

10. **Interferes with the iron metabolism of microbes**

11. **Specific marker of neutrophil activation**

12. **Proteolysis of complement and coagulation factors**

13. **Index of increased monocyte/macrophage turnover**
    A. Cathepsin G
    B. Lysozyme
    C. Human neutrophil lipocalin
    D. Lactoferrin

14. **Eosinophil granules are rich in acid phosphatase, peroxidase, and lysozyme.**
    A. True   B. False

15. **All of the following statements regarding the function of eosinophils are true *except***
    A. antagonizing the effects of the mediators released from basophils
    B. enhancing the effects of the mediators released from mast cells
    C. ingestion of immune complexes
    D. clearance of parasites

16. **All of the following statements regarding natural killer (NK) cells are true *except***
    A. NK cells do not recirculate between blood and lymph.
    B. NK cells secrete interferon-γ (IFN-γ).
    C. Killer (K) cells appear to represent a particular stage of NK cell development or activation.
    D. Activation of NK cells induces immunologic memory.

17. **All of the following statements regarding C-reactive protein (CRP) are true *except***
    A. CRP activates complement via the classic pathway.
    B. Many similarities exist between CRP and antibodies.
    C. CRP does not increase in viral infections.
    D. Deficiency states of CRP are uncommon.

18. **All of the following statements regarding erythrocyte sedimentation rate (ESR) are true** *except*

    A. ESR elevations are slower and much more prolonged compared with CRP.
    B. ESR measurements are directly proportional to the plasma level of haptoglobin.
    C. Systemic lupus erythematosus (SLE) demonstrates marked elevations in CRP, but not ESR.
    D. Rheumatoid arthritis demonstrates elevations in both ESR and CRP.

Match each of the following with the corresponding type of complement receptor (each answer may be used more than once).

19. **CD21**

20. **CD11c/CD18**

21. **Receptor for phagocytosis**

22. **Receptor for Epstein-Barr virus**

23. **Clearance of immune complexes**

    A. Complement receptor type 1
    B. Complement receptor type 2
    C. Complement receptor type 3
    D. Complement receptor type 4

24. **All of the following statements regarding measuring the complement in the clinical laboratory are true** *except*

    A. The solid-phase assay (CH_{100}) is much easier to perform compared with the fluid phase (CH_{50}).
    B. Complement deficiencies are rare.
    C. The solid-phase assay (CH_{100}) does detect the heterozygous complement deficiencies.
    D. The solid- and fluid-phase complement assays are hemolysis-based methods.

25. **Quantitation of C3 and C4 is a much more sensitive measure of complement consumption** *in vivo* **than hemolytic assays.**

    A. True   B. False

Match each of the following cytokines with the corresponding primary functions.

26. **Interleukin-5 (IL-5)**

27. **Platelet-derived growth factor (PDGF)**

28. **IL-13**

29. **IL-12**

    A. Activates T cells and NK cells
    B. Promotes B-cell growth and differentiation
    C. Eosinophil growth factor
    D. Activate fibroblasts to synthesize collagen

30. **All of the following statements regarding cytokines in disease are true except**

    A. IL-13 plays a critical role in the development of asthma.
    B. IL-1 and tumor necrosis factor-α (TNF-α) induce cartilage degeneration in rheumatoid arthritis.
    C. TNF-α, IL-1β, IL-6, and IL-8 are elevated in human sepsis.
    D. Using anti–TNF-α for treatment of sepsis has been successful.

31. **All of the following substances are products of the cyclooxygenase pathway except**

    A. Prostaglandin E_2 (PGE_2)
    B. Prostacyclin
    C. Leukotriene B_4 (LTB_4)
    D. Thromboxane A_2 (TXA_2)

32. **All of the following statements regarding apoptosis are true except**

    A. IL-1β–converting enzyme (ICE) inhibits apoptosis.
    B. Expression of bcl-2 inhibits apoptosis.
    C. The only mechanism to initiate apoptosis is via surface-receptor stimulation.
    D. Fas (CD95) is a proapoptotic molecule.

33. **All of the following statements regarding the role of apoptosis in diseases of the immune system are true except**

    A. Mutations in CD95 inhibit apoptosis.
    B. The bcl-2 antagonists might be used to treat follicular lymphoma.
    C. The eye and testis express low levels of CD95L.
    D. Death of $CD4^+$ cells in human immunodeficiency virus (HIV) occurs by apoptosis.

64

MONOCLONAL GAMMOPATHIES

QUESTIONS

Match each of the following clinical condition with the corresponding feature.

1. **Amyloid (AL)**

2. **Cryoglobulin type II**

3. **Light chain disease**

4. **Monoclonal gammopathy of undetermined significance (MGUS)**
   A. Constitutes 15% of cases of multiple myeloma
   B. Most common cause of serum M protein
   C. 20% have multiple myeloma or Waldenström macroglobulinemia.
   D. Associated with hepatitis C

5. **All of the following statements regarding patient evaluation for monoclonal gammopathy are true *except***
   A. Both urine and serum protein electrophoresis should be included in the initial evaluation of patients.
   B. If protein electrophoresis is negative, immunofixation should be the next step.
   C. For the initial evaluation of patients, protein electrophoresis should be performed using high-resolution methods.
   D. A negative result on spot urine sample cannot be used to rule out the presence of monoclonal free light chains.

6. **Approximately 20% to 25% of patients with MGUS followed for 20 to 35 years will develop clinically significant B-cell lymphoproliferative disorders.**
   A. True   B. False

7. **A high-resolution method for protein electrophoresis is one that permits crisp separation of transferrin and C3 in the β-region.**
   A. True   B. False

8. **All of the following statements regarding multiple myeloma are true *except***
   A. Patients with light chain tetramers have no Bence Jones proteins in urine.
   B. The malignancy involves, not only the plasma cells, but the entire B-cell lineage.
   C. Renal failure is a common finding in multiple myeloma patients.
   D. Plasma cells produce an osteoclast-activating factor.

9. **All of the following statements regarding POEM-SIQ1 syndrome are true *except***
   A. Patients may develop hyperpigmentation of the skin.
   B. Patients present mainly with polyneuropathy.
   C. It comprises >5% of the multiple myeloma cases.
   D. Organomegaly usually involves the heart.

10. **All of the following statements regarding the immunoglobulin isotypes in multiple myeloma are true *except***
    A. The ratio of kappa to lambda light chains is 1:9 in immunoglobulin D (IgD) myeloma.
    B. Patients with IgE myeloma present with hyperviscosity symptoms.
    C. IgM myeloma is more common than IgE myeloma.
    D. IgA myeloma may be difficult to diagnose on serum protein electrophoresis.

11. **All of the following statements regarding biclonal gammopathies are true *except***
    A. Two different light chain types are present in the urine.
    B. There is no special clinical significance of biclonal gammopathies.
    C. The presence of two different heavy chains with the same light chain isotype does not establish the diagnosis of biclonal gammopathy.
    D. Molecular studies must be performed to confirm the diagnosis.

12. **The following findings are consistent with Waldenström macroglobulinemia** *except*

    A. monoclonal spike that is located close to the β-globulin band
    B. IgM >20 g/dL
    C. bone marrow infiltration by lymphoplasmacytoid lymphocytes
    D. rouleaux formation

13. **All of the following statements regarding MGUS are true** *except*

    A. Relatively large gammopathies, up to 3 g/dL, may represent a benign lymphoplasmacytic lesion.
    B. Decreased γ-globulin component denotes worse prognosis.

    C. About 20% of patients will develop malignant B-cell lymphoproliferative disease over a 10-year period.
    D. Approximately 70% of monoclonal gammopathy cases are due to MGUS.

14. **All of the following statements regarding amyloidosis are true** *except*

    A. Biopsy of the rectum might establish the diagnosis of amyloidosis.
    B. The AA type of amyloid consists of immunoglobulin light chain.
    C. Patients do not have bone pain.
    D. Patients sometimes present with macroglossia.

65

PRIMARY IMMUNODEFICIENCY DISEASES

QUESTIONS

Select the one best answer of the choices offered.

1. **Which of the following is a common presentation of immunodeficiency disorders?**

   A. Failure to thrive
   B. Chronic infections
   C. Infections by uncommon organisms
   D. Mental retardation

2. **All of the following statements regarding immunodeficiency disorders are true *except***

   A. Frequency and severity of infections tend to parallel the extent of immunologic deficit.
   B. Isolated immunoglobulin G (IgG) subclass deficiencies typically present with bacterial meningitis.
   C. Patients with cellular immune defects often exhibit fungal, protozoal, mycobacterial, and viral infections.
   D. Recurrent pyogenic infections are typical of hypogammaglobulinemia.

3. **All of the following statements regarding disorders of the complement system are true *except***

   A. They may be hereditary or acquired.
   B. They account for 40% of immune deficiency disorders.
   C. They result from either deficiency of a particular component or production of a nonfunctional molecule.
   D. Not all complement components exhibit a known deficiency syndrome.

4. **All of the following statements regarding C3 deficiency are true *except***

   A. C3b inactivator deficiency results in a pseudo C3 deficiency that is asymptomatic.
   B. Patients exhibit reduced serum opsonization capacity.

   C. It is associated with an increased risk of severe bacterial infections, especially by encapsulated organisms.
   D. C3 deficiency may occur as a primary genetic defect or through deficiency of factor I.

5. **All of the following statements regarding C5, C6, C7, or C8 deficiency are true *except***

   A. It exhibits impaired bacteriolysis.
   B. It exhibits impaired opsonization.
   C. It is associated with frequent disseminated neisserial infections.
   D. C8-β deficiency occurs primarily in whites and α-γ deficiency is more common in blacks.

6. **All of the following statements regarding C1 esterase inhibitor (C1-INH) deficiency are true *except***

   A. Deficiency is due to either a silent C1-INH allele or to an allele encoding a dysfunctional molecule.
   B. It can be associated with systemic lupus erythematosus (SLE) or lupus-like syndromes.
   C. Roughly 50% of patients exhibit hereditary angioneurotic edema (HANE).
   D. HANE typically affects the face and respiratory tract.

7. **Paroxysmal nocturnal hemoglobinuria (PNH) is associated with defects in**

   A. spectrin
   B. decay accelerating factor (DAF) and CD59
   C. CD40 ligand
   D. glycophorins C and D

8. **All of the following statements regarding chronic granulomatous disease (CGD) are true *except***

   A. It results from a heterogeneous group of molecular defects resulting in a variable spectrum of clinical presentations.
   B. It usually presents in children with recurrent or recalcitrant soft tissue, lymph node, and respiratory infections most commonly due to *Staphylococcus aureus*.

C. It results from defects in NADH reductase.

D. Type 1 CGD is X-linked, accounting for two thirds CGD cases.

9. **All of the following are associated with Chediak-Higashi syndrome *except***

A. giant cytoplasmic granules in neutrophils, monocytes, and lymphocytes

B. persistent neutrophilia

C. storage pool-type platelet defect with a prolonged bleeding time

D. oculocutaneous albinism

10. **All of the following are true of X-linked agammaglobulinemia *except***

A. It usually presents in infants in the first 3 months of life.

B. It exhibits a high incidence of infection, particularly by encapsulated pyogenic bacteria.

C. Patients are particularly susceptible to viral hepatitis.

D. Lymph nodes are hypoplastic with absence of germinal centers.

11. **All of the following statements regarding common variable immunodeficiency are true *except***

A. It is composed of a heterogeneous group of disorders characterized by a deficiency of γ-globulins.

B. It is associated with autoimmune and neoplastic disorders, including gastric carcinoma, lymphoma, and amyloidosis.

C. Number of circulating B lymphocytes is normal.

D. γ-Globulin levels usually are undetectable.

12. **Wiskott-Aldrich syndrome (WAS) has been mapped to a chromosome mutation on**

A. 11p13

B. Xp11.22

C. 6q21.3

D. Xq26.3

13. **All of the following statements regarding Job syndrome are true *except***

A. autosomal dominant, hyper-IgE disorder

B. defect in neutrophil motility

C. recurrent staphylococcal abscesses involving the skin, lungs, joints, and soft tissues

D. peripheral blood basophilia

14. **Patients with ataxia-telangiectasia are at increased risk of developing**

A. hematopoietic malignancies

B. sarcomas

C. melanomas

D. carcinomas

15. **All of the following are chromosomal instability syndromes *except***

A. Bloom syndrome

B. Fanconi anemia

C. DiGeorge syndrome

D. Ataxia-telangiectasia

Indicate whether each of the following statements is true (T) or false (F).

16. **C3b plays an important role in immune complex solubilization and clearance.**

17. **SLE patients deficient in C2 have prominent cutaneous features and are more frequently ANA and anti-dsDNA positive than their complement sufficient counterparts.**

18. **Myeloperoxidase (MPO)-deficient patients cannot produce O_2^- and H_2O_2 in their granulocytes.**

19. **Biopsies of lymphoid tissues reveal hypoplasia, absence of germinal centers, and diminished plasma cells.**

20. **IgA deficiency is the most common primary immunodeficiency, with prevalence between 1:350 and 1:3,000.**

21. **Patients with adenosine deaminase (ADA) deficiency suffer from both humoral and cellular immunodeficiency.**

22. **HLA class I molecule deficiency is uniformly associated with an increased susceptibility to recurrent pyogenic infections.**

23. **WAS is an X-linked immunodeficiency disorder characterized by thrombocytopenia and eczema.**

24. **Cytomegalovirus (CMV) infection causes significant mortality in patients with Duncan disease.**

25. **Patients with ataxia-telangiectasia variant suffer from microcephaly and ataxia.**

66

ALLERGIC CONDITIONS

QUESTIONS

Select the one best answer of the choices offered.

1. **Histamine, leukotrienes, and platelet-activating factor correspond with which of the following types of hypersensitivity reaction?**
   A. Immediate
   B. Cytotoxic
   C. Immune complex
   D. Cell mediated

2. **Goodpasture disease belongs to which category of hypersensitivity reaction?**
   A. Type I
   B. Type II
   C. Type III
   D. Type IV

3. **All of the following statements regarding allergy are true *except***
   A. It is an acute inflammatory condition that occurs rapidly on exposure to an allergen and is associated with systemic eosinophilia.
   B. It is an acquired hypersensitivity that has an immune basis.
   C. It shows positivity on skin testing to one or more aeroallergens and may exhibit elevation of total immunoglobulin E (IgE).
   D. It is a hypersensitivity reaction mediated by IgE.

4. **All of the following statements regarding rhinitis are true *except***
   A. Allergic rhinitis is defined by positive skin tests to inhaled aeroallergen(s) and symptoms that correspond with exposure to the allergen.
   B. Allergic rhinitis may be seasonal or perennial.
   C. Nonallergic rhinitis includes vasomotor type and nonallergic rhinitis with eosinophilia.
   D. Presence of eosinophils in the nasal mucosa and mucus differentiates allergic from nonallergic rhinitis.

5. **All of the following statements regarding asthma are true *except***
   A. It is a condition of reversible obstructive airway disease with airway hyperirritability to histamine that is suppressed by methacholine.
   B. The best method for asthma diagnosis is spirometry.
   C. The prevalence of asthma and death from asthma has been increasing in all age groups.
   D. Allergy is diagnosed less frequently in adult asthmatics than in children.

6. **All of the following statements regarding asthmatics who are sensitive to nonsteroidal antiinflammatory drugs (NSAIDs) are true *except***
   A. Patients may require oral or inhaled corticosteroids.
   B. Patients may develop nasal polyps.
   C. Sensitivity occurs in 40% of chronic asthmatics.
   D. Patients are inflicted with chronic sinusitis.

7. **All of the following statements regarding urticaria or angioedema are true *except***
   A. The specific cause of chronic or recurrent urticaria usually cannot be determined.
   B. Urticaria may be associated with an IgE-mediated response in some cases of food and insect sting hypersensitivity.
   C. Most cases of angioedema are caused by mast cell degranulation in deep dermal tissues.
   D. Systemic mastocytosis does not cause urticaria.

8. **Which skin condition often is associated with gluten sensitive enteropathy?**
   A. Erythema multiforme
   B. Dermatitis herpetiformis
   C. Systemic lupus erythematosus
   D. Psoriasis

9. **All of the following statements regarding dermatitis are true *except***
   A. Atopic dermatitis often is associated with IgE-mediated hypersensitivity.

B. Atopic dermatitis often is associated with allergic rhinitis and asthma.

C. Atopic dermatitis typically appears in adults and improves with antistreptococcal antibiotics.

D. Allergic contact dermatitis is due to a type IV hypersensitivity response and typically takes 48 hours for a significant response to occur.

10. **All of the following are common causes of allergic contact dermatitis *except***

   A. urushiols derived from plants of the *Rhus* genus
   B. nickel
   C. chromates
   D. fungal antigens of *Alternaria*

11. **Thermophilic actinomycetes in grains is associated with which type of hypersensitivity pneumonitis?**

   A. Farmer's lung
   B. Bird fancier's disease
   C. Malt worker's lung
   D. Woodworker's lung

12. **All of the following statements regarding skin testing are true *except***

   A. Skin testing is the most accurate and cost-effective method to diagnose patients with IgE-mediated disorders.
   B. A positive test is indicated by a wheal-and-flare response.
   C. Percutaneous testing should be attempted before intradermal testing in patients with IgE-mediated hypersensitivity.
   D. Intradermal testing is more specific than the percutaneous test.

13. **All of the following statements regarding allergy testing are true *except***

   A. The most popular method for measuring total serum IgE is the noncompetitive RIST (radioimmunosorbent test).
   B. RIST assays may be competitive or noncompetitive.
   C. RAST (radioallergosorbent test) assay measures binding of specific IgE to allergen.
   D. RAST assay is a competitive immunoassay.

14. **All of the following statements regarding cytologic examination of nasal secretions are true *except***

   A. Absence of eosinophils does not rule out an allergic condition.

B. Nonallergic rhinitis with eosinophilia may be diagnosed if >50% of the inflammatory cells are eosinophils and skin tests to aeroallergens are negative.

C. Cytology is not useful to differentiate allergic rhinitis from acute viral rhinitis.

D. Lower respiratory mucus is more difficult to examine for inflammatory cells than nasal mucus.

15. **The photomicrograph depicted in Figure 66.1F shows**

   A. Charcot-Leyden crystals
   B. Churchman spirals
   C. asbestos body
   D. monosodium urate

Indicate whether each of the following statements is true (T) or false (F).

16. **Asthma is best diagnosed by ventilation-perfusion (V/Q) scan.**

17. **Dermatographisms are characterized wheal-and-flare reaction triggered by scratching the skin.**

18. **At work, performance of spirometry is more practical than peak expiratory flow rate measurements.**

19. **A percutaneous skin testing is more sensitive and specific than intradermal skin tests.**

20. **Allergic bronchopulmonary mycosis (ABPM) include the presence of asthma, positive immediate skin test reaction to the fungus, and elevation of total IgE and precipitins to the fungus.**

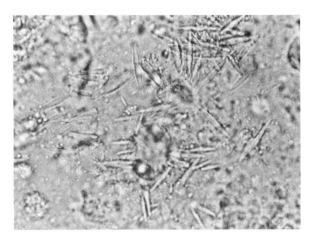

FIGURE 66.1F.

RECEPTOR ASSAYS OF THE CLINICAL LABORATORY

QUESTIONS

Select the one best answer of the choices offered.

1. **All of the following bind to intracellular receptors** *except*

   A. gonadal steroids
   B. vitamin D
   C. thyroid hormones
   D. somatostatin

2. **All of the following are peptide regulator factors** *except*

   A. glucagon
   B. gonadotropin-releasing hormone
   C. transforming-growth factor
   D. somatostatin

3. **All of the following statements regarding cellular receptors are true** *except*

   A. Intracellular cytosolic receptors are closely associated with chromatin.
   B. Most regulators of cell function are hydrophobic molecules that locate to cellular membranes.
   C. Some steroid hormones bind to transcription regulator regions of DNA and affect gene expression.
   D. Membrane receptors include allosterically activated enzymes, receptors coupled to an enzyme via a G protein and membrane receptors that form a channel.

4. **All of the following statements regarding cellular receptors for steroid hormones are true** *except*

   A. All steroid hormone receptors are present in the cytoplasm, and, when the steroid binds, the complex is translocated into the nucleus.
   B. Estrogen (ER) and progesterone (PR) receptors are confined to the nucleus.
   C. Unoccupied gonadal steroid receptors are located in the nucleus.

   D. Steroid receptors are composed of a single polypeptide that contains hormone-binding, DNA-binding, and N-terminus domains.

5. **All of the following are receptor-associated enzymes that may be activated by membrane-bound receptors** *except*

   A. adenylate cyclase
   B. protein kinase
   C. retinoic receptor
   D. phosphodiesterases

6. **All of the following statements regarding tyrosine kinase receptors are true** *except*

   A. They include insulin and epidermal growth factor receptor (EGFr).
   B. They consist of only single membrane-spanning receptors.
   C. They contain cytoplasmic tyrosine kinase activity.
   D. They include disulfide bound heterotetramer ligand-binding properties.

7. **All of the following are true of ER and PR receptors** *except*

   A. Presence of PR in human breast cancer is indicative of ER responsiveness.
   B. Roughly 60% of breast cancers are ER positive and two thirds of ER-positive tumors respond to endocrine therapy.
   C. ER-negative breast tumors are resistant to endocrine therapy.
   D. Determination of both ER and PR does not increase the prognostic value over either ER or PR alone.

8. **All of the following statements regarding epidermal growth factor or its receptor EGFr are true** *except*

   A. 50% of EGFr-positive breast cancer patients display a positive correlation between levels of EGFr and ER and PR receptors.

B. EGFr overexpression has been demonstrated in a variety of tumors.

C. Demonstration of EGFr overexpression may have clinical utility and prognostic significance, but there is no consensus on the value of this finding.

D. EGFr is involved in fetal growth and developmental events.

9. **Proteins that bind EGFr include all of the following *except***

A. virus growth factor EGF-like protein
B. transforming growth factor-α
C. c-*erb*-b2
D. amphiregulin

10. **All of the following are statements of c-*erb*-b2 onco-protein are true *except***

A. It is localized to chromosome 7.
B. EGFr cytoplasmic region is homologous to protein product of c-*erb*-b2.
C. It contains a highly protease-resistant extracellular domain.
D. It demonstrates intrinsic tyrosine kinase activity.

11. **All of the following are true of dextran-coated charcoal assay *except***

A. It uses the adsorptive properties of charcoal to remove small and large molecular weight compounds from solution at different rates.
B. Dextran is used to enhance the adsorptive properties of charcoal.
C. The method is widely used for quantification of most steroid receptors.
D. It forms the basis for most proficiency testing programs.

12. **All of the following methods may be used to measure steroid receptors *except***

A. sucrose density-gradient ultracentrifugation
B. hydroxyapatite assay
C. atomic absorption
D. high-performance liquid chromatography (HPLC)

13. **All of the following statements regarding immunoassays are true *except***

A. Development of monoclonal antibodies to receptors has facilitated development of clinical receptor assays.
B. Immunoassays give good correlation to biochemical methods for ER receptors.
C. Immunoassay results are independent of binding of E2 to the receptor.

D. Enzyme immunoassays (EIA) are the most sensitive and universally standardized ER receptor assays.

14. **All of the following are true of membrane-bound receptor analysis *except***

A. It requires tissue specimens for a sample.
B. Residual cytosol will produce artificially low results for some receptors (EGFr).
C. Western blot analysis is the most commonly used method.
D. Saturation and displacement assays require a relatively large amount of tissue.

15. **All of the following may cause errors in receptor measurements due to interference by nonreceptor binders *except***

A. albumin
B. corticosteroid-binding globulin
C. dithiothreitol
D. sex-hormone-binding globulin

16. **All of the following are true of familial hypercholesterolemia (FH) *except***

A. Mutations in the low-density lipoprotein (LDL) receptor gene can prevent expression of a normal LDL receptor.
B. About 1 of 500 people are heterozygous for an FH gene.
C. Patients with homozygous FH often have no LDL receptor and succumb to their disease by adolescence.
D. Heterozygous individuals for FH exhibit normal cholesterol levels and do not require treatment.

17. **All of the following are good features of prognostic markers *except***

A. provide information on tumor cell proliferation rate.
B. attainable by invasive surgery.
C. metastatic potential
D. responsiveness to chemotherapy

18. **All of the following may be associated with a favorable prognosis in breast cancer *except***

A. ER/PR positivity
B. negative lymph nodes
C. EGFr negativity
D. c-*erb*-b2 oncogene amplification

19. **All of the following are true of prostate cancer *except***

A. Hormone therapy produces a successful response in 80% of patients.
B. Androgen ablation may be accomplished through orchiectomy or ER therapy.

C. All tumors eventually become resistant to hormone therapy.

D. Receptors for androgens, ER, and PR are significant prognostic markers that need to be measured at the time of diagnosis.

20. Family history of diabetes mellitus is much more frequent in

A. type I

B. type II

C. insulin-dependent diabetes

D. infants

Indicate whether each of the following statements is true (T) or false (F).

21. Binding specificity describes the strength of attraction between ligand and receptor.

22. Samples for hormone receptor assay are heat-labile proteins and should be stored immediately in 4°C if they will be assayed within 1 hour.

23. Errors in receptor measurement may be caused by interference with nonreceptor binders such as albumin.

24. Metastatic endometrial carcinomas typically have low concentrations of ER and PR receptors.

25. Type I diabetes occurs in 80% to 90% of all diabetics and is the most common form of diabetes.

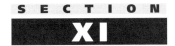

SECTION XI

BLOOD BANK/TRANSFUSION MEDICINE

68 Organization, Functions, Regulation, and Legal Concerns of Blood Banks
69 Blood Collection
70 Pretransfusion Testing
71 Blood Component Therapy
72 Transfusion Therapy
73 Neonatal Transfusion
74 Complications of Blood Transfusions
75 Immune Hemolysis

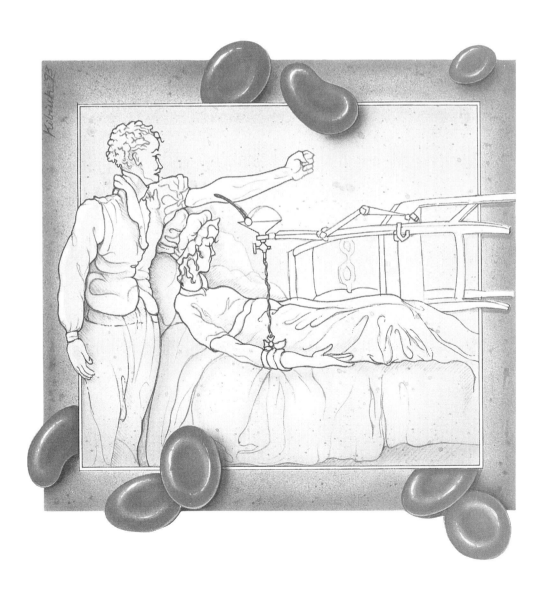

68

ORGANIZATION, FUNCTIONS, REGULATION, AND LEGAL CONCERNS OF BLOOD BANKS

QUESTIONS

Select the one best answer of the choices offered.

1. **Prior to 1945, which of the following blood group systems were known?**
   A. ABO, Rh, P, and MNS
   B. ABO, Duffy, P, MNS
   C. ABO, Kell, Rh, P
   D. ABO, Duffy, Lewis, MNS

2. **The Standards of the American Association of Blood Banks (AABB) defines a blood bank as an organization with the following responsibilities** *except*
   A. collection and storage of blood
   B. blood component preparation
   C. transfusion of blood and its components
   D. interstate distribution of blood components

3. **Therapeutic plasma exchange with fresh frozen plasma (FFP) is the treatment of choice for which of the following diseases?**
   A. Thyroid storm
   B. Thrombotic thrombocytopenic purpura (TTP)
   C. Disseminated intravascular coagulation (DIC)
   D. Systemic lupus erythematosus (SLE)

4. **The director of a hospital transfusion service is directly responsible for all of the following** *except*
   A. marketing and distribution of blood products
   B. quality control/quality improvement programs
   C. compliance with accrediting agencies
   D. consultant to clinical colleagues

5. **The AABB accreditation and inspection program is**
   A. mandatory by the Food and Drug Administration (FDA)
   B. required by the College of American Pathologists (CAP) for accreditation
   C. conducted every year, unannounced
   D. voluntary and conducted every 2 years

6. **Annual inspections by which agency are necessary for maintaining a transfusion medicine license?**
   A. AABB
   B. FDA
   C. Joint Commission on Accreditation of Healthcare Organizations (JCAHO)
   D. CAP

7. **Elements of a malpractice lawsuit include all of the following** *except*
   A. invasive procedures
   B. lack of compliance with the standard of care
   C. negligence by the defendant
   D. compensatory damages to plaintiff

8. **All of the following statements regarding informed consent for transfusion are true** *except*
   A. It is the physician's responsibility to explain risks and benefits of the transfusion.
   B. Patients are allowed to make an informed decision.
   C. Documentation is necessary to demonstrate the patient's awareness of the risks of transfusion.
   D. A progress note in the medical record is the most desirable to documentation.

Indicate whether each of the following statements is true (T) or false (F).

9. **Landsteiner recognized the ABO blood group system at the outset of the twentieth century.**

10. **The problems of anticoagulation, preservation, and storage of blood had to be solved before indirect transfusion could be accomplished.**

11. The advent of plastic transfusion equipment has not circumvented the complications of transfusion, such as pyrogen-related reactions and air embolism.

12. The American Red Cross and America's Blood Centers collect >90% of the blood transfused in the country.

13. Pretransfusion testing and issuance of blood to the patient for transfusion are the responsibility of the hospital transfusion service.

14. All transfusion facilities are required to register with the FDA and regulated by the Code of Federal Regulations.

15. FDA annual inspections of blood banks are announced as compared with the peer-conducted inspections of the AABB.

16. The JCAHO inspects all hospital laboratories, including blood banks.

17. Legislation defines blood transfusion as a sale of a product; therefore, blood banks may be held responsible in a malpractice lawsuit in the absence of proof of negligence.

18. The physician responsible for the patient's care is the one who bears the responsibility for explaining the risks and benefits of transfusion to the patient.

19. The consent form for a transfusion is the responsibility of the transfusion service.

20. A competent patient has the right to refuse transfusion.

69

BLOOD COLLECTION

QUESTIONS

Select the one best answer of the choices offered.

1. **The estimated American population is 270 million people. Approximately how many million people donate blood?**
   A. 150
   B. 50
   C. 8
   D. 1

2. **The minimal age requirement according to the American Association of Blood Banks (AABB) standards for allogeneic blood donation is ___ years old.**
   A. 16
   B. 17
   C. 21
   D. 25

3. **The maximum number of times allogeneic blood can be donated is**
   A. once every 3 days
   B. once every 2 weeks
   C. once every 4 weeks
   D. once every 8 weeks

4. **A prospective donor with a history of hepatitis before age 11 should be**
   A. eligible to donate blood
   B. deferred for 3 months
   C. deferred for 12 months
   D. permanently deferred

5. **All the following statements will result in 12-month deferral *except***
   A. exposure to hepatitis in household or by sex
   B. incarceration for >72 hours
   C. donor with antibody to hepatitis B surface antigen (HBsAg)
   D. skin or body piercing

6. **Which of the following medications is a cause for permanent deferral?**
   A. Acitretin (Soriatane)
   B. Etretinate (Tegison)
   C. Finasteride (Proscar)
   D. Isotretinoin (Accutane)

7. **The typical blood volume collected from a donor weighing >50 kg is ___ mL.**
   A. 300 to 350
   B. 350 to 400
   C. 450 to 500
   D. 600 to 650

8. **The AABB standards on blood donations requires all of the following tests *except***
   A. alanine aminotransferase (ALT)
   B. syphilis
   C. human immunodeficiency virus types 1 and 2 (HIV-1/HIV-2)
   D. human T-cell lymphotrophic virus types I and II (HTLV I/II)

9. **Severe vasovagal reactions from donors are characterized by**
   A. hypotension and bradycardia
   B. hypertension and bradycardia
   C. hypotension and tachycardia
   D. hypertension and tachycardia

10. **The minimal hemoglobin concentration for autologous blood donation is ___ g/dL.**
    A. 9.0
    B. 10.0
    C. 11.0
    D. 12.5

11. **Adenine-enriched anticoagulant solutions (AS-1) allow storage of red blood cells (RBCs) for ___ days.**
    A. 35
    B. 42

C. 53
D. 60

12. RBCs can be stored in a frozen state (less than −120°C) for

A. 1 year
B. 5 years
C. 10 years
D. indefinitely

13. Current leukoreduction filters can effectively reduce leukocytes from RBCs by

A. one log
B. two logs
C. three logs
D. four logs

14. Benefits of leukoreduction include all of the following *except*

A. prevention of graft versus host disease
B. reduce febrile transfusion reactions
C. provide "cytomegalovirus-safe" blood
D. decrease disease transmission of HTLV

15. Maximum storage time for platelets in a 20° to 24°C rotary incubator is ___ days.

A. 3
B. 5
C. 7
D. 10

16. Quality control requirements for platelets include

A. pH >5.2 and platelet count <5.5×10^9 in 50% of the platelet units tested
B. pH <6.2 and platelet count >4.0×10^9 in 75% of the platelet units tested
C. pH <6.2 and platelet count >5.5×10^{10} in 50% of the platelet units tested
D. pH >6.2 and platelet count >5.5×10^{10} in 75% of the platelet units tested

17. Cryoprecipitate is rich in all of the following *except*

A. von Willebrand factor (vWF)
B. fibrinogen
C. factor VII
D. factor VIII

18. A plateletpheresis donor complains of perioral numbness and tingling after the procedure. This is most likely due to

A. hypotension
B. hypertension
C. hypocalcemia
D. hypercalcemia

19. Plateletpheresis product should contain ___ platelets.

A. 3.0×10^{11}
B. 3.0×10^{10}
C. 5.5×10^{10}
D. 5.5×10^{11}

20. Therapeutic plasma exchange has been effective for all of the following *except*

A. disseminated intravascular coagulation (DIC)
B. Guillain-Barré syndrome
C. thrombotic thrombocytopenic purpura (TTP)
D. myasthenia gravis

Indicate whether each of the following statements is true (T) or false (F).

21. Two key components to the support of blood donation are convenient sites and a personal request.

22. It is easier to recruit a new blood donor than to retain a regular blood donor.

23. Blood donors can be deferred with a body temperature >37.5°C.

24. Blood from directed donations demonstrate greater safety with lower frequency of positive markers for infectious disease than the general blood donor pool.

25. Storage of RBCs leads to depletion of 2,3-diphosphoglycerate (2,3-DPG).

26. Washed RBCs have been used to treat patients with paroxysmal nocturnal hemoglobinuria.

27. A unit of fresh frozen plasma can be stored for a year below −18°C without appreciable loss of activity.

28. Cryoprecipitate should contain at least 80 mg of fibrinogen.

29. Apheresis donors can be drawn as often as every 48 hours, but no more than 24 times a year.

30. Granulocyte recovery in cytapheresis is improved with the administration of hydroxyethyl starch.

PRETRANSFUSION TESTING

QUESTIONS

Select the one best answer of the choices offered.

1. Elements of routine compatibility testing include all of the following *except*

   A. ABO and Rh typing of donor blood
   B. ABO and Rh typing of the intended recipient's blood
   C. recognition of unexpected antibodies to red blood cell (RBC) antigens in donor white cells
   D. comparison of current test results with records of previous tests

2. Antihuman globulin (AHG) tests are used to detect and antibodies that coat RBCs, but do not agglutinate them directly

   A. Immunoglobulin G (IgG) and anti-C3d
   B. IgG and anti-C3b
   C. IgM and anti-C3d
   D. IgM and anti-C3b

3. The indirect antiglobulin test (IAT) is used to detect and identify all of the following *except*

   A. unexpected antibodies in the serum of blood donors
   B. prospective transfusion recipients
   C. prenatal patients
   D. autoantibodies

4. The direct antiglobulin test (DAT) is used to detect antibodies bound to RBCs *in vivo* in all of the following *except*

   A. drugs
   B. infants with hemolytic disease of the newborn
   C. alloimmune response to a previous transfusion
   D. plateletpheresis donors

5. All the following statements regarding the ABO blood group are true *except*

   A. ABO locus is on chromosome 6.
   B. A and B genes are expressed codominantly.
   C. The four common ABO blood group phenotypes are A, B, AB, and O.
   D. O gene is an amorph.

6. Pretransfusion testing results of the forward and reverse reaction are depicted below. What is/are the possible phenotype(s)?

anti-A	anti-B	A RBCs	B RBCs
4+	4+	0	0

   A. A
   B. O or Bombay
   C. B
   D. AB

7. All of the following statements regarding the Lewis (Le) blood group are true *except*

   A. Anti-Le^a antibodies are present in Le^{a-b+} people
   B. Le^b individuals are secretors.
   C. Lewis antibodies are cold reacting IgMs.
   D. Le locus is present on chromosome 19.

8. Which Rh antigen in pretransfusion testing is routinely screened for?

   A. C
   B. E
   C. D
   D. f

9. Labeling of blood samples at the bedside must include all of the following *except*

   A. patient's first and last names
   B. unique hospital identification number
   C. date of collection and phlebotomists initials
   D. Do not resuscitate (DNR) status of patient

10. Transfusion of packed RBCs is requested by the medicine service. The patient has a history of being transfused 2 months prior at an outside hospital. Pretransfusion testing using blood collected no more than ___ days in advance may be used for serologic studies.

A. 3
B. 5
C. 7
D. 14

11. **Gel column technology for detecting RBC antigen–antibody interactions**

    A. requires centrifugation and addition of AHG reagent
    B. has higher sensitivity and specificity than standard tube method with low ionic strength saline (LISS)
    C. has a lower sensitivity and higher specificity than standard tube method with LISS
    D. is a more time-consuming procedure

12. **All the following statements regarding solid-phase adherence assays are true *except***

    A. RBCs pellet at the bottom of a well indicates a positive reaction.
    B. Antibodies or RBC membranes are coated on the wells.
    C. Direct and indirect solid-phase adherence assays are available for RBC serologic testing.
    D. Indirect tests detect unexpected antibodies to RBC antigens.

13. **Use of polyspecific AHG reagent with anticomplement activity may facilitate the detection of**

    A. Le^a and Le^b antibodies
    B. jk^a and jk^b antibodies
    C. Rh antibodies
    D. MNS antibodies

14. **All of the following statements regarding autocontrol are correct *except***

    A. It consists of testing the patient's serum against his or her own RBCs.
    B. It is a DAT.
    C. It may identify an alloimmune response.
    D. It is a routine component of pretransfusion testing.

15. **Major cross-match involves test between**

    A. donor's serum or plasma and recipient's RBCs
    B. donor's RBCs and recipient's serum or plasma
    C. recipient's serum or plasma with R1R1 screen cells
    D. donor's serum or plasma and A_1 RBCs

Indicate whether each of the following statements is true (T) or false (F).

16. **IgMs are naturally acquired antibodies found normally in plasma.**

17. **Landsteiner's law is the reciprocal relationship between antigens on RBCs and antibodies in the serum.**

18. **Blood from a weak D (D^u) positive donor is labeled Rh negative.**

19. **Blood samples used for compatibility testing must be kept at 1° to 6°C for 3 days after each transfusion.**

20. **LISS solution permits adequate detection of clinically significant antibodies after short incubation times (10 to 15 minutes).**

21. **DAT/autocontrol is a good predictive test for immune-mediated hemolysis in patients with clinical manifestations of hemolytic anemia.**

22. **The American Association of Blood Banks (AABB) does not require checking against previous compatibility testing records prior to release of blood for transfusion.**

23. **Electronic cross-match to detect ABO incompatibility is acceptable by the AABB.**

24. **A record of visual inspection of a unit of blood for transfusion should be performed prior to its release.**

25. **Verification of recipient identification, unit identification, ABO/Rh, and expiration date must be performed at the bedside before transfusion.**

71

BLOOD COMPONENT THERAPY

QUESTIONS

Select the one best answer of the choices offered.

1. The costs of obtaining a unit of blood have increased in recent years because of all of the following *except*

   A. transfusion safety issues
   B. cost of donor recruitment
   C. interstate taxes
   D. donor tests mandated by regulations

2. The development that revolutionized the practice of transfusion medicine was

   A. glass bottles
   B. sterile techniques
   C. universal precautions
   D. plastic, multiple-bag, closed system

3. Coagulation factors VIII and XIII and fibrinogen are precipitated when plasma is frozen at

   A. −1°C
   B. −8°C
   C. −12°C
   D. −18°C

4. Most methods for the freezing of red cells use

   A. citrate
   B. glycerol
   C. cadmium
   D. magnesium phosphate

5. Blood cells should be frozen within ___ days after collection.

   A. 2
   B. 4
   C. 6
   D. 10

6. Solvent detergent treatment is not effective in inactivating

   A. Parvovirus B19
   B. hepatitis B virus (HBV)
   C. human immunodeficiency virus (HIV)
   D. human T-cell lymphotrophic virus (HTLV)

7. A unit of whole blood has a total volume of approximately ___ mL.

   A. 350
   B. 500
   C. 650
   D. 850

8. The hematocrit value is about ___% in a unit of whole blood.

   A. 25
   B. 30
   C. 35
   D. 40

9. It is generally accepted that most healthy humans do not experience a compensatory significant increase in cardiac output until the hemoglobin value is below ___ g/dL.

   A. 3
   B. 7
   C. 9
   D. 12

10. There is no evidence that wound healing is impaired until a hematocrit value of ___% is reached.

    A. 38
    B. 28
    C. 20
    D. 17

11. For a red blood cell product to be designated "leukocyte poor," ___% of the white blood cells must be removed.

    A. 20
    B. 30
    C. 50
    D. 70

12. The standards of the American Association of Blood Banks (AABB) state that platelet preparations from whole blood shall contain a minimum of ___ platelets in at least 75% of the units.
    A. 5.5×10^{10}
    B. 5.5×10^5
    C. 4.5×10^8
    D. 3.2×10^6

13. Each bag of platelet concentrate contains ___ mL of platelets and plasma.
    A. 50 to 60
    B. 70 to 90
    C. 110 to 140
    D. 130 to 170

14. Each unit of platelet concentrate will increase the circulating platelet count by approximately ___/μL in an average 70-kg person.
    A. 2,000
    B. 4,500
    C. 7,500
    D. 9,500

15. In general, if the platelet count exceeds ___/μL, the patient is unlikely to bleed intraoperatively.
    A. 6,000
    B. 18,000
    C. 28,000
    D. 50,000

16. All of the following clinical situations are associated with platelet dysfunction *except*
    A. uremia
    B. anemia
    C. aspirin use
    D. semisynthetic penicillin

17. Platelet dysfunction in uremia is a defect in ___
    A. thrombin
    B. platelet factor 3
    C. platelet factor 1
    D. fibrin

18. Indications for use of leukocyte-poor platelets include all of the following *except*
    A. ameliorate the symptoms of febrile nonhemolytic reactions in sensitized patients
    B. ameliorate febrile nonhemolytic reaction in non-sensitized patients
    C. prevent development of a refractory state
    D. decrease exposure to viruses known to reside in white blood cells

19. Platelets can be successfully frozen and then thawed for transfusion up to ___ years later.
    A. 3
    B. 5
    C. 7
    D. 9

20. Fresh frozen plasma (FFP) is defined as plasma separated from the red blood cells of a donor within ___ hours after donation and held at −18°C or lower.
    A. 2
    B. 4
    C. 6
    D. 8

21. According to the Food and Drug Administration (FDA), a unit of FFP should be transfused within ___ hours.
    A. 2
    B. 4
    C. 6
    D. 8

Indicate whether each of the following statements is true (T) or false (F).

22. Granulocyte transfusions are indicated for severely and persistently neutropenic patients (<250 granulocytes/μL).

23. Adoptive immunotherapy is an attempt to reconstitute immune competence.

24. Lymphokine-activated killer (LAK) cells are generated after short-term incubation with interleukin-2 (IL-2).

25. FFP that has been thawed at 30° to 37°C and then not transfused within 48 hours can be relabeled " single donor plasma."

26. If cryoprecipitate is removed from a unit of whole blood or FFP, such plasma is deficient in factors VIII and XIII, fibrinogen, and fibronectin.

27. The protein largely found in a plasma protein fraction is fibrinogen.

28. About 15 g of albumin is synthesized in the steady state.

29. The most common causes of hypoalbuminemia are burns, chronic hepatic disease, chronic protein-losing enteropathy, and acute nephroses.

30. Serious bleeding episodes generally are associated with factor VIII levels <13% of normal.

72

TRANSFUSION THERAPY

QUESTIONS

Select the one best answer of the choices offered.

1. **Patients with platelet counts <5,000 to 10,000 μL are at ___ risk of hemorrhage.**

   A. no
   B. insignificant (slight)
   C. moderate
   D. significant

2. **A formula to evaluate response of platelet transfusion is the corrected count increment (CCI), which is given by**

   A. [(posttransfusion platelet count/μL − pretransfusion platelet count/μL)] ÷ number of platelets transfused $\times 10^{11}$
   B. [(posttransfusion platelet count/μL − pretransfusion platelet count/μL) × body surface area (BSA)] ÷number of platelets transfused $\times 10^{11}$
   C. [(posttransfusion platelet count/μL − pretransfusion platelet count/μL) × BSA] ÷ number of platelets transfused $\times 10^{10}$
   D. [(posttransfusion platelet count/μL) × BSA] ÷ number of platelets transfused $\times 10^{11}$

3. **A practical definition of massive transfusion in adults is**

   A. transfusion of ≥10 units of red blood cells (RBC)s within 24 hours
   B. transfusion of 30% of the patient's blood volume
   C. transfusion of ≥6 units of RBCs within 24 hours
   D. transfusion of 50% of the patient's blood volume

4. **A 26-year-old woman in a motor vehicle accident (MVA) has a hemoglobin of 6 g/dL. Until type and cross-match are performed, the best treatment option is**

   A. give colloids and transfuse with O-positive blood
   B. transfuse with O-positive blood
   C. give crystalloids until ABO-compatible blood is available
   D. transfuse with O-negative blood

5. **Every unit of RBCs contains about ___ mg of iron.**

   A. 20 to 40
   B. 40 to 80
   C. 120 to 180
   D. 200 to 250

6. **Autologous blood transfusion is transfusion of**

   A. blood from unrelated donors
   B. recipient's own blood
   C. blood from family members
   D. blood from wife or husband

7. **Acute normovolemic hemodilution refers to the collection of units of blood immediately prior to surgery with simultaneous**

   A. homologous transfusion of red cells
   B. transfusion of platelets
   C. autologous blood transfusion
   D. volume replacement using crystalloid or colloid solutions

8. **Individuals with posttransfusion purpura classically are**

   A. HPA-1a (PL^{A1}) antigen positive
   B. nulliparous females
   C. HPA-1a (PL^{A1}) antigen negative
   D. males with no history of previous transfusion

9. **A patient receives 6 units of random donor platelets. There is no increase in 24-hour posttransfusion platelet count. The next best step is**

   A. transfuse 6 units of random donor platelets every 12 hours
   B. transfuse with compatible single donor platelets
   C. transfuse with HLA-matched platelets
   D. perform platelet count 1 hour posttransfusion

10. **In the HLA matching nomenclature, a match grade of C is**

    A. Two donor antigens are identical to recipient antigens; third and fourth donor antigens are both cross-reactive with recipient antigens.
    B. All four donor antigens are identical to those of the recipient.
    C. Three donor antigens are identical to those of the recipient; fourth donor and recipient antigens are nonidentical and non–cross-reactive.
    D. Three donor antigens are identical to recipient antigens; fourth donor antigen is unknown.

11. **Intravenous administration of vitamin K will reverse anticoagulant effects of warfarin within ___ hours.**

    A. Immediately
    B. 6 to 8
    C. 12 to 24
    D. 48 to 72

12. **von Willebrand factor (vWF) synthesized by endothelial cells is stored in**

    A. dense granules of platelets
    B. Weibel-Palade bodies
    C. Nemaline bodies
    D. Russell bodies

13. **Desmopressin (DDAVP) is contraindicated in which subtype of von Willebrand disease?**

    A. Type I
    B. Type IIA
    C. Type IIB
    D. Type III

14. **Prophylaxis of transfusion-associated graft versus host disease (TA-GVHD) is achieved by**

    A. ultraviolet light (UVB)
    B. β-radiation
    C. leukoreduction filters
    D. γ-radiation

15. **The maximum time 1 unit of RBCs typically can be transfused in a patient without evidence of congestive heart failure (CHF) is ___ hours.**

    A. 1 to 2
    B. 4 to 6
    C. 8 to 10
    D. >10

Indicate whether each of the following statements is true (T) or false (F).

16. **One unit of RBCs will raise the hemoglobin by approximately 3 g/dL.**

17. **The approximate level for many coagulation factor required for hemostasis is 20% to 30%.**

18. **A typical dose of cryoprecipitate is One unit per 10 kg of body weight.**

19. **Immunoglobulin M (IgM) antibodies typically cause warm autoimmune hemolytic anemia (WAIHA).**

20. **Platelet transfusion in immune thrombocytopenic purpura (ITP) is of limited value.**

21. **Platelet transfusions are contraindicated in thrombotic thrombocytopenic purpura (TTP).**

22. **Hemolysis, elevated liver enzymes, and low platelet count (HELLP) syndrome develops in 4% to 12% of women with preeclampsia or eclampsia at the end of pregnancy.**

23. **Proteins C and S are vitamin-K–independent coagulation proteins synthesized by the liver.**

24. **A patient with blood group AB transplanted with stem cells from a blood group B donor can be transfused with group O blood.**

25. **Generally, normal (0.9%) saline, lactated Ringer, and glucose solutions all can be added to blood components during infusion.**

NEONATAL TRANSFUSION

QUESTIONS

Select the one best answer of the choices offered.

1. **Pretransfusion testing for infants <4 months of age should include**

   A. forward and reverse typing
   B. forward typing only
   C. antibody identification
   D. direct antiglobulin test (DAT)

2. **The prevalence of the Rh-negative genotype is ___% in Caucasians.**

   A. 1
   B. 6
   C. 10
   D. 15

3. **The prevalence of the Rh-negative genotype is ___% in African-Americans**

   A. 0.3
   B. 5.0
   C. 8
   D. 15

4. **Fetal maternal hemorrhage (FMH) >30 mL may occur in ___% of pregnancies.**

   A. 1
   B. 10
   C. 30
   D. 50

5. **Patients at risk for large FMH include all of the following *except***

   A. amniocentesis
   B. twin gestation
   C. manual removal of placenta
   D. ectopic pregnancy

6. **All of the following statements regarding the Kleihauer-Betke test are true *except***

   A. Fetal hemoglobin cells resists acid elution.
   B. It is a screening test that provides a qualitative index of FMH.
   C. It quantifies fetal red cells in the maternal blood.
   D. It is useful in calculating the dose of Rh immune globulin (RhIG) to administer.

7. **In a term infant, exchange transfusion should be performed in all of the following situations *except***

   A. cord hemoglobin >110 g/dL
   B. serum bilirubin >20 mg/dL
   C. cord bilirubin >4 mg/dL
   D. increase of bilirubin ≥0.5 mg/dL/h

8. **Factors that are known to decrease bilirubin binding and predispose to kernicterus include all of the following *except***

   A. low birth weight
   B. hypothermia
   C. hyperthermia
   D. sepsis

9. **All of the following statements regarding neonatal alloimmune thrombocytopenia (NAIT) are true *except***

   A. Adjuvant therapy with steroids and/or intravenous immunoglobulins may be beneficial.
   B. Transfusion of washed maternal platelets to infant may be necessary.
   C. HPA-1a (PL^{A1}) antibodies is the most common cause in Caucasians.
   D. First-born infants are not affected.

10. **All the following statements regarding transfusion-associated graft versus host disease are true *except***

    A. It is reported in infants following transfusions of blood products from relatives.
    B. Hypercellular bone marrow is commonly present.
    C. Human immunodeficiency virus (HIV)-infected patients are not at risk.
    D. γ-Irradiation is an effective prophylaxis.

Indicate whether each of the following statements is true (T) or false (F).

11. **Very-low-birth-weight infants is defined as <1,500 g.**

12. **Physiologic indicators of significant anemia, such as tachypnea, tachycardia, and lethargy, correlate well to hemoglobin levels and response to blood transfusions.**

13. **All blood components obtained from biologic parents and siblings should be irradiated prior to transfusion.**

14. **Infants with kernicterus have deposits of lipid-soluble free bilirubin in the basal ganglion and cerebellum.**

15. **An infant with blood type B born to a mother with blood type AB is at an increased risk of ABO hemolytic disease of the newborn (HDN).**

16. **Thrombocytopenia is defined as a platelet count <100×10^9/L.**

17. **Fresh frozen plasma (FFP) is indicated for treatment of hypovolemic shock in neonates.**

18. **A neonate with necrotizing enterocolitis (NEC) is at increased risk of T-antigen activation.**

19. **Transmission of hepatitis G virus after neonatal transfusion causes significant liver disease and mortality.**

20. **γ-Irradiation is effective in preventing cytomegalovirus (CMV) transmission.**

COMPLICATIONS OF BLOOD TRANSFUSIONS

QUESTIONS

Select the one best answer of the choices offered.

1. The most common cause of transfusion-related fatalities reported to the Food and Drug Administration (FDA) during 1990 to 1998 is

   A. bacterial contamination
   B. hemolysis
   C. transfusion-associated graft versus host disease (TAGVHD)
   D. transfusion-related acute lung injury (TRALI)

2. Initial laboratory evaluation of transfusion reaction should include all of the following steps *except*

   A. direct antiglobulin test (DAT)
   B. clerical check
   C. antibody identification
   D. visual inspection

3. Febrile nonhemolytic transfusion reaction in the first phase demonstrates all of the following *except*

   A. cough
   B. tachycardia
   C. neutrophilic leukocytosis
   D. palpitations

4. TRALI is associated with all of the following signs and/or symptoms except

   A. Respiratory distress
   B. Pulmonary edema
   C. Hypotension
   D. Increased pulmonary capillary wedge pressure

5. All of the following statements regarding urticarial transfusion reaction are true *except*

   A. It is a type IV hypersensitivity reaction.
   B. It is an immunoglobulin E (IgE)-mediated response.
   C. Transfusion may be continued in most instances.

   D. It is characterized by hives and pruritus in the absence of fever.

6. Severe allergic reactions that culminate in acute anaphylaxis is mediated by anti-___ antibodies

   A. IgG
   B. IgA
   C. IgE
   D. IgM

7. The most common microorganism contaminating red blood cells (RBCs) is

   A. *Escherichia coli*
   B. *Proteus mirabilis*
   C. *Yersinia enterocolitica*
   D. *Staphylococcus epidermidis*

8. The classic definition of delayed hemolytic transfusion reactions includes all of the following findings *except*

   A. compatible cross-match with pretransfusion serum
   B. negative antibody screen on the recipient pretransfusion serum
   C. history of blood transfusion
   D. nulliparous

9. Posttransfusion purpura (PTP) is a syndrome of profound thrombocytopenia occurring ____ days after transfusion.

   A. 1 to 2
   B. 3 to 5
   C. 5 to 14
   D. 14 to 21

10. Nucleic acid testing (NAT) would reduce the window period of human immunodeficiency virus (HIV) types 1 and 2 to ____ days.

    A. 6 to 11
    B. 11 to 22

C. 35 to 47

D. 41 to 53

Indicate whether each of the following statements is true (T) or false (F).

11. **Elevation of 1°C accompanied by chills is indicative of an acute hemolytic transfusion reaction.**

12. **Prestorage leukocyte reduction decreases the frequency of febrile nonhemolytic transfusion reactions (FNHTRs).**

13. **The most effective way to prevent FNHTRs is bedside leukocyte filtration.**

14. **Hypotensive reactions occur more frequently following platelet transfusions than red cell transfusions.**

15. **Delayed hemolytic transfusion reactions refer to nonimmune hemolysis of red cells days to weeks after transfusion.**

16. **TAGVHD has been reported in immunocompetent and immunosuppressed patients.**

17. **Solvent detergent treatment of blood donor components is an effective treatment for inactivation of viral hepatitis A.**

18. **Transfusion-transmitted hepatitis C accounts for approximately 7% of the 3.9 million infected persons, with a 1:120,000 risk per unit transfused prior to NAT.**

19. **Hepatitis D is a defective RNA passenger virus that requires hepatitis C as a "helper" for assembling envelope proteins.**

20. **The P blood group antigen is a Parvovirus B19 receptor.**

IMMUNE HEMOLYSIS

QUESTIONS

Select the one best answer of the choices offered.

1. **All of the following are common laboratory findings in immune hemolysis** *except*

   A. decrease in hematocrit and hemoglobin
   B. increase in serum lactate dehydrogenase (LDH)
   C. decrease in serum haptoglobin
   D. peripheral blood smear with macrocytosis

2. **Paroxysmal cold hemoglobinuria (PCH) is caused by**

   A. anti-i
   B. anti-P
   C. anti-I
   D. anti-e

3. **Cold agglutinin syndrome due to autoanti-I is seen most commonly after**

   A. platelet transfusion
   B. Epstein-Barr virus (EBV) infection
   C. *Mycoplasma pneumoniae* infection
   D. cytomegalovirus (CMV) infection

4. **All of the following statements regarding Donath-Landsteiner antibody are true** *except*

   A. It is an immunoglobulin M (IgM) alloantibody with wide thermal amplitude.
   B. It is a biphasic hemolysin autoantibody.
   C. Transfusions rarely are necessary.
   D. It is an anti-P antibody.

5. **The prototype drug to induce hapten-dependent immune hemolysis is**

   A. procainamide
   B. quinidine
   C. α-methyldopa
   D. penicillin

6. **Which type of drug-related immune hemolysis would have a positive eluate?**

   A. Type I
   B. Type II
   C. Type III
   D. None of the above

7. **A patient receiving a high dose of penicillin is noted to have a decreasing hemoglobin and hematocrit (H&H). Routine serum testing will show**

   A. increased serum haptoglobin
   B. hypobilirubinemia
   C. positive direct antiglobulin test (DAT)
   D. negative DAT

8. **Symptoms of an acute hemolytic transfusion reaction (HTR) include all of the following except**

   A. fever and chills
   B. hypotension
   C. bone marrow hypoplasia
   D. respiratory distress

9. **Which of the following blood group systems is notorious for delayed HTR?**

   A. Kidd
   B. MNS
   C. Chido
   D. Lewis

10. **All of the following are commonly occurring antibodies that are not known to cause hemolytic disease of the newborn (HDN) except**

    A. anti-Le^a
    B. anti-Le^b
    C. anti-K
    D. anti-P

11. **A reading in zone three of the Liley graph indicates**

    A. low level of bilirubin in the amniotic fluid
    B. high level of bilirubin in the amniotic fluid
    C. mild or no significant destruction of fetal red blood cells (RBCs)
    D. low risk of hydrops fetalis

12. **A standard dose of Rh immune globulin (RhIG) consists of 300 μg of anti-D, which is able to cover**

    A. 15 mL of fetal whole blood
    B. 30 mL of fetal whole blood
    C. 30 mL of fetal RBCs
    D. 50 ml of fetal RBCs

13. **A 76kg, 28-year-old, G2P1, O-negative mother delivers a healthy term B-positive baby girl. Rosette test is positive. The Kleihauer-Betke test is 3.0%. What dose of RhIG should the mother receive?**

    A. 2
    B. 3
    C. 4
    D. 5

14. **Routine administration of RhIG after delivery has reduced the production of anti-D in pregnant women from 13% to**

    A. 0.1%
    B. 1.0%
    C. 5.0%
    D. 10.0%

15. **Antepartum (28 weeks and of gestation) and postpartum administration of RhIG to nonsensitized Rh-negative women will reduce the risk of developing anti-D to:**

    A. 0.05%
    B. 0.1%
    C. 1.0%
    D. 5.0%

Indicate whether each of the following statements is true (T) or false (F).

16. **IgM antibodies bound to red blood mediate extravascular immune hemolysis cells (RBCs) that are subsequently removed from the circulation by the reticuloendothelial system.**

17. **Cold autoimmune hemolytic anemia (AIHA) is the most common form of AIHA.**

18. **Warm autoimmune hemolytic anemia (WAIHA) may occur with no underlying disease or as a secondary phenomenon associated with chronic lymphocytic leukemia (CLL).**

19. **The presence of an alloantibody can be ruled out in a patient with WAIHA.**

20. **Autologous adsorption removes autoantibody from sensitized RBCs.**

21. **A patient with fever and chills during transfusion has an acute HTR.**

22. **Monitoring a rise in antibody titration for the risk of hemolytic disease of the newborn is an excellent predictor of disease severity.**

23. **Percutaneous umbilical sampling (PUBS) is the most accurate way to determine the severity of hemolysis.**

24. **Cord blood sample collected from the infant usually is stored in the blood bank/transfusion service for a minimum of 7 days.**

25. **Blood used for intrauterine transfusions should be as fresh as possible, irradiated, and CMV negative.**

ANSWERS TO THE QUESTIONS

CHAPTER 1

1. C (P. 3, Column 2)
2. B (p. 3, column 2)
3. B (p. 4, column 2)
4. B (p. 5, column 1)
5. D (p. 5, column 2, Fig. 1.1)
6. B (p. 6, column 1)
7. B (p. 6, column 2, Fig. 1.4)
8. D (p. 8, column 1)
9. B (p. 9, column 1)
10. A (p. 9, column 2, Fig. 1.9)
11. A (p. 10, column 1)
12. C (p. 10, column 1)
13. C (p. 10, column 2)
14. C (p. 11, column 2)
15. B (p. 12, column 2)
16. D (p. 14, column 1, Table 1.2)

17. A (p. 15, column 2)
18. D (p. 15, column 2, Fig. 1.14)
19. C (p. 16, column 2)
20. A (p. 17, column 1)
21. B (p. 17, column 1)
22. D (p. 17, column 2)
23. D (p. 18, column 2)
24. C (p. 18, column 2)
25. D (p. 20, Fig. 1.18)
26. B (p. 22, column 1)
27. A (p. 22, column 2)
28. C (p. 23, column 1)
29. A (p. 24, column 1)
30. D (p. 24, column 2)
31. T (p. 24, column 1)
32. F (p. 28, column 1)
33. F (p. 28, column 2)
34. T (p. 29, column 1)

	Management		
Elements	**Ideas**	**Things**	**People**
Tasks	Conceptual thinking	Administration	Leadership
Continuous Functions	Analyze problems	Make decisions	Communicate
Definitions of continuous functions	Gather facts, ascertain causes. develop alternatives	Arrive at conclusions and judgements	Ensure understanding
Sequential functions	**Plan**	**Organize and staff**	**Direct** / **Control**
Activities	Set objectives — Define performance standards — Develop strategies — Prepare budgets	Organize work-flow and tasks — Establish organizational structure — Select and schedule staff	Monitor performance against established standards — Take actions to bring system under control

FIGURE 1.1. The management process. (From Hartwick DF. *Directing the clinical laboratory.* New York: Field and Wood, 1990:2, with permission.)

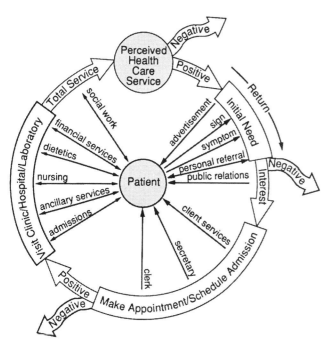

FIGURE 1.9. Patient health care provider "life cycle." (Modified from Gronroos C. *Service management and marketing.* Lexington, MA: DC Heath, 1990:130.)

35. F (p. 29, column 2, Table 1.4)
36. T (p. 29, column 2, Table 1.4)
37. T (p. 31, column 2, Table 1.7)
38. F (p. 32, column 2)
39. T (p. 35, column 1, Figs. 1.A1 and 1.A3)
40. T (p. 37, column 2)

CHAPTER 2

1. C (p. 49, column 1)
2. A (p. 49, column 2)
3. C (p. 51, column 2)
4. D (p. 51, Table 2.1)
5. B (p. 52, column 1)
6. B (p. 53, column 2, Table 2.2)
7. A (p. 55, column 2)
8. D (p. 57, column 1, Table 2.4)
9. C (p. 60, column 2, Table 2.5)
10. A (p. 65, column 1)
11. B (p. 66, column 2)
12. F (p. 49, column 2)
13. T (p. 51, column 2)
14. F (p. 51, column 2)
15. F (p. 54, column 1)
16. T (p. 54, column 1)
17. F (p. 57, column 1)
18. T (p. 58, column 1)
19. T (p. 59, column 1)
20. F (p. 60, column 1)

TABLE 2.2. KEY ELEMENTS NECESSARY FOR DEVELOPMENT OF AN INTEGRATED DELIVERY SYSTEM (IDS)

An IDS requires these qualities to allow it to be clinically and fiscally responsible for the health of the defined population:

- The organization must be patient centered.
- Physicians and nonphysician providers who order tests and service must be directly involved.
- The hub of the IDS needs to be the whole system, not one site.
- Information systems must link each operating site.
- The organization must be able to assess the needs of the population it serves.
- The system must adapt quickly when conditions warrant change.
- The system must be based on a cross-function/cross-service line structure.
- Those affiliated with the system must be multiskilled.
- The organization's focus needs to be on the continuum of care, not in the acute care hospital.
- The system must be able to improve continuously.
- Clinical decision making must be based on the clinical staff's approved evidence-based protocols.
- Incentives and compensation must reward appropriate behavior.

CHAPTER 3

1. D (p. 78, column 2)
2. C (p. 79, column 1)
3. D (p. 80, column 1)
4. D (p. 82, column 1, Fig. 3.1)

TABLE 2.5. DEFINITION OF A PROVIDER

An entity authorized to receive direct (or indirect "incident to" reimbursement) such as a

Hospital Rural care primary hospital Skilled nursing facility Home health agency Hospice	with an agreement to participate in Medicare

or a

Clinic Rehabilitation agency Public health agency	with an agreement to furnish outpatient services

or a practitioner who is a

Physician
Nonphysician practitioner
  (e.g., optometrist, podiatrist)
Nurse (clinician, practitioner,
  specialist)
Physician's assistant
Clinical psychologist
Clinical social worker
Medical nutrition support
Physical occupational therapist
	with a provider number furnished by the Health Care Financing Administration (HCFA) or a managed care organization

FIGURE 3.1. Informational signs for accident prevention formatted according to regulations of the Occupational Safety and Health Administration.

5. A (p. 84, column 1)
6. B (p. 83, column 1)
7. D (p. 82, column 2)
8. D (p. 84, column 1, Fig. 3.3)
9. A (p. 84, column 2, Table 3.2)
10. B (p. 84, column 2)
11. F (p. 84, column 2)
12. T (p. 85, column 2)
13. F (p. 87, column 1)
14. T (p. 90, column 2)
15. F (p. 91, column 1)
16. T (p. 91, column 2)
17. F (p. 92, column 2)
18. T (p. 94, column 1)
19. T (p. 94, column 2)
20. F (p. 95, column 1)

CHAPTER 4

1. A (p. 97, column 1)
2. A (p. 97, column 1)
3. B (p. 97, column 2)

TABLE 3.2. MAXIMUM ALLOWABLE SIZES OF CONTAINERS OF IGNITABLE LIQUIDS

Ignitability Class	Glass	Metal or Approved Plastic	Safety Can
IA	1 pt (0.473 L)	1 gal (3.8 L)	2 gal (7.9 L)
IB	1 gal (3.8 L)	5 gal (19.0 L)	5 gal (19.0 L)
IC	1 gal (3.8 L)	5 gal (19.0 L)	5 gal (19.0 L)
II	1 gal (3.8 L)	5 gal (19.0 L)	5 gal (19.0 L)
III	5 gal (19.0 L)	5 gal (19.0 L)	5 gal (19.0 L)

Adapted from NFPA 30. *Flammable and combustible liquids code,* 1996. Quincy, MA: National Fire Protection Association, 1996, with permission. This reprinted material is not the complete and official position of the National Fire Protection Association on the referenced subject, which is represented only by the standard in its entirety.

4. C (p 97, column 2)
5. B (p 99, column 1)
6. B (p. 99, Table 4.2)
7. D (p. 100, column 2)
8. B (p. 101, column 1)
9. E (p. 101, column 1)
10. C (p. 101, column 2)
11. A (p. 101, column 2)
12. A (p. 101, column 2)
13. B (p. 102, column 1)
14. A (p. 102, column 2)
15. D (p. 103, column 1)
16. E (p. 103, Table 4.3)
17. B (p. 104, Table 4.4)
18. A (p. 104, column 1)
19. D (p. 104, Table 4.5)
20. B (p. 105, column 1)
21. B (p. 105, column 2)
22. C (p. 105, column 2)
23. C (p. 107, column 2)
24. A (p. 107, column 2)

TABLE 4.2. CIRCADIAN RHYTHMS IN SELECTED ANALYTES

Analyte[a]	Time of Peak Concentration[b]	Percent Change[c]
Serum		
Sodium	1300	2
Potassium	1100	19
Glucose	1800	59
Phosphorus	2200	38
Urea nitrogen	2300	25
Cholesterol	2200	11
Total bilirubin	0700	62
Total protein	1800	8
γ-glutamyltransferase	1000	960
Thyroid-stimulating hormone	0200	206
Cortisol	0730	1111
Melatonin	0300	211
Iron	1208	32
Aldosterone	0800	95
Whole blood		
Total white blood cells	1900	38
Red blood cells	0430	10
Lymphocytes	0130	67
Neutrophils	1700	61
CD4+ cells	0030	51
Urine		
Volume	0300	278
Specific gravity	1600	193
Calcium	1600	333
Creatinine	2108	30
Sodium	2012	54

[a]All analytes demonstrated statistically significant circadian rhythms in healthy middle-aged male subjects (11).
[b]Peak times are given as local clock times.
[c]Percentage of changes in analyte concentration are calculated as [(peak concentration – trough concentration)/daily mean concentration)] × 100.
Data from reference 11.

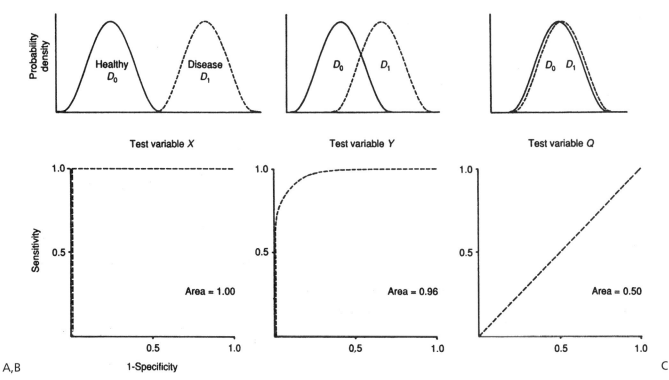

FIGURE 4.10. Receiver operating characteristic (ROC) curves for three tests of differing discriminatory power. The distribution of analyte values in healthy and diseased groups and the corresponding ROC curves are shown for a perfect test (i.e., with 100% clinical accuracy) **(A)**, a typical test that has adequate discriminatory power but will give some false-positive and F-negative results **(B)**, and a test that does no better than chance at discriminating healthy and diseased subjects **(C)**. (Redrawn from Strike PW. *Measurement in laboratory medicine.* Oxford, UK: Butterworth-Heinemann, 1996.)

25. C (p. 109, column 2)
26. B (p. 109, column 2)
27. A (p. 110, column 1)
28. B (p. 110, column 2)
29. B (p. 113, column 2)
30. A (p. 113, column 2)
31. B (p. 113, column 2)
32. D (p. 114, column 2)
33. B (p. 115, Fig. 4.10)

34. B (p. 117, column 1)
35. A (p. 117, column 2)

CHAPTER 5

1. B (p. 123, column 1, Fig. 5.6)
2. B (p. 123, column 1)
3. B (p. 126, column 2)

Integrated report example

Patient demographics	Case worker
Gross pictures	Gross description
Microscopic picture	Microscopic description or comment
Molecular or Flow cytometry studies and special procedures.	
Final Diagnosis (with integrated comment)	

FIGURE 5.6. Integrated report example.

4. B (p. 128, column 1)
5. D (p. 130, column 1)
6. A (p. 130, column 2)
7. B (p. 130, column 2)
8. B (p. 130, column 2)
9. A (p. 132, column 1)
10. B (p. 132, column 1)

CHAPTER 6

1. 1. B (p. 134, column 1)
2. B (p. 134, column 2)
3. B (p. 135, column 1)
4. A (p. 135, column 1)
5. C (p. 135, column 1)
6. C (p. 135, column 1)
7. A (p. 136, column 1)
8. A (p. 136, column 1)
9. B (p. 136, column 1)
10. D (p. 136, column 2)
11. B (p. 137, column 1)
12. A (p. 137, column 2)
13. A (p. 137, column 2)
14. B (p. 137, column 2)
15. A (p. 138, column 1)
16. C (p. 138, column 1)
17. A (p. 138, column 2)
18. C (p. 138, column 2)
19. D (p. 139, column 2)
20. B (p. 139, column 2)
21. D (p. 140, column 2)
22. A (p. 141, column 1)

CHAPTER 7

1. D (p. 145, column 1, Fig. 7.5)
2. D (p. 145, column 2)
3. B (p. 146, column 2)
4. A (p. 147, column 1)
5. C (p. 147, column 2)
6. A (p. 148, column 1)
7. C (p. 148, column 1)
8. D (p. 149, column 1)
9. C (p. 151, column 1)
10. A (p. 151, column 1)
11. B (p. 151, column 1)
12. D (p. 152, column 1)
13. C (p. 153, column 2)
14. B (p. 155, column 1)
15. A (p. 156, column 2)
16. A (p. 156, column 2)
17. B (p. 156, column 2)
18. C (p. 156, column 2)

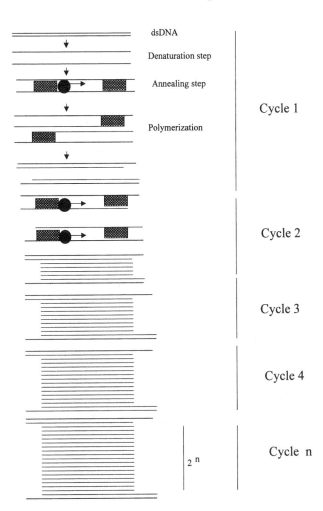

FIGURE 7.5. Polymerase chain reaction (PCR). Each cycle of the PCR is composed of denaturation of double-stranded DNA by heat, followed by annealing of primers (checkered boxes) to the complementary target sequence. Annealing is favored by lowering the temperature of the reaction below the melting temperature (Tm) of the primer pair. The last step in the cycle is extension by a thermostable DNA polymerase. After one cycle, the number of target copies is doubled. After two cycles, the number of copies of the target sequence is quadruplicated. After 20 cycles, the number of target copies could reach one million.

CHAPTER 8

1. C (p. 164, column 1)
2. A (p. 165, column 1)
3. B (p. 165, column 2)
4. E (p. 167, Table 8.3)
5. C (p. 167, Table 8.3)
6. D (p. 167, Table 8.3)
7. B (p. 167, Table 8.3)
8. A (p. 167, Table 8.3)
9. E (p. 167, Table 8.3)
10. B (p. 167, Table 8.3)
11. D (p. 167, Table 8.3)
12. A (p. 167, Table 8.3)

TABLE 8.3. RANGE OF MUTATION TYPES IN THE CFTR GENE

Mutation	Type	Description
R117H, G551D	Point (missense)	Amino acid codon to new amino acid codon in exons 4 and 11; R117H is phenotypically mild, G551D severe
G542X, W1282X	Point (nonsense)	Amino acid codon to stop codon in exons 11 and 20
ΔF508	Deletion (nonframeshift)	Loss of amino acid phenylalanine at CFTR residue 508
3659delC[a]	Deletion (frameshift)	Amino acid codon to frameshift in exon 19
3100insA	Insertion (frameshift)	Amino acid codon to frameshift in exon 16
621 + 1G > T[a]	Splice junction	G > T at first nucleotide of intron 4
3849+ 10kbG > T[a]	Splice junction	Mutation at considerable distance (10 kb) from splice junction activates cryptic splicing in intron 19
CF50kbdel#1	Large deletion	Complex deletion involving exons 4–7 and 11–18

[a]For these mutations, the numbers used are nucleotides numbered from the 5′ end of mature mRNA, not amino acid numbers; "silent" nucleotide polymorphisms that do not lead to a change of amino acid are also numbered using nucleotide numbers.
CFTR, cystic fibrosis transmembrane conductance regulator.

TABLE 8.4. COMMON DISORDERS ASSOCIATED WITH DIFFERENT TYPES OF GENETIC MUTATIONS

Type of Mutation	Disease	Genes Affected
"Point" mutations (to include small insertions or deletions of one or more nucleotides)	α Thalassemia	α-globin
	β Thalassemia	β-globin
	Cystic fibrosis	CFTR
	Duchenne/Becker muscular dystrophy	Dystrophin
	Gaucher disease	Glucocerebrosidase
	Hemophilia A	Factor VIII
	Hereditary hemochromatosis	HFE
	Hypercoagulability—factor V Leiden	Factor V
	Hypercoagulability—factor II	Prothrombin (factor II)
	Neurofibromatosis, type I	Neurofibromin
	Sickle cell anemia	β-globin
Splice junction mutations	β Thalassemia	β-globin
	Cystic fibrosis	CFTR
Intragenic inversion	Hemophilia A	Factor VIII
Partial or full gene deletion	α Thalassemia	α-globin
	β Thalassemia	β-globin
	AR spinal muscular atrophy (SMA)	Survival motor neuron (SMN)-telomeric
	Duchenne/Becker muscular dystrophy	Dystrophin
	Hemophilia A	Factor VIII
	Neurofibromatosis, type I	Neurofibromin
Partial or full gene duplication	Charcot-Marie Tooth disease, type 1A	Peripheral myelin protein 22 (PMP22)
	Duchenne/Becker muscular dystrophy	Dystrophin
Trinucleotide repeat expansion	Dentatorubro-pallidoluysian atrophy (DRPLA)	Atrophin (CAG)[b]
	Fragile X syndrome	FMR-I (CGG)
	Friedreich ataxia	Frataxin (GAA)
	Huntington disease	Huntington (CAG)
	Myotonic dystrophy	Myotonin kinase (CTG)
	Spinocerebellar ataxia, type I	Ataxin (CAG)
	X-linked SMA (Kennedy disease)	Androgen receptor (CAG)
Hybrid genes due to chromosomal crossover	β Thalassemia	β- and γ-globin
Imprinted genes[a]	Prader-Willi syndrome (PWS), maternal imprint	? Several
	Angelman syndrome (AS), paternal imprint	? Several
	Beckwith-Wiedemann syndrome	Unknown

[a]Imprinting is believed to be associated with methylation and lack of expression of a critical gene(s). Loss of a functional paternal (PWS) or maternal gene (AS) by deletion, uniparental disomy, abnormal methylation, or possibly point mutation leads to disease.
[b]Repeated trinucleotide given in parentheses.
AR, autosomal recessive; CFTR, cystic fibrosis transmembrane conductance regulator; HFE, hemochromatosis.

TABLE 9.1. CLASSIFICATION OF ONCOGENES

Class	Type	Examples
1	Growth factors	*sis*, α-TGF
2	Growth factor receptors	*erb* (EGFR), *HER2/neu*
3	Cytoplasmic signal transduction modulators	H-, K-, N-*ras, src, raf*
4	Nuclear transcription factors	N-, c-, L-*myc*, c-*jun, fos*
5	Cell cycle enhancers	PRAD1 (cyclin D)
6	Inhibitors of apoptosis	bcl-2, bcl-X

13. C (p. 167, Table 8.3)
14. B (p. 169, Table 8.4)
15. A (p. 169, Table 8.4)
16. C (p. 169, Table 8.4)
17. D (p. 169, Table 8.4)
18. C (p. 169, Table 8.4)
19. C (p. 169, column 1)
20. D (p. 170, column 1)
21. A (p. 170, column 2)
22. B (p. 171, column 1)
23. A (p. 171, column 2)
24. C (p. 172, column 1)

CHAPTER 9

1. E (p. 176, Table 9.1)
2. F (p. 176, Table 9.1)
3. B (p. 176, Table 9.1)
4. C (p. 176, Table 9.1)
5. A (p. 176, Table 9.1)
6. D (p. 176, Table 9.1)
7. A (p. 176, column 1)
8. C (p. 176, column 1)
9. A (p. 176, column 1)
10. B (p. 176, column 1)
11. C (p. 176, column 2)
12. B (p. 178, Table 9.3)
13. D (p. 178, Table 9.3)
14. C (p. 178, Table 9.3)
15. A (p. 178, Table 9.3)
16. D (p. 178, column 1)
17. B (p. 179, Table 9.4)
18. D (p. 179, Table 9.4)
19. E (p. 179, Table 9.4)
20. A (p. 179, Table 9.4)
21. C (p. 179, Table 9.4)

TABLE 9.4. ASSOCIATIONS BETWEEN MOLECULAR CHANGES AND PROGNOSIS

Tumor	Alteration	Association	References
Bladder cancer	LOH RB	High grade/muscle invasion	86
	Genomic alterations 2q–, 5p+, 5q–, 6q–, 8p–, 10q–, 18q–, 20q+	Higher grade	87
Breast cancer	Plasma DNA similar to tumor DNA	Poor prognosis?	88
	Allelic loss at 1p22–p31	Lymph node metastasis, tumor size >2 cm	89
Cervical carcinoma	LOH on chromosome 1	Advanced stage	90
Colorectal cancer	LOH at 18q21	Recurrence/poor survival (Dukes B and C)	91, 92
	p53 expression	Recurrence/poor survival (Dukes A)	92
	M1 and K-*ras* mutations in normal-appearing colonic mucosa micrometastases	Predictive of colorectal cancer	93
		Decreased survival (50% vs. 91%)	94
	P16-hypermethylation	Shorter survival in T3N0M0 tumors	95
Gastric cancer	LOH p53	Invasive potential	96
	LOH of 7q (D7S95)	Poor prognosis	97
Gliomas	Chromosome 22q loss	Astrocytoma progression	98
HNSCC	LOH of 14q	Poor outcome	99
	LOH on 2q	Poor prognosis	100
	LOH at 17p	Chemoresistance	101
Melanoma	LOH in plasma	Advanced stage/tumor progression	102
Neuroblastoma	N-*myc* amplification	Poor prognosis	103
	TRK-A expression	Good prognosis	103
Neuroblastomas, 4s	N-*myc* amplification, 1p deletion, 17q gains, elevated telomerase activity	Poor outcome (*not independent*)	104
NSCLC	Allelic imbalances on 9p	Poor prognosis	105
	Reduced Fhit protein expression	Poor prognosis (stage I)	106
	LOH 11p13	Poor prognosis	107
PNET	LOH of 17p	Metastatic disease	108
	c-*myc* amplification	Poor prognosis	108
Prostate cancer	LOH on 13q	Advanced stage	109
Retinoblastoma	LOH at RB1 locus	Tumoral differentiation, absence of choroidal invasion	110

HNSCC, head and neck squamous cell carcinoma; LOH, loss of heterozygosity; NSCLC, non-small cell lung cancer; PNET, primitive neuroectodermal tumor; RB, retinoblastoma gene.
Modified from Table 1 in reference 85.

TABLE 9.5. GENES ASSOCIATED WITH INHERITED CANCER SYNDROMES

Condition	Gene(s)	Gene Classification	Location/Type of Tumor	References
Breast and/or ovarian cancer	BRCA1 and BRCA2	Tumor suppressor	Breast,[a] ovary,[a] colon, prostate	128
Familial adenomatous polyposis (FAP)	APC	Tumor suppressor	Colon,[a] small bowel, stomach, bone, CNS, soft tissue	128–130
Hereditary nonpolyposis colorectal cancer (HNPCC)	hMSH2, hMLH1, PMS1, PMS2, hMSH3, hMSH6	Mismatch repair	Right side of colon,[a] endometrium,[a] stomach, ovary, small bowel, transitional cell, sebaceous, CNS	128–130
Renal cancer	VHL	Tumor suppressor	Kidney,[a] hemangioblastoma, pheochromocytoma	128
Neurofibromatosis types I/II	NF1, NF2	Tumor suppressor	CNS,[a] myeloid leukemia	128
Nevoid basal cell carcinoma	PTC	Development and cellular proliferation	Skin,[a] CNS	128
Inherited prostate cancer	BRCA1, HPC1, others	Tumor suppressor	Prostate[a]	128, 131
Familial melanoma	MLM1, CDKN2A, CDK4	Cell cycle regulator, oncogene (CDK4)	Skin,[a] pancreas	128, 132
Multiple endocrine neoplasia (MEN2A/B)	RET	Oncogene	Thyroid[a] and adrenal glands	128, 133, 134
Li Fraumeni syndrome	P53	Tumor suppressor	Bone, soft tissue, breast, brain, adrenal gland, leukemia	128, 135, 136
Tuberous sclerosis	TSC1, TSC2	Tumor suppressor	Hamartomas of skin, CNS, heart, kidney	128
Retinoblastoma	RB1	Tumor suppressor	Eye,[a] bone, soft tissue, brain, skin	128
Rhabdoid predisposition	HSNF5/INI 1	Tumor suppressor	CNS, kidney	137
Xeroderma pigmentosum	XP	DNA repair	Skin	128
Bloom syndrome	BLM	Helicase (DNA ligation)	Leukemia, GI carcinoma	128
Ataxia telangiectasia	ATM	Cell cycle regulator	Leukemia, lymphoma, GI carcinoma	128

[a]Most common location of tumors.
CNS, central nervous system; GI, gastrointestinal.

22. D (p. 181, Table 9.5)
23. C (p. 181, Table 9.5)
24. B (p. 181, Table 9.5)
25. A (p. 181, Table 9.5)
26. E (p. 181, Table 9.5)
27. A (p. 181, column 1)

CHAPTER 10

1. A (p. 190, column 1)
2. C (p. 190, column 1)
3. B (p. 190, column 1)
4. A (p. 190, column 1)
5. A (p. 190, column 1)
6. B (p. 190, column 1)
7. C (p. 190, column 1)
8. D (p. 190, column 1)
9. A (p. 190, column 1)
10. E (p. 190, column 2)
11. B (p. 190, column 2)
12. A (p. 190, column 2)
13. C (p. 190, column 2)
14. B (p. 191, column 1)
15. B (p. 192, Table 10.8)
16. A (p. 192, column 1)
17. C (p. 192, column 2)

18. D (p. 193, Table 10.10)
19. C (p. 193, Table 10.11)
20. D (p. 195, Table 10.13)
21. B (p. 198, column 2)
22. B (p. 200, column 1)
23. C (p. 200, column 1)
24. A (p. 200, column 1)
25. A (p. 200, column 1)
26. B (p. 201, Table 10.19)
27. C (p. 203, column 1)
28. D (p. 205, Table 10.24)

CHAPTER 11

1. B (p. 211, column 2)
2. B (p. 212, column 1)
3. C (p. 212, column 2)
4. A (p. 212, column 2)
5. A (p. 213, column 2)
6. C (p. 214, column 2)
7. A (p. 215, column 1)
8. B (p. 215, column 2)
9. D (p. 216, column 1)
10. B (p. 218, column 1)
11. B (p. 218, column 1)
12. D (p. 220, Table 11.1)

TABLE 10.10. ADVANTAGES AND DISADVANTAGES OF THE TWO-TUBE OR TWO-STEP NESTED PCR (TSNP)

Advantages
  Increased sensitivity
    Addition of new enzyme and reagents allows for longer maintenance of the reaction in the "exponential" phase
    Target DNA used in nested (second) step is the amplicon from the first round, which is many fold greater in number than original target in clinical sample
    Smaller size of final amplicon produced by second round of amplification increases efficiency of reaction
    Inhibitors of PCR in clinical sample are decreased during second round due to dilution as new reagents are added during the second step
  Increased specificity
    Decrease in nonspecific banding ("dirty background") over traditional PCR following 40 or more cycles of amplification. These bands are a result of coamplification of genomic sequences (reference 63)
    Decreased false positives from concatenation of fragmented DNA (reference 64)
Disadvantages
  Greater expense than straight PCR as twice as much enzyme and reagents are used
  Extra manipulations and length of the assay as cycling blocks cannot be programmed for all cycles from the start
  Increased risk of contamination unless three rooms are used for setup instead of two (pre-PCR, PCR, and internest transfer rooms)

PCR, polymerase chain reaction.
Adapted and updated from Sandin RL. Polymerase chain reaction and other amplification techniques in mycobacteriology. In: Heifitz L, ed. *Clinics in laboratory medicine. Clinical mycobacteriology.* Philadelphia: WB Saunders, 1996:617, with permission.

13. E (p. 220, Table 11.1)
14. B (p. 220, Table 11.1)
15. A (p. 220, Table 11.1)
16. C (p. 220, Table 11.1)
17. C (p. 220, Table 11.1)
18. D (p. 220, Table 11.1)

TABLE 10.11. ADVANTAGES AND DISADVANTAGES OF THE ONE-STEP (ONE-TUBE) NESTED PCR (OSNP)

Advantages
  Less expensive than TSNP
  Faster than TSNP as there is no internest transfer step and instrument can be programmed from the start
  Less contamination risks than TSNP and less manipulations
  Addition of twice the amount of enzyme from the start may help approximate the level of sensitivity of TSNP
Disadvantages
  No added advantages of diluting out inhibitors
  May never approximate the extreme sensitivity of TSNP

PCR, polymerase chain reaction; TSNP, two-step nested PCR.
From Sandin RL. Polymerase chain reaction and other amplification techniques in mycobacteriology. In: Heifitz L, ed. *Clinics in laboratory medicine. Clinical mycobacteriology.* Philadelphia: WB Saunders, 1996:617, with permission.

TABLE 11.1. COMMON RECURRING CHROMOSOMAL TRANSLOCATIONS IN NON-HODGKIN LYMPHOMA

Lymphoma	Translocation	Oncogene Involved
Small lymphocytic	(14;19)(q32;q13.1)	bcl-3
Mantle cell	t(11;14)(q13;q32)	CCNDI (cyclin D1)
Lymphoplasmacytic	t(9;14)(p13;q32)	PAXS
Marginal zone	t(11;18)(q21;q21)	Unknown
Follicle center cell	t(14;18)(q32;q31)	bcl-2
Burkitt	t(8;14)(q24;q32)	c-*myc*
	t(2;8)(q12;q24)	c-*myc*
	t(8;22)(q24;q11)	c-*myc*
Diffuse large cell	t(3;-)(q27;-)	bcl-6
Anaplastic large cell	t(2;5)(q23;q35)	NPM-ALK

19. E (p. 220, Table 11.1)
20. A (p. 220, Table 11.1)
21. B (p. 220, Table 11.1)
22. D (p. 220, column 1)
23. D (p. 220, column 2)
24. A (p. 221, column 1)
25. A (p. 221, column 2)
26. B (p. 221, column 2)
27. C (p. 222, column 2)
28. D (p. 222, column 2)
29. A (p. 224, column 1)
30. A (p. 224, column 1)
31. B (p. 224, column 1)
32. B (p. 224, column 2)
33. C (p. 225, column 2)
34. A (p. 226, Table 11.2)
35. C (p. 226, Table 11.2)
36. D (p. 226, Table 11.2)
37. E (p. 226, Table 11.2)
38. B (p. 226, Table 11.2)

TABLE 11.2. COMMON RECURRING CHROMOSOMAL TRANSLOCATIONS ENCOUNTERED IN ACUTE LEUKEMIAS

Disease	Translocation	Genes Involved
AML	t(6;9)(p23;q34)	DEK-CAN
AML-M2	t(8;21)(q22;q22)	AML1-ETO
AML-M3	t(15;17)(q22;q21)	PML-RARα
AML-M4Eo	inv(16)(p13;q22)	CBFβ-MYH
AML-M4/M5, biphenotypic	t(11;19)(q23;p13)	MLL-ENL
AML-M5, biphenotypic	t(9;11)(p21;q23)	MLL-AF9
CML	t(9;22)(q34;q11)	BCR-ABL
Precursor B-ALL	t(12;21)(p13;q22)	ETV6-AML1
	t(9;22)(q34;q11)	BCR-ABL
	t(4;11)(q21;q23)	MLL-AF9
Pre–B-ALL	t(1;19)(q23;p13)	E2A-PBX1
B-ALL	t(8;14)(q24;q32)	MYC-IgH

ALL, acute lymphoblastic leukemia; AML, acute myelogenous leukemia; CML, chronic myelogenous leukemia.

39. B (p. 226, Table 11.2)
40. C (p. 226, Table 11.2)
41. D (p. 226, Table 11.2)
42. E (p. 226, Table 11.2)
43. A (p. 226, Table 11.2)
44. C (p. 226, column 2)
45. C (p. 229, column 1)
46. C (p. 230, column 1)
47. A (p. 230, column 1)
48. B (p. 230, column 2)
49. B (p. 231, column 1)
50. B (p. 232, column 1)
51. B (p. 232, column 2)
52. D (p. 233, column 1)
53. A (p. 233, column 2)

CHAPTER 12

1. C (p. 242, column 1)
2. C (p. 242, column 1, Fig. 12.1)

3. A (p. 242, column 1)
4. B (p. 243, column
5. A (p. 244, column 1)
6. C (p. 244, column 1)
7. C (p. 244, column 2)
8. A (p. 245, column 1)
9. D (p. 245, column 2)
10. C (p. 246, column 1, Fig. 12.4)
11. B (p. 247, column 1)
12. B (p. 247, column 1)
13. A (p. 247, column 1)
14. C (p. 247, column 1)
15. A (p. 247, column 2)
16. A (p. 248, column 1)
17. A (p. 248, column 2, Fig. 12.6)
18. D (p. 249, column 2)
19. C (p. 251, column 2)
20. A (p. 252, column 2)
21. A (p. 252, column 2)
22. B (p. 253, column 2)
23. A (p. 253, column 2)

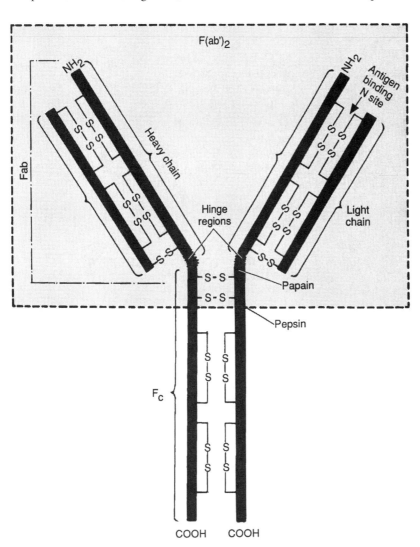

FIGURE 12.1. Schematic representation of immunoglobulin G (IgG) antibody. Papain digestion releases two Fab fragments and one Fc fragment. Pepsin digestion releases one F(ab')$_2$ fragment. Both enzyme digestions conserve antigen-binding sites.

TABLE 12.1. ENZYMES COMMONLY USED IN ENZYME IMMUNOASSAY

Enzyme	Some Substrates
Alkaline phosphatase	4-Methylumbelliferone phosphate *p*-nitrophenyl phosphate
Glucose-6-phosphate dehydrogenase	Glucose-6-phosphate + NADP$^+$
Glucose oxidase	Glucose
Peroxidase	H_2O_2
β-Galactosidase	β-Galactosides

24. A (p. 254, column 2)
25. B (p. 255, column 2, Table 12.1)
26. A (p. 255, column 1)
27. B (p. 255, column 2)
28. A (p. 256, column 2)
29. D (p. 257, column 2)
30. D (p. 259, column 2)
31. F (p. 241, column 2)
32. F (p. 247, column 1)
33. T (p. 254, column 1)
34. F (p. 255, column 2)
35. T (p. 257, column 2)

CHAPTER 13

1. D (p. 263, column 1)
2. B, C, E, A, D (p. 264, column 2, Table 13.2)
3. D (p. 263, column 2)
4. C (p. 265, column 1)
5. B (p. 265, column 2)
6. D (p. 265, column 2)
7. A (p. 265, column 2, Table 13.3)
8. B (p. 267, column 1)
9. C, D, A, E, G, B, F (p. 267, column 2, Fig. 13.2)
10. A (p. 267, column 2)
11. C (p. 268, column 1)
12. A (p. 268, column 2)
13. B (p. 268, column 2)
14. D (p. 269, column 1)
15. D (p. 269, column 2)
16. C (p. 270, column 1)
17. C (p. 271, column 2)
18. A (p. 271, column 2)
19. B (p. 271, column 1)
20. B (p. 269, column 2)
21. B (p. 272, column 1)
22. C (p. 273, column 1)
23. A, C, B (p. 273, column 2)
24. C (p. 274, column 1)
25. D (p. 274, column 2)
26. A (p. 275, column 1)
27. B (p. 275, column 2)

TABLE 13.2. CLASSIFICATION OF SELECTED MAJOR[a] AND MINOR PLASMA PROTEINS BY ELECTROPHORETIC MOBILITY

Albumin zone
  Albumin
  Prealbumin
α$_1$ Zone
  α$_1$-Antitrypsin
  High-density lipoprotein (α-lipoproteins)
  α$_1$-Antichymotrypsin
  Orosomucoid
  α-Fetoprotein
α$_2$ Zone
  α$_2$-Macroglobulin
  Haptoglobin
  Ceruloplasmin
  Gc-Globulin
β Zone
  Low-density lipoprotein (β-lipoproteins)
  Transferrin
  C3
  β$_2$-Microglobulin
  Hemopexin
  Fibrinogen (may be in γ zone)
γ Zone
  Immunoglobulins
  C-Reactive protein
  Fibrinogen
  Lysozyme

[a]In bold face.

28. B (p. 276, column 1)
29. D (p. 277, column 1)
30. A (p. 278, column 1)
31. T (p. 265, column 2)
32. F (p. 267, column 1)
33. F (p. 269, column 2)
34. T (p. 272, column 1)
35. F (p. 272, column 2, Table 13.3)
36. T (p. 274, column 1)
37. F (p. 274, column 2)
38. T (p. 278, column 2)
39. T (p. 278, column 2)
40. F (p. 279, column 2)

CHAPTER 14

1. A (p. 281, column 1)
2. D (p. 281, column 2, Fig. 14.1)
3. B (p. 282, column 1)
4. C (p. 282, column 2)
5. D (p. 283, column 1, Fig. 14.2)
6. C (p. 283, column 2)
7. A (p. 284, column 1)
8. B (p. 285, column 1)
9. C (p. 284, column 2)

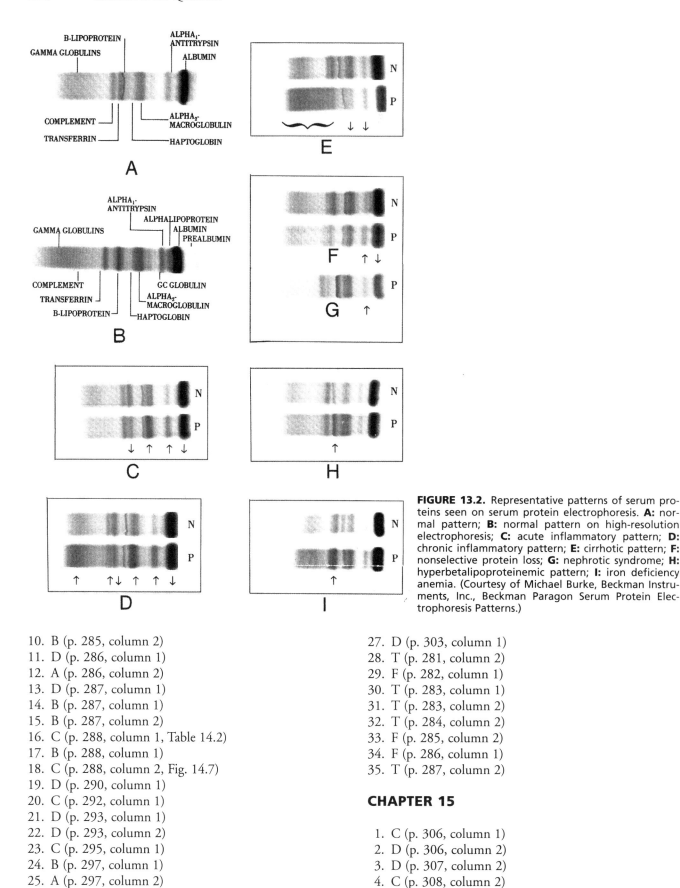

FIGURE 13.2. Representative patterns of serum proteins seen on serum protein electrophoresis. **A:** normal pattern; **B:** normal pattern on high-resolution electrophoresis; **C:** acute inflammatory pattern; **D:** chronic inflammatory pattern; **E:** cirrhotic pattern; **F:** nonselective protein loss; **G:** nephrotic syndrome; **H:** hyperbetalipoproteinemic pattern; **I:** iron deficiency anemia. (Courtesy of Michael Burke, Beckman Instruments, Inc., Beckman Paragon Serum Protein Electrophoresis Patterns.)

10. B (p. 285, column 2)
11. D (p. 286, column 1)
12. A (p. 286, column 2)
13. D (p. 287, column 1)
14. B (p. 287, column 1)
15. B (p. 287, column 2)
16. C (p. 288, column 1, Table 14.2)
17. B (p. 288, column 1)
18. C (p. 288, column 2, Fig. 14.7)
19. D (p. 290, column 1)
20. C (p. 292, column 1)
21. D (p. 293, column 1)
22. D (p. 293, column 2)
23. C (p. 295, column 1)
24. B (p. 297, column 1)
25. A (p. 297, column 2)
26. B (p. 301, column 2)

27. D (p. 303, column 1)
28. T (p. 281, column 2)
29. F (p. 282, column 1)
30. T (p. 283, column 1)
31. T (p. 283, column 2)
32. T (p. 284, column 2)
33. F (p. 285, column 2)
34. F (p. 286, column 1)
35. T (p. 287, column 2)

CHAPTER 15

1. C (p. 306, column 1)
2. D (p. 306, column 2)
3. D (p. 307, column 2)
4. C (p. 308, column 2)
5. B (p. 308, column 2, Fig. 15.8)

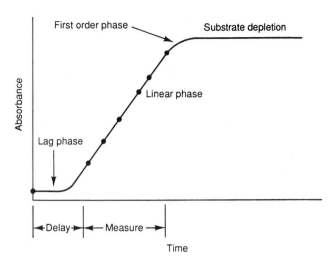

FIGURE 14.2. Absorbance versus time curve for a single-reagent assay system. The lag phase is the time necessary for activation of the enzyme. The linear phase (zero-order kinetics) is where the reaction rate is proportional to enzyme activity. The end of the first-order phase is where the substrate is depleted and the reaction ends.

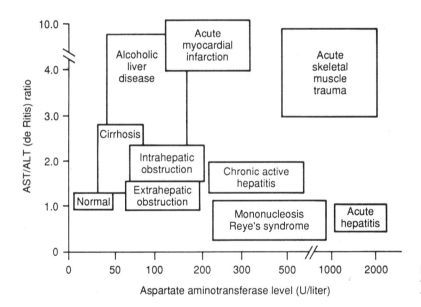

FIGURE 14.7. Ratio of aspartate aminotransferase to alanine aminotransferase verus aspartate aminotransferase levels in various liver diseases.

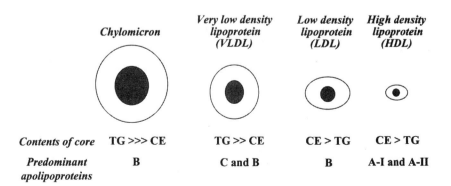

FIGURE 15.8. Comparison of size and composition of the core in the four major classes of lipoproteins. Apo, apolipoprotein; CE, cholesterol ester; TG, triglyceride.

TABLE 15.6. CLASSIFICATION OF PATIENTS ACCORDING TO SERUM CHOLESTEROL LEVEL

Total Cholesterol Level	Initial Classification
<200 mg/dL (5.2 mmol/L)	Desirable blood cholesterol
200–239 mg/dL (5.2–6.2 mmol/L)	Borderline-high blood cholesterol
≥240 mg/dL (6.2 mmol/L)	High blood cholesterol
<35 mg/dL (0.9 mmol/L)	Low high-density lipoprotein cholesterol

6. A (p. 308, column 2, Fig. 15.8)
7. B (p. 308, column 2)
8. D (p. 313, column 1)
9. C (p. 313, column 2)
10. A (p. 313, column 2)
11. A (p. 313, column 2)
12. C (p. 314, column 2, Table 15.5)
13. B (p. 314, column 2, Fig. 15.16)
14. B (p. 315, column 1, Table 15.6)
15. C (p. 315, column 1, Fig. 15.15)
16. A (p. 318, column 1)
17. D (p. 318, column 1)
18. C (p. 318, column 2)
19. D (p. 318, column 2)
20. D (p. 319, column 2)
21. C (p. 320, column 1)
22. B (p. 320, column 1)
23. F (p. 306, column 2)
24. T (p. 307, column 1)
25. T (p. 307, column 2)
26. T (p. 311, column 1)

27. T (p. 311, column 2)
28. F (p. 314, column 2, Fig. 15.16)
29. T (p. 319, column 1)
30. F (p. 220, column 1)

CHAPTER 16

1. B (p. 322, column 2)
2. A (p. 324, column 1)
3. C (p. 324, column 1)
4. C (p. 325, column 1)
5. D (p. 326, column 1)
6. B (p. 326, column 2)
7. A (p. 327, column 1)
8. D (p. 328, Table 16.2)
9. C (p. 328, column 1)
10. A (p. 328, column 1)
11. B (p. 328, column 2)
12. D (p. 329, column 1)
13. B (p. 329, column 2)

TABLE 16.2. GROWTH HORMONE REFERENCE INTERVALS

Condition	Preparation	Collection Time	Results	Increased Levels	Decreased Levels
Normal 　Child 　Adult 　　Female 　　Male	Fasting	Early a.m.	1–10 µg/L <10 µg/L <2 µg/L	Giantism, acromegaly, ectopic secretion, stress, exercise, prolonged fasting	Growth hormone deficiency Hypopituitarism Adrenal cortical hyperfunction
Dopa stimulation	500 mg adult 10 mg/kg child	0, 30, 60, 90, 120, 180 min	>10 µg/L or >5 µg/L above baseline		No response if glucose >120 mg/dL; poor response in hypopituitarism
Arginine stimulation	Child 0.5 g/kg Adult 30 g/kg 30 min	0, 30, 60 min	Fasting <5 µg/L Peak >10 µg/L at 30–60 min		Hypopituitarism no response
Insulin stimulation	0.1 U/kg adult 0.05 U/kg child IV	0, 15, 30, 45, 60, 90 min	>10 µg/L or >5 µg/L above baseline Glucose level ≤50% of baseline		Poor response in hypopituitarism, hypothyroidism
Exercise (vigorous)	20 min		>5 µg/L		
Glucose suppression	75 g or 1.75 g/kg after fast	0, 30, 60, 90, 120 min	Decrease to <5 µg/L	None to poor suppression in acromegaly, giantism, and ectopic secretion	

TABLE 16.5. URINE OSMOLALITY FOR DIABETES INSIPIDUS OF DIFFERENT ORIGINS AND POLYDIPSIA

	Neurogenic Diabetes Insipidus	Nephrogenic Diabetes Insipidus	Psychogenic Polydipsia
Random plasma osmolality	↑	↑	↓
Random urine osmolality	↓	↓	↓
Urine osmolality during mild water deprivation	No change	No change	↑
Urine osmolality during nicotine or hypertonic saline	No change	No change	↑
Urine osmolality after vasopressin intravenously	↑	No change	↑
Plasma vasopressin	Low	Normal or high	Low

From Greenspan PS. *Basic endocrinology,* 3rd ed. Norwalk, CT: Appleton & Lange, 1991, with permission.

14. C (p. 330, column 1)
15. B (p. 330, column 2)
16. B (p. 330, column 2)
17. B (p. 331, column 1)
18. A (p. 331, column 1)
19. D (p. 331, column 2)
20. A (p. 332, Table 16.5)
21. B (p. 332, Table 16.5)
22. C (p. 332, Table 16.5)
23. A (p. 332, Table 16.5)
24. B (p. 332, Table 16.5)
25. A (p. 332, Table 16.5)
26. B (p. 332, Table 1
27. B (p. 332, Table 16.5)
28. B (p. 332, Table 16.5)
29. A (p. 332, Table 16.5)
30. D (p. 332, column 1)
31. D (p. 332, column 2)
32. C (p. 333, column 1)
33. D (p. 333, column 2)
34. A (p. 333, column 2)
35. A (p. 335, Table 16.6)
36. B (p. 336, column 1)
37. A (p. 336, column 1)
38. A (p. 336, column 1)
39. C (p. 336, column 1)
40. D (p. 336, column 2)
41. B (p. 337, column 1)
42. A (p. 337, column 1)
43. C (p. 337, column
44. B (p. 337, column 1)
45. A (p. 337, column 1)
46. B (p. 337, column 1)
47. C (p. 337, column 1)
48. B (p. 337, column 1)
49. A (p. 337, column 1)
50. A (p. 337, column 2)
51. C (p. 338, column 1)
52. A (p. 338, column 1)
53. B (p. 338, column 1)
54. C (p. 338, column 1)
55. B (p. 338, column 2)

56. D (p. 339, column 1)
57. B (p. 339, column 2)
58. A (p. 340, column 1)
59. D (p. 340, column 1)
60. D (p. 340, column 2)
61. C (p. 340, column 2)
62. A (p. 340, column 2)
63. E (p. 341, column 1)
64. B (p. 341, column 1)
65. B (p. 341, Table 16.9)
66. C (p. 341, Table 16.9)
67. A (p. 341, Table 16.9)
68. B (p. 342, column 1)
69. D (p. 342, column 1)
70. B (p. 342, column 2)
71. C (p. 343, column 1)
72. B (p. 343, column 2)
73. A (p. 343, column 2)
74. A (p. 343, column 2)
75. A (p. 343, column 2)
76. B (p. 343, column 2)
77. A (p. 343, column 2)
78. A (p. 346, column 1)

CHAPTER 17

1. B (p. 347, column 1, Table 17.1)
2. C (p. 347, column 2)
3. A (p. 347, column 2)

TABLE 17.1. WATER DISTRIBUTION IN A 70-KG PERSON

Component	Volume (L)
Total body water (60% of lean body mass)	42
Intracellular fluid (66% of total body water)	28
Extracellular fluid (34% of total body water)	14
Interstitial fluid	10.5
Vascular compartment (including blood cells)	3.5

4. A (p. 347, column 2)
5. B (p. 347, column 2)
6. A (p. 348, column 1)
7. C (p. 348, column 2)
8. C (p. 349, column 1)
9. C (p. 349, column 2)
10. B (p. 349, column 2)
11. B (p. 350, column 2)
12. B (p. 350, column 2)
13. A (p. 350, column 2)
14. D (p. 350, column 2, Fig. 17.1)
15. B (p. 352, column 1)
16. A (p. 353, column 2, Fig. 17.2)
17. D (p. 353, column 2, Fig. 17.2)
18. B (p. 352, column 2, Fig. 17.3)
19. A (p. 352, column 2)
20. C (p. 353, column 1)
21. A (p. 353, column 2)
22. A (p. 355, column 2, Table 17.3)
23. D (p. 356, column 1)
24. D (p. 357, column 1)
25. A (p. 357, column 1)
26. B (p. 357, column 2)
27. D (p. 358, column 1)
28. C (p. 359, column 2)
29. B (p. 359, column 2)
30. C (p. 360, column 2)
31. A (p. 361, column 1, Table 17.5)
32. C (p. 361, column 1, Fig. 17.6)
33. D (p. 361, column 2, Table 17.6)
34. C (p. 362, column 1, Table 17.7)
35. D (p. 362, column 2, Table 17.7)
36. D (p. 363, column 2)
37. A (p. 363, column 2)
38. C (p. 364, column 1)
39. C (p. 364, column 1)

40. A (p. 365, column 1)
41. F (p. 347, column 1)
42. F (p. 348, column 1)
43. F (p. 348, column 2)
44. T (p. 350, column 1)
45. F (p. 360, column 1)
46. T (p. 364, column 1)
47. T (p. 364, column 2)
48. T (p. 364, column 2)
49. F (p. 350, column 1)
50. F (p. 350, column 1)

CHAPTER 18

1. A (p. 366, column 2)
2. B (p. 366, column 2)
3. A (p. 367, column 2)
4. D (p. 367, column 2)
5. C (p. 368, column 2)
6. C (p. 368, column 2)
7. D (p. 370, column 1)
8. B (p. 370, column 2)
9. B (p. 371, column 1)
10. C (p. 372, Table 18.2)
11. D (p. 372, Table 18.2)
12. B (p. 372, Table 18.2)
13. A (p. 372, Table 18.2)
14. D (p. 373, column 1
15. B (p. 373, Table 18.3)
16. C (p. 373, Table 18.3)
17. D (p. 373, Table 18.3)
18. B (p. 373, Table 18.3)
19. A (p. 373, Table 18.3)
20. B (p. 375, column 2)
21. A (p. 375, column 2)

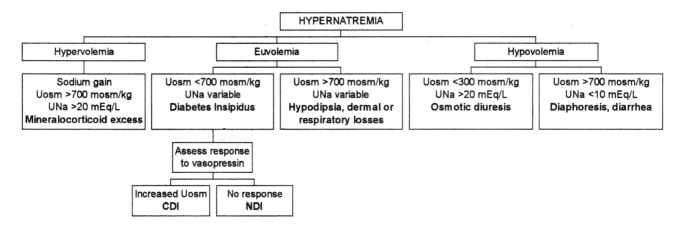

FIGURE 17.2. Selective differential diagnosis and laboratory approach to hypernatremia. CDI, central diabetes insipidus; NDI, nephrogenic diabetes insipidus; UOsm, urine osmolality; UNa, urine sodium.

TABLE 18.2. METHODOLOGIES USED IN POINT-OF-CARE INSTRUMENT

Analytes	Electrochemical	Optical
P_{O_2}	Amperometric Clark-type electrode	Optode based on • Fluorescence quenching, or • Absorbance change of O_2 binding molecules
P_{CO_2}	Potentiometric Severinghaus-type electrode	Optode based on pH sensor and gas-permeable membrane
pH	Glass or polymer membrane electrodes	Optode based on fluorescence or absorbance measurement of immobilized pH indicator
Electrolytes	ISEs (potentiometric)	Solution phase complexing reagents or colorimetric strip test
Hematocrit	Conductivity cell or ISEs (measure change in electrolytes after RBC lysis)	Microcentrifuge or cell counter
Total hemoglobin	—	Direct absorbance measurement or colorimetric measurement of pseudoperoxidase activity
Glucose	Amperometric enzyme electrodes based	Colorimetric measurement of glucose on immobilized glucose oxidase metabolite

ISE, ion selective electrode.
Adapted from Misiano DR, Meyerhoff ME, Collison ME. Current and future directions in the technology relating to bedside testing of critically ill patients. *Chest* 1990;97[Suppl]:2045–2145.

22. A (p. 375, column 2)
23. B (p. 375, column 2)
24. B (p. 376, column 1)
25. D (p. 376, column 1)
26. A (p. 376, column 2)
27. C (p. 375, column 2)
28. B (p. 376, column 2)
29. C (p. 377, column 1)

CHAPTER 19

1. D (p. 378, column 1)
2. D (p. 378, column 1)
3. B (p. 378, column 2, Fig. 19.1)
4. C (p. 380, column 1)
5. C (p. 381, column 1)
6. A (p. 381, column 1)
7. B (p. 381, column 2)
8. D (p. 381, column 2)
9. D (p. 382, column 1)

10. A (p. 382, column 2)
11. B (p. 383, column 1, Table 19.2)
12. B (p. 383, column 1, Table 19.2)
13. A (p. 383, column 2)
14. D (p. 383, column 2)
15. B (p. 384, column 1)
16. B (p. 384, column 1)
17. C (p. 384, column 1)
18. A (p. 384, column 1)
19. A (p. 384, column 2)
20. D (p. 384, column 2)
21. A (p. 384, column 2)
22. C (p. 385, column 1)
23. D (p. 385, column 2)
24. B (p. 386, column 1)
25. A (p. 386, column 1)
26. D (p. 386, column 2, Table 19.4)
27. C (p. 387, column 1)
28. C (p. 387, column 1)
29. D (p. 387, column 1)
30. D (p. 387, column 2)

TABLE 18.3. PATHOPHYSIOLOGIC CLASSIFICATION OF RESPIRATORY FAILURE

Mechanism	Blood Gas Values	A-a O2 Gradient	Response to O_2
Low inspired oxygen	Low P_{O_2} and low/normal P_{CO_2}	Normal	Increased P_{O_2}
Hypoventilation	Low P_{O_2}, elevated P_{CO_2}	Normal	Increased P_{O_2}
Ventilation/perfusion ($\dot{V}/\dot{Q}$) mismatch	Low P_{O_2}, elevated P_{CO_2} when severe	Increased	Increased P_{O_2}
Right to left shunt	Low P_{O_2} and normal P_{CO_2}	Increased	Minimal improvement
Diffusion impairment	Low P_{O_2} and elevated P_{CO_2}	Increased	Minimal improvement

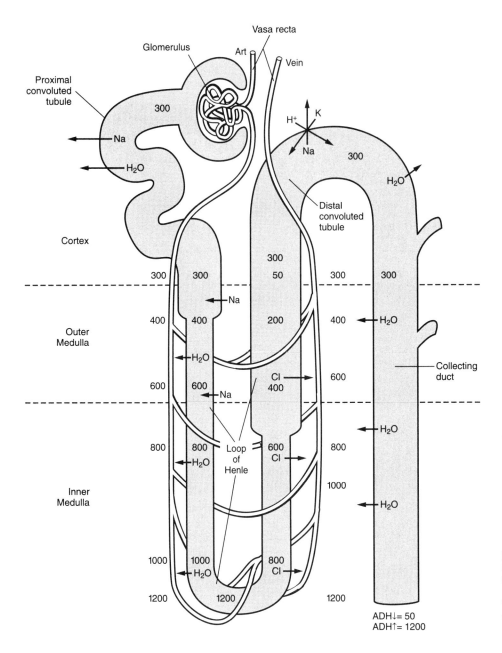

FIGURE 19.1. Diagram of the renal nephron. The numbers indicate the changes in osmolality (mOsm/kg H₂O) in the interstitium and tubular fluid. Tubular exchanges of water and ions during the course of the production of urine are indicated.

TABLE 19.2. ETIOLOGIES OF ELEVATED SERUM UREA

Prerenal
  Increased synthesis of urea
    Catabolic states: fever, stress, burns
    High-protein diet
    Gastrointestinal bleeding
    Hyperthyroidism
    Cushing syndrome
    Hemolysis
    Antianabolic drugs/tetracycline
    Steroid therapy
    Low-calorie diet
    Malignancy
    Sepsis
  Decreased perfusion of kidney
    Congestive heart failure
    Hypotension, shock
    Renal vein thrombosis
    Dehydration
    Cirrhosis, ascites
Intrinsic renal disease
  Glomerular disease
  Tubular disease (acute tubular necrosis)
  Interstitial disease
Postrenal
  Urinary tract obstruction
    Benign prostatic hyperplasia
    Prostatic carcinoma
    Carcinoma of bladder of bilateral ureters
    Retroperitoneal tumor
    Calculi
  Extravasation of urine into tissues

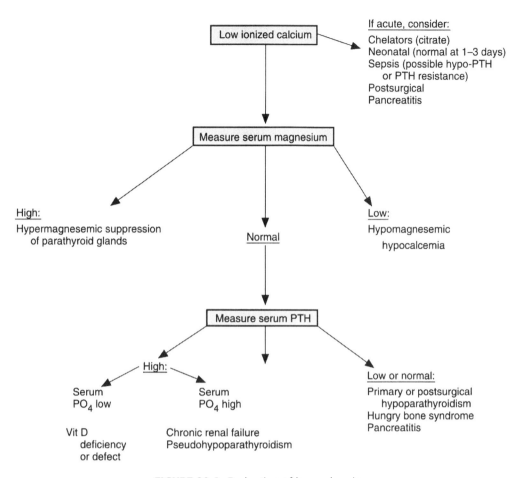

FIGURE 20.4. Evaluation of hypocalcemia.

CHAPTER 20

1. D (p. 392, column 1)
2. D (p. 394, column 1, Fig. 20.3)
3. B (p. 394, column 1)
4. A (p. 394, column 2)
5. B (p. 394, column 2)
6. D (p. 395, column 1)
7. D (p. 395, column 1)
8. B (p. 395, column 2, Fig. 20.4)
9. C (p. 395, column 2)
10. B (p. 395, column 2, Fig. 20.4)
11. A (p. 395, column 2)
12. D (p. 395, column 2)
13. A (p. 397, column 1)
14. D (p. 397, column 1)
15. C (p. 398, column 1)
16. A (p. 398, column 1)
17. A (p. 398, column 2)
18. B (p. 398, column 2)
19. D (p. 399, column 1)

20. C (p. 395, column 2, Table 20.3)
21. A (p. 401, column 1)
22. B (p. 401, column 1)
23. A (p. 401, column 2)
24. D (p. 404, column 1, Fig. 20.7)
25. A (p. 404, column 1, Fig. 20.7)

TABLE 20.3. CAUSES OF HYPOMAGNESEMIA

Diarrhea
Diuretics, especially loop diuretics (furosemide)
Diabetes
Dietary
Alcoholism
Drugs, especially cyclosporine and cisplatin
Cellular hypoxia
Toxemia or eclampsia of pregnancy
Skin loss from burns

CHAPTER 21

1. F (p. 407, column 1, Table 21.4)
2. T (p. 407, column 2)
3. E (p. 408, column 1)
4. T (p. 409, column 1)
5. E (p. 409, column 1)

CHAPTER 22

1. C (p. 418, column 1)
2. D (p. 418, column 1)
3. D (p. 418, column 2)
4. A (p. 419, column 1)
5. B (p. 419, column 2)
6. D (p. 419, column 2)
7. D (p. 419, column 2)
8. D (p. 419, column 2)
9. B (p. 420, column 1)
10. A (p. 420, column 1)
11. C (p. 420, column 1, Table 22.1)
12. A (p. 420, column 2)
13. C (p. 421, column 1)
14. B (p. 421, column 2)
15. D (p. 422, column 1)
16. D (p. 422, column 2)
17. B (p. 423, column 1)
18. B (p. 423, column 2)
19. A (p. 424, column 1)
20. C (p. 425, column 1, Fig. 22.2)
21. B (p. 426, column 1)
22. D (p. 429, column 1)
23. C (p. 430, column 1)
24. A (p. 434, column 1)
25. C (p. 434, column 1)
26. T (p. 421, column 2)
27. T (p. 422, column 2)

TABLE 21.4. THE "SECOND HIT": EXAMPLES OF UNSAFE AND SAFE AGENTS AND DRUGS

Unsafe	Safe
Ethanol	Acetaminophen
Antiepilepsy drugs	Aspirin
Barbiturates	Atropine
Birth control pills	Bromides
Calcium channel blockers	Chloral hydrate
Carbamazepine	Penicillin
Clonazepam	Phenothiazines
Danazol	Narcotic analgesics
Diclofenac	Cimetidine
Ergots	Insulin
Rifampine	Glucocorticoids
Sulfonamides	Streptomycin

TABLE 22.1. SPOT TESTS

Drug(s)	Test	Comments
Volatiles (U, S)	Dichromate	Alcohols and aldehydes
Salicylates (U, S)	Trinder	Positive after therapeutic doses
Acetaminophen (U)	Cresol-ammonia	Positive after therapeutic doses
Phenothiazines (U)	FPN	Color and sensitivity vary with phenothiazine
Imipramine/ desipramine, trimipramine (U)	Forrest	Interfered with by some phenothiazines
Ethchlorvynol (U,S)	Diphenylamine	Good sensitivity and specificity

FPN, fixed pattern noise; S, serum; U, urine.
From Stevens HM. Colour tests. In: Moffet AC, ed. *Clark's isolation and identification of drugs,* 2nd ed. London: The Pharmaceutical Press, 1986:128–147.

28. F (p. 423, column 2)
29. T (p. 424, column 1)
30. F (p. 424, column 1)
31. T (p. 428, column 1)
32. F (p. 428, column 2)
33. T (p. 430, column 1)
34. T (p. 432, column 2)
35. T (p. 433, column 1)

CHAPTER 23

1. C (p. 439, column 2)
2. C (p. 439, column 2)
3. A (p. 440, column 1)
4. C (p. 440, column 2)
5. C (p. 441, column 1)
6. B (p. 443, column 1)
7. D (p. 443, column 1)
8. A (p. 443, column 2)
9. D (p. 444, column 1)
10. B (p. 446, column 1)
11. A (p. 446, column 1)
12. C (p. 448, column 1)
13. B (p. 448, column 2)
14. A (p. 450, column 1)
15. B (p. 450, column 2)
16. D (p. 454, column 1)
17. D (p. 457, column 1, Table 23.7)
18. C (p. 459, column 2, Table 23.8)
19. B (p. 460, column 1)
20. A (p. 460, column 1)
21. F (p. 440, column 2)
22. F (p. 441, column 1)
23. T (p. 444, column 2)

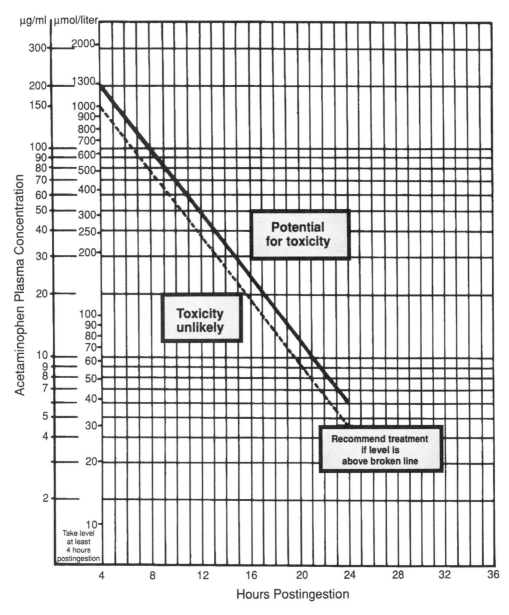

FIGURE 22.2. Nomogram relating acetaminophen plasma concentration, time since ingestion, and risk of toxicity. (Modified from Rumack BH, Matthew H. Acetaminophen poisoning and toxicity. *Pediatrics* 1975;55:871–876.)

24. T (p. 450, column 1)
25. F (p. 450, column 1)
26. F (p. 455, column 1)
27. T (p. 457, column 1)
28. F (p. 457, column 2)
29. F (p. 458, column 1)
30. T (p. 459, column 1)

CHAPTER 24

1. A (p. 464, column 1)

2. A (p. 464, column 2, Table 24.1)
3. D (p. 464, column 2, Table 24.1)
4. A (p. 466, column 1, Table 24.2)
5. B (p. 467, column 1, Table 24.3)
6. C (p. 467, column 2)
7. A (p. 468, column 1)
8. D (p. 468, column 2, Table 24.4)
9. B (p. 468, column 2)
10. D (p. 470, column 2, Table 24.5)
11. B (p. 473, column 2, Table 24.6)
12. A (p. 476, column 2, Table 24.7)
13. C (p. 476, column 2, Table 24.8)

14. B (p. 478, column 1, Table 24.9)
15. C (p. 479, column 1, Table 24.9)
16. F (p. 464, column 2)
17. T (p. 466, column 2)
18. T (p. 471, column 2)
19. F (p. 472, column 1)
20. F (p. 472, column 2)
21. T (p. 472, column 2)
22. F (p. 473, column 2)
23. T (p. 475, column 2)
24. T (p. 479, column 1, Table 24.9)
25. T (p. 481, column 2)

CHAPTER 25

1. B (p. 483, column 2)
2. A (p. 484, column 1, Table 25.3)
3. A (p. 484, column 2, Table 25.4)
4. D (p. 485, column 2, Table 25.5)
5. C (p. 487, column 1)
6. D (p. 487, column 1, Table 25.6)
7. B (p. 487, column 2, Table 25.7)
8. F (p. 483, column 2)
9. T (p. 484, column 2)
10. T (p. 485, column 1)
11. F (p. 485, column 2)
12. T (p. 487, column 1)
13. F (p. 487, column 2)

CHAPTER 26

1. B (p. 490, column 1)
2. D (p. 490, column 2)
3. C (p. 490, column 2)
4. B (p. 491, column 2)
5. A (p. 492, column 1)
6. A (p. 496, column 2)
7. B (p. 497, column 1)

CHAPTER 27

1. C (p. 501, column 1)
2. B (p. 501, column 1)
3. A (p. 501, column 2)
4. D (p. 501, column 2)
5. B (p. 501, column 2)
6. A (p. 502, column 1)
7. B (p. 502, column 2)
8. B (p. 502, column 2)
9. D (p. 502, column 2)
10. C (p. 503, column 1, Table 27.1)
11. D (p. 503, column 2)

TABLE 27.1. LABORATORY EXAMINATION OF SYNOVIAL FLUID

Macroscopic examination
  Volume
  Viscosity
  Clarity
  Color
Cell counting
  Leukocyte count
  Erythrocyte count
Microscopic examination
  Wet preparation
  Stained preparation
  Polarized microscopy for crystals
Microbiologic examination
  Gram stain
  Culture
Special studies
  Chemical examination
  Immunologic examination

12. A (p. 504, column 2, Table 27.2)
13. A (p. 505, column 1)
14. C (p. 505, column 2)
15. C (p. 508, column 2)
16. D (p. 510, column 2, Fig. 27.15)
17. B (p. 512, column 1)
18. C (p. 512, column 2)
19. A (p. 514, column 1)
20. B (p. 515, column 2)
21. F (p. 502, column 1)
22. T (p. 502, column 1)
23. T (p. 502, column 2)
24. F (p. 503, column 2, Fig. 27.3)
25. T (p. 504, column 1)
26. F (p. 506, column 2, Fig. 27.9)
27. T (p. 507, column 1, Table 27.4)
28. T (p. 507, column 1)
29. T (p. 508, column 2)
30. F (p. 508, column 2)

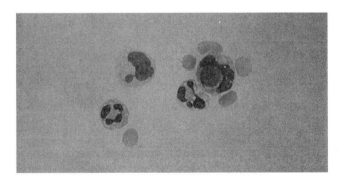

FIGURE 27.9. Tart cell is a macrophage containing a phagocytized nucleus that retains some nuclear detail (Wright-Giemsa stain).

31. T (p. 511, column 2)
32. F (p. 513, column 2, Table 27.6)
33. F (p. 514, column 2)
34. T (p. 515, column 2)
35. T (p. 516, column 1)

CHAPTER 28

1. C (p. 520, column 1)
2. A (p. 521, column 1)
3. B (p. 521, column 2)
4. B (p. 522, column 1)
5. D (p. 522, column 1)
6. A (p. 523, column 1)
7. C (p. 523, column 1)
8. B (p. 524, column 1)
9. D (p. 525, column 2)
10. B (p. 527, column 1)
11. A (p. 529, column 2)
12. C (p. 530, column 1)
13. A (p. 533, column 1, Fig. 28.5)
14. D (p. 534, column 1, Fig. 28.9)
15. B (p. 536, column 2, Fig. 28.14)
16. C (p. 541, column 2, Fig. 28.28)
17. B (p. 542, column 2, Fig. 28.32)
18. D (p. 546, column 2)
19. B (p. 547, column 1, Fig. 28.45)
20. A (p. 549, column 2, Fig. 28.50)
21. T (p. 521, column 1)
22. T (p. 521, column 2)
23. T (p. 522, column 2)
24. F (p. 522, column 2, Fig. 27.3)

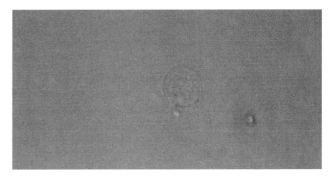

FIGURE 28.50. *Trichomonas vaginalis* in urine. Note the flagella and the spherical character of this parasite. These organisms are easily misdiagnosed as white blood cells (bright-field microscopy, ×400).

25. F (p. 524, column 1)
26. T (p. 524, column 2)
27. T (p. 525, column 1)
28. F (p. 526, column 1)
29. T (p. 526, column 2)
30. T (p. 527, column 1)
31. T (p. 527, column 2)
32. F (p. 528, column 2)
33. F (p. 531, column 1)
34. F (p. 535, column 1, Table 28.4)
35. F (p. 535, column 2)
36. F (p. 539, column 2, Fig. 28.25)
37. T (p. 540, column 2)
38. F (p. 540, column, Fig. 28.26)
39. F (p. 543, column 2)
40. T (p. 549, column 1)

CHAPTER 29

1. B (p. 555, column 2)
2. C (p. 558, column 2, Fig. 29.5)
3. B (p. 559, column 2)
4. C (p. 559, column 2)
5. A (p. 561, column 2)
6. B (p. 561, column 1
7. D (p. 562, column 2)
8. C (p. 564, column 2)
9. D (p. 564, column 2)
10. B (p. 564, column 1)
11. B (p. 567, column 1, Fig. 29.14)
12. A (p. 568, column 2)
13. B (p. 569, column 2, Table 29.1)
14. C (p. 571, column 1, Table 29.1)
15. D (p. 579, column 2)
16. C (p. 580, column 1)
17. C (p. 582, column 1)
18. A (p. 584, column 1)

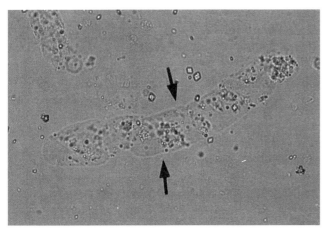

FIGURE 28.14. Granular cast. This type of cast is fundamentally a hyaline cast to which granules have attached along its surface. In the example shown here *(arrows)*, the granules do not cover the entire surface of the cast but are relatively evenly dispersed (bright-field microscopy, ×160.) (From the College of American Pathologists, with permission.)

19. D (p. 585, column 1)
20. D (p. 585, column 2)
21. F (p. 555, column 2)
22. F (p. 555, column 2, Fig. 29.1)
23. F (p. 555, column 2, Table 29.2)
24. T (p. 558, column 1)
25. T (p. 561, column 1)
26. F (p. 561, column 2)
27. F (p. 561, column 2)
28. T (p. 562, column 1)
29. T (p. 562, column 1)
30. T (p. 564, column 2)
31. F (p. 566, column 2)
32. F (p. 568, column 1)
33. T (p. 570, column 1)
34. F (p. 580, column 1)
35. T (p. 583, column 2)

CHAPTER 30

1. D (p. 589, column 1, Table 30.7)
2. D (p. 589, column 1)
3. D (p. 589, column 1)
4. C (p. 589, column 2)
5. C (p. 589, column 2)
6. C (p. 589, column 2)
7. A (p. 589, column 2)
8. B (p. 589, column 2)
9. B (p. 593, column 1)
10. B (p. 593, column 1)
11. A (p. 593, column 1)
12. D (p. 596, column 1)

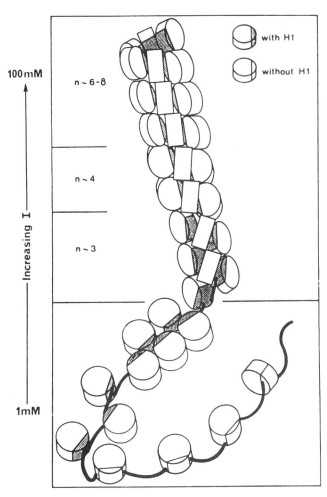

FIGURE 29.5. Idealized drawing of the solenoid structure of a chromosome showing the open zigzag of nucleosomes that form the solenoid. (From Thomas E, Koller TH, Klieg A. *J Cell Biol* 1979;83:403–427, with permission.)

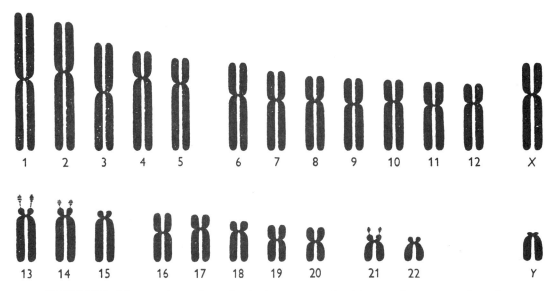

FIGURE 29.1. Idiogram drawn from standard measurements of human chromosomes from the 1960 Denver conference. (From Editorial comments. *Ann Hum Genet* 1960;24:319, with permission.)

TABLE 30.7. CONTIGUOUS GENE SYNDROMES

Autosomal	
Obesity, hyperphagia, MR	1p36
Vander Woude syndrome, MR	1q32–q41
Piebald trait, MR	2q34–q36
Albright's hereditary osteodystrophy like with obesity	2q37
Rieger syndrome, MR	4q25–q27
Adenomatous polyposis, MR	5q21
Craniosynostosis, MR	7p21.2–p21.3
Greig cephalopolysyndactyly, MR	7p13
Russell-Silver syndrome	upd7mat
Williams syndrome	7q11.23
Spherocytosis I, MR	8p11.2–p21.1
Langer-Giedeon syndrome[a]	8q24.11–24.13
Trichorhinophalangeal, type I	8q24.12
DiGeorge syndrome	10p13
Beckwith-Wiedemann syndrome[a]	dup 11p15.5
Wilms tumor, aniridia (WAGR)[a]	11p13
Retinoblastoma, MR[a]	13q14
Angelman, syndrome	15q11–q12 mat; upd15pat
Prader-Willi syndrome[a]	15q11–q12 pat; upd15mat
Rubinstein-Taybi syndrome	16p13.3
Miller-Dieker syndrome[a]	17p13.3
Smith-Magenis syndrome	17p11
Alagille syndrome (arteriohepatic dysplasia), MR	20p11.23–p12.1
DiGeorge syndrome, MR	22q11.2
Velocardiofacial syndrome	22q11.2
X chromosomal	
Ichthyosis, chondrodysplasia punctata, and Kallmann syndrome, MR	Xp22.3
Microphthalmia, iridoschisis, goiter, labium synechia, and craniotabes	Xp22
Choroideremia, deafness, MR	Xp21.1–21.3
Duchenne and Becker dystrophy, MR	Xp21
DMD, CGD, McLeod phenotype, retinitis, MR	Xp21
DMD, glycerol kinase deficiency, Aland eye disease, MR	Xp21
Glycerol kinase deficiency, adrenal hypoplasia, hypogonadotropic hypogonadism, MR	Xp11.2–p21

[a]"Classic" contiguous gene syndromes. All of the contiguous gene syndromes are deletions except Beckwith-Wiedemann and Charcot-Marie-Tooth syndromes.
CGD, chronic granulomatous disease; DMD, Duchenne muscular dystrophy; MR, mental retardation.

13. B (p. 596, column 2)
14. D (p. 596, column 2)
15. D (p. 599, column 2)
16. B (p. 602, column 1)
17. A (p. 602, column 1)
18. C (p. 605, column 1)
19. B (p. 605, column 2)
20. C (p. 607, column 1)
21. B (p. 608, column 1)
22. B (p. 608, column 2)
23. B (p. 608, column 1)
24. C (p. 610, column 2)
25. C (p. 612, column 1)
26. C (p. 612, column 2)
27. D (p. 613, column 2)
28. D (p. 614, column 1)
29. A (p. 614, column 1)
30. C (p. 616, column 2)
31. B (p. 618, column 2)

32. C (p. 619, column 1)
33. C (p. 620, column 1)
34. D (p. 621, column 1)
35. A (p. 621, column 1)
36. C (p. 622, column 2)
37. C (p. 623, column 1)
38. A (p. 625, column 1)
39. B (p. 625, column 2)
40. A (p. 627, column 2)
41. T (p. 593, column 1)
42. T (p. 600, column 2)
43. F (p. 609, column 2)
44. T (p. 610, column 2)
45. T (p. 612, column 1)
46. F (p. 615, column 2)
47. F (p. 624, column 2)
48. T (p. 625, column 2)
49. T (p. 626, column 1)
50. F (p. 628, column 1)

CHAPTER 31

1. C (p. 636, column 1, Table 31.1)
2. A (p. 636, column 1)
3. D (p. 638, column 2)
4. C (p. 638, column 2)
5. B (p. 638, column 2, Table 31.4)
6. A (p. 640, column 1)
7. C (p. 640, column 1)
8. D (p. 640, column 1)
9. A (p. 642, column 1)
10. C (p. 642, column 2)
11. B (p. 642, column 2)
12. D (p. 643, column 1, Fig. 31.2)
13. B (p. 643, column 1, Table 31.8)
14. C (p. 643, column 2)
15. C (p. 646, column 2, Fig. 31.4)
16. D (p. 647, column 1)
17. A (p. 650, column 2)
18. D (p. 651, column 1, Table 31.11)
19. B (p. 652, column 2)
20. A (p. 653, column 1)
21. T (p. 636, column 1)
22. F (p. 636, column 2)
23. F (p. 637, column 1)
24. F (p. 639, column 1)
25. T (p. 640, column 1)
26. T (p. 642, column 1)
27. F (p. 642, column 1)
28. T (p. 645, column 1)
29. T (p. 649, column 2)
30. T (p. 652, column 1)
31. F (p. 653, column 1)
32. T (p. 653, column 2)
33. T (p. 653, column 2)
34. F (p. 654, column 1)
35. T (p. 655, column 2)

TABLE 31.1. INDICATIONS FOR PRENATAL CYTOGENETIC OR AFP DIAGNOSIS

Advanced maternal age
One parent carries a chromosome rearrangement
Previous offspring with a chromosome abnormality
Previous offspring with a neural tube defect or hydrocephalus
High maternal serum AFP
Low maternal serum AFP (or similar screening result)
Fetal abnormality detected by ultrasound examination
Fetus at risk for X-linked or prenatally diagnosable inherited disease

AFP, α-fetoprotein.

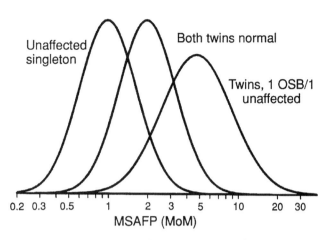

FIGURE 31.2. Distribution of maternal serum α-fetoprotein values for singleton and twin pregnancies. Median multiple of median (MoM) is 1.0 for normal singletons, 2.0 for normal twins, and 4.8 for twins [one twin normal and one with open spina bifida (OSB)] is 4.8 MoM. (From Palomaki G. Foundation of Blood Research, Scarborough, ME, with permission.)

CHAPTER 32

1. B (p. 658, column 1)
2. C (p. 661, column 1)
3. C (p. 662, column 1)
4. D (p. 662, column 1)
5. A (p. 662, column 2)
6. A (p. 664, column 1)
7. A (p. 664, column 2)
8. D (p. 664, column 2)
9. C (p. 664, column 2)
10. B (p. 664, column 2)
11. D (p. 666, column 1)
12. C (p. 666, column 1)
13. A (p. 666, column 1, Figure 32.2)
14. B (p. 666, column 1)
15. B (p. 667, column 2)
16. A (p. 678, column 1)
17. C (p. 678, column 1)
18. C (p. 678, column 2)
19. D (p. 678, column 2)
20. B (p. 678, column 1)
21. A (p. 678, column 2)
22. C (p. 679, column 1)
23. D (p. 679, column 1)
24. A (p. 679, column 2)
25. B (p. 679, column 2)
26. C (p. 681, column 1)
27. A (p. 681, column 2)
28. C (p. 683, column 1)
29. B (p. 683, column 2)
30. C (p. 683, column 2)
31. D (p. 683, column 1)

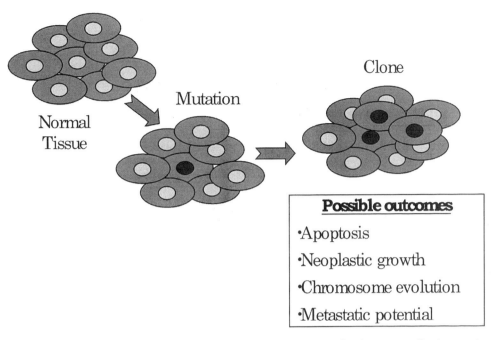

FIGURE 32.2. Formation of a clone. In the early stages, the cells of a chromosomally abnormal clone may die as a consequence of genetic imbalance or may be destroyed by the immune system. If not, the clone may proliferate and form a malignant tumor, and subclones may form as a result of chromosome evolution.

32. A (p. 682, column 2)
33. E (p. 682, column 1)
34. B (p. 683, column 2)

CHAPTER 33

1. D (p. 686, column 1)
2. A (p. 686, column 2, Table 33.1)

TABLE 33.1. FEATURES OF BLOOM SYNDROME

Clinical
  Pre- and postnatal growth deficiency, with relatively normal body proportions
  Telangiectatic erythema of face, sun sensitive
  Microcephaly with dolichocephaly
  Malar and mandibular hypoplasia
  Relative prominence of nose and ears
  High-pitched squeaky voice
  Hypo- and hyperpigmented areas of skin
  Immunodeficiency
    Increased otitis media and pneumonia
    Bronchiectasia and chronic lung failure
  Male infertility; female subfertility and premature menopause
  Diabetes mellitus, usually adult onset
  Increased incidence of neoplasia of many types and sites
Cytogenetic
  Excessive spontaneous chromosomal breakage
  Homologous quadriradial configurations
  Elevated sister-chromatid exchange frequency

3. C (p. 686, column 2)
4. A (p. 687, column 2, Fig. 33.1)
5. D (p. 691, column 2, Table 33.2)
6. B (p. 691, column 2)
7. D (p. 692, column 1)
8. C (p. 694, column 1, Table 33.3, Figure 33.1)
9. A (p. 694, column 1)
10. D (p. 694, column 2)
11. B (p. 696, column 1)
12. D (p. 697, column 1, Table 33.4)
13. B (p. 697, column 2)
14. C (p. 698, column 1, Table 33.5)
15. A (p. 698, column 2)
16. B (p. 700, column 1, Table 33.7)
17. F (p. 686, column 1)
18. F (p. 686, column 1)
19. T (p. 691, column 2)
20. F (p. 695, column 1)
21. T (p. 695, column 2)
22. T (p. 700, column 1)
23. T (p. 700, column 2, Table 33.7)
24. F (p. 700, column 2)
25. F (p. 701, column 1)

CHAPTER 34

1. B (p. 704, column 1)
2. C (p. 705, column 2)

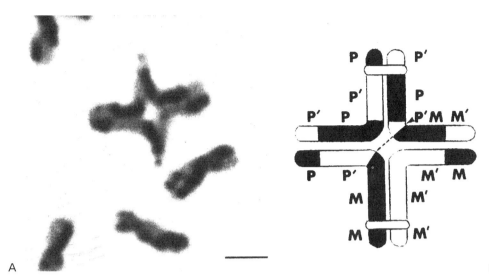

FIGURE 33.1. A: Qr configuration formed between two apparently homologous chromosomes in a BS T lymphocyte. Chromosomes are differentially stained as a result of growth for two cell cycles in BrdU-containing medium. **B:** Diagrammatic representation of event that led to Qr formation in **(A)**. Chromatids arbitrarily have been designated P and P′ for the paternally derived chromosome and M and M′ for the maternally derived chromosome. The presence of P′ segments on P chromatids and P segments on P′ chromatids indicates that exchanges have taken place between the sister chromatids of the paternal chromosome. This also is T for M′ and M chromatids of maternal origin. The presence of M/M′ segments on P/P′ chromatids and P/P′ segments on M/M′ chromatids signifies the exchange of DNA segments between nonsister chromatids of the homologous chromosomes that led to the formation of Qr. The point at which the nonsister chromatid exchange occurred is designated by the *dashed line*. Bar represents 2 μm. (Ray JH, German J. The chromosome changes in Bloom's syndrome, ataxia-telangiectasia, and Fanconi's anemia. In: Arrighi FE, Rao PN, Strubblefield E, eds. *Genes, chromosomes and neoplasia*. New York: Raven Press, 1981:351–378, with permission.)

3. B (p. 707, column 1)
4. C (p. 715, column 1)
5. D (p. 715, column 2)
6. A (p. 716, column 2)
7. D (p. 718, column 2)
8. A (p. 719, column 2)
9. C (p. 721, column 1, Figure 34.5)
10. B (p. 721, column 1)
11. D (p. 721, column 2)
12. D (p. 722, column 1)
13. C (p. 725, column 2)
14. A (p. 726, column 1)
15. B (p. 726, column 1)
16. A (p. 728, column 1)
17. T (p. 707, column 1)
18. T (p. 708, column 2)
19. T (p. 711, column 2)
20. T (p. 712, column 2)
21. F (p. 715, column 1)
22. T (p. 715, column 2)
23. F (p. 718, column 1)
24. T (p. 718, column 1)
25. T (p. 718, column 2)
26. F (p. 720, column 2)

27. T (p. 721, column 1)
28. T (p. 722, column 1)
29. T (p. 728, column 2)
30. T (p. 728, column 2)

CHAPTER 35

1. T (p. 733, column 2)
2. A (p. 733, column 2)
3. B (p. 734, column 1, Figure 35.3)
4. T (p. 739, column 1)
5. D (p. 740, column 1)
6. F (p. 741, column 1)
7. E (p. 741, column 2)
8. T (p. 743, column 1)
9. T (p. 743, column 2)
10. E (p. 750, column 2)

CHAPTER 36

1. D (p. 758, column 1, Table 36.1)
2. T (p. 761, column 2)

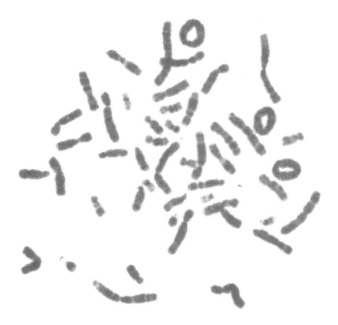

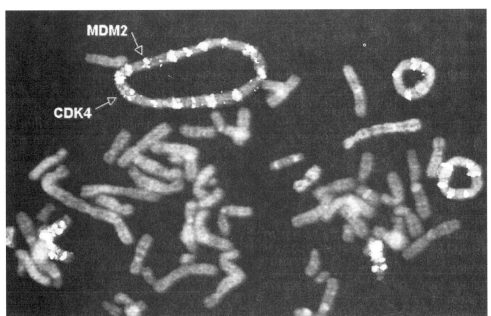

FIGURE 34.5. Top: G-banded metaphase spread showing supernumerary ring chromosomes in an atypical lipomatous tumor. These ring chromosomes characteristically contain amplified chromosome 12 sequences **(bottom)** as shown by two-color fluorescence *in situ* hybridization using probes for MDM2 and CDK4. (Courtesy of Dr. David Gisselsson, Department of Clinical Genetics, Lund University Hospital, Lund Sweden.)

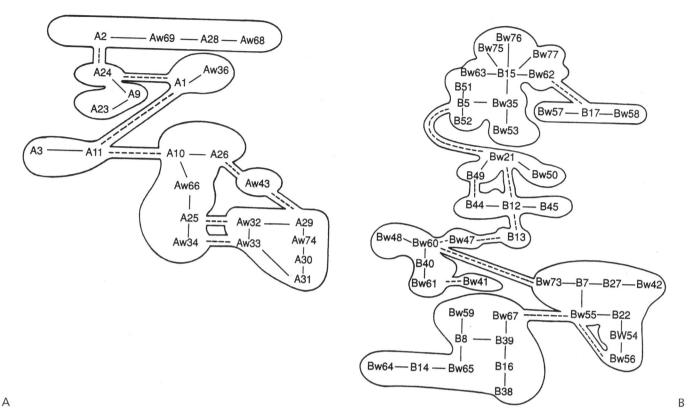

FIGURE 35.3. Prominent cross-reactive groups (CREGs) of the HLA antigens. **A:** CREGs of the HLA-A antigens. **B:** CREGs of the HLA-B antigens. The antigens form tightly bound clusters that are strongly cross-reactive. In addition, some weaker cross-reactivity *(dotted lines)* exists between the clusters.

TABLE 36.1. GENERIC AND GROUP-SPECIFIC (ALLELE GROUP DRB1*O1) PRIMERS USED FOR AMPLIFICATION OF EXON 2 OF DRB ALLELES

Amplification Type	Intron-Exon	Nucleotide Sequence[a]	Orientation
DRB generic			
		Intron 1 NUC/Exon-2 CODONS[c]	Forward
2DRBAMP-A[b]	**Intron1**	−8 −1 5 6 7 8	Mixture
	TO	5′ CCCCACAG CA CGT TTC TTG 3′	
	Exon2	5′ ——————— —— —— C — 3′	
2DRBAMP-B	Exon2	93 92 91 90 89 88 87	Reverse
		5′ CCG CTG CAC TGT GAA GCT CT 3′	
DRB1*01 group specific			
2DRBAMP-1[d]	**Exon2**	7 8 9 10 11 12 13	Forward
		5′ TTC TTG TGG CAG CTT AAG TT 3′	
2DRBAMP-B	Exon2	93 92 91 90 89 88 87	Reverse
		5′ CCG CTG CAC TGT GAA GCT CT 3′	

[a]Nucleotide sequences of oligonucleotide primers used for amplification of DRB alleles. Primer pairs were selected to match the sequences of alleles of the locus (generic primers) or groups of alleles (group-specific primers).

[b]A mixture of primers is required to amplify all the DRB alleles. Note Codon 8 in Figure 36.1, which shows similarity of DRB1*07011, *15011, and *16011 (and their difference from *0101) necessitating the use of a different primer in the mixture.

[c]Relative positions are shown as codons for nucleotides from exons. The sequences shown in Figure 35.1 can be used for comparison. Please notice that the sequence alignment in Figure 35.1 shows only coding DNA (exon sequences). Therefore, for comparison with Figure 35.1, the exon segments of the primer should be used. The nucleotide sequence of the forward primers can be visualized directly; the sequence of the reverse primers can be matched by converting the sequence to the complementary nucleotide and by inverting the orientation of the complementary bases.

[d]For amplification of the DRB1*01 alleles, group specificity is obtained with the forward primer 2-DRBAMP-1; the nucleotide sequence of this primer matches only DRB1*01 alleles; in bold and underlined are shown polymorphic nucleotide positions.

TABLE 37.2. CADAVER KIDNEY GRAFT SURVIVAL ACCORDING TO HAPLOTYPE MATCHES

Level of HLA Mismatch	1-Year Survival (%)	5-Year Survival (%)
0	95.2	82.1
1	96.1	82.2
2	94.8	82.0
3	95.0	81.8
4	94.9	81.0
5	94.4	80.1
6	93.8	78.8

Data from United Network for Organ Sharing 1998 (2).

11. E (p. 770, column 2)
12. T (p. 774 Table 37.4)
13. T (p. 774, column 1)
14. E (p. 776, column 2)
15. T (p. 778, column 1, Table 37.2)

CHAPTER 38

1. E (p. 779, column 2)
2. D (p. 781, column 1)
3. F (p. 783, column 2)
4. T (p. 784, column 1)

CHAPTER 37

1. T (p. 763, column 1)
2. C (p. 764, column 2)
3. T (p. 764, column 2)
4. A (p. 765, column 1)
5. T (p. 766, column 1)
6. T (p. 766, column 1)
7. T (p. 766, column 2)
8. E (p. 768, column 1)
9. T (p. 770, column 2)
10. T (p. 770, column 2)

CHAPTER 39

1. C (p. 791, column 1)
2. A (p. 791, column 2)
3. A (p. 793, column 2)
4. B (p. 794, column 1)
5. C (p. 794, column 1)
6. B (p. 749, column 1)
7. B (p. 794, column 2, Figure 39.1)
8. C (p. 794, column 2)
9. A (p. 794, column 2)
10. C (p. 794, column 2)

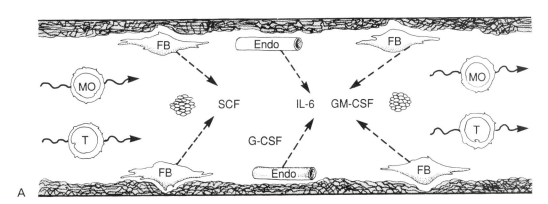

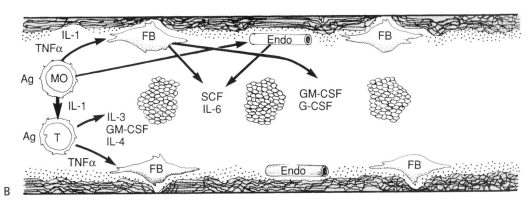

FIGURE 39.1. A: Basal hematopoiesis. **B:** Antigen-amplified hematopoiesis.

CHAPTER 40

1. B (p. 797, column 2)
2. B (p. 797, column 2)
3. A (p. 799, column 1)
4. D (p. 801, column 2)
5. C (p. 802, column 1)
6. B (p. 804, column 1)
7. A (p. 806, column 2)
8. C (p. 807, column 1)
9. B (p. 808, Table 40.6)
10. D (p. 810, column 1)
11. C (p. 814, Table 40.9)
12. A (p. 821, column 1)
13. B (p. 821, Table 40.14)
14. D (p. 821, Table 40.15)
15. C (p. 823, Table 40.18)
16. C (p. 825, Table 40.22)
17. A (p. 825, column 1)
18. C (p. 827, column 2)
19. D (p. 826, column 1)
20. A (p. 826, column 2)
21. B (p. 828, column 1)

CHAPTER 41

1. A (p. 830, column 1)
2. D (p. 831, Table 41.1)
3. C (p. 831, Table 41.1)
4. D (p. 833, column 1)
5. A (p. 833, column 1)
6. C (p. 835, column 1)
7. B (p. 835, column 2)
8. D (p. 836, column 2)
9. B (p. 838, column 1)
10. A (p. 839, column 1)
11. A (p. 839, column 2)
12. C (p. 839, column 2)
13. B (p. 840, column 1)
14. A (p. 840, column 2)
15. D (p. 841, column 1)
16. D (p. 842, column 1)
17. C (p. 842, column 2)
18. B (p. 843, column 1)
19. A (p. 843, column 2)
20. D (p. 844, column 1)
21. A (p. 844, column 2)
22. A (p. 844, column 2)
23. D (p. 846, column 1)
24. C (p. 847, column 1)
25. B (p. 848, column 1)
26. C (p. 848, column 1)
27. B (p. 848, column 1)
28. C (p. 848, column 1)
29. A (p. 848, column 1)
30. D (p. 852, Table 41.8)
31. C (p. 852, column 2)
32. B (p. 854, column 1)
33. B (p. 855, column 1)
34. C (p. 857, column 2)
35. A (p. 859, column 1)
36. B (p. 859, column 2)
37. A (p. 860, column 2)
38. B (p. 860, column 2)
39. B (p. 861, column 1)
40. A (p. 861, column 1)
41. D (p. 861, column 2)
42. C (p. 861, column 2)
43. D (p. 861, column 2)
44. A (p. 861, column 2)
45. B (p. 861, column 2)
46. A (p. 862, column 1)
47. C (p. 862, column 1)

CHAPTER 42

1. C (p. 867, Table 42.1)
2. A (p. 867, Table 42.1)
3. D (p. 867, Table 42.1)
4. B (p. 867, Table 42.1)
5. B (p. 866, column 2)
6. A (p. 868, column 1)
7. C (p. 872, column 1)
8. A (p. 872, column 1)
9. C (p. 872, column 1)
10. B (p. 872, column 1)
11. D (p. 872, column 1)
12. C (p. 872, column 2)
13. A (p. 872, column 2)
14. D (p. 872, column 2)
15. B (p. 872, column 2)
16. A (p. 879, column 2)
17. B (p. 880, column 2)
18. C (p. 882, column 1)
19. A (p. 882, column 2)
20. C (p. 883, column 1)
21. D (p. 883, column 2)
22. D (p. 885, column 2)
23. B (p. 886, Table 42.8)
24. D (p. 886, Table 42.8)
25. C (p. 886, Table 42.8)
26. A (p. 886, Table 42.8)
27. C (p. 887, column 1)
28. B (p. 887, column 2)
29. A (p. 888, column 2)
30. D (p. 888, column 2)
31. A (p. 888, column 2)
32. A (p. 889, column 1)

TABLE 43.3. FAB CLASSIFICATION OF ACUTE LYMPHOBLASTIC LEUKEMIA

Cytologic Feature	L1	L2	L3
Size	Predominant small cells	Heterogeneous, intermediate to large cells	Large cells
Cytoplasm	Scant	Variable to moderately abundant	Moderately abundant
Nucleoli	Small/inconspicuous	≥1; prominent to large	≥1; prominent and large
Nuclear chromatin	Homogeneous and intermediate reticular	Heterogeneous, with some having finely reticular chromatin	Finely reticular
Nuclear shape	Regular and round	Irregular	Regular to round
Basophilic cytoplasm	Slight to none	Slight to none	Intense
Vacuolation	Slight to none	Slight to none	Prominent; sharply punched

FAB, French-American-British.

CHAPTER 43

1. B (p. 896, column 1)
2. B (p. 896, column 2)
3. D (p. 896, column 2)
4. C (p. 896, column 2)
5. A (p. 896, column 2)
6. C (p. 898, column 2)
7. B (p. 898, column 2)
8. B (p. 899, Table 43.3)
9. A (p. 899, Table 43.3)
10. C (p. 899, Table 43.3)
11. A (p. 899, Table 43.3)
12. C (p. 899, Table 43.3)
13. B (p. 899, Table 43.3)
14. C (p. 901, column 1)
15. D (p. 902, column 2)
16. A (p. 902, column 2)
17. B (p. 903, column 2)
18. B (p. 904, column 2)
19. C (p. 904, column 2)
20. C (p. 904, column 2)
21. B (p. 904, column 2)
22. D (p. 904, column 2)
23. A (p. 904, column 2)
24. D (p. 905, column 1)
25. A (p. 905, column 2)
26. C (p. 906, Table 43.10)
27. D (p. 906, Table 43.10)
28. A (p. 906, Table 43.10)
29. B (p. 906, Table 43.10)
30. C (p. 906, column 2)
31. D (p. 907, Table 43.12)
32. C (p. 907, Table 43.12)
33. A (p. 907, Table 43.12)
34. B (p. 907, Table 43.12)
35. C (p. 907, column 1)
36. D (p. 907, column 1)
37. E (p. 907, column 1)
38. A (p. 907, column 1)
39. B (p. 907, column 1)
40. B (p. 907, column 2)
41. A (p. 908, column 1)
42. C (p. 908, column 2)
43. C (p. 910, column 1)
44. D (p. 910, column 1; and p 906, Table 43.10)
45. B (p. 911, column 1)
46. A (p. 918, Table 43.16)
47. C (p. 918, Table 43.17)
48. C (p. 920, Table 43.19)

CHAPTER 44

1. B (p. 923, column 2)
2. D (p. 927, column 2)
3. B (p. 928, column 2)
4. C (p. 928, column 2)
5. A (p. 929, column 2)
6. B (p. 930, column 2)
7. B (p. 930, column 2)
8. D (p. 925, Table 44.2)

TABLE 43.10. INCIDENCE OF ACUTE MYELOGENOUS LEUKEMIA ACCORDING TO FAB SUBTYPE

FAB Subtype	Incidence (%)
M0	1–2
M1	18
M2	28
M3	8
M4	27
M5	10
M6	4
M7	5

FAB, French-American-British classification.

9. C (p. 933, column 2)
10. B (p. 934, column 2)
11. C (p. 934, column 2)
12. A (p. 935, column 1)
13. A (p. 935, column 1)
14. D (p. 935, column 2)
15. C (p. 937, Table 44.9)
16. D (p. 938, column 2)
17. A (p. 938, column 2)
18. C (p. 942, column 1)
19. A (p. 944, column 1)
20. E (p. 950, Table 44.20)
21. D (p. 950, Table 44.20)
22. A (p. 950, Table 44.20)
23. B (p. 950, Table 44.20)
24. C (p. 950, Table 44.20)
25. B (p. 951, Table 44.21)
26. B (p. 951, Table 44.21)
27. C (p. 951, Table 44.21)
28. C (p. 951, Table 44.21)
26. B (p. 952, Table 44.23)
27. C (p. 952, Table 44.23)
28. A (p. 952, Table 44.23)
29. D (p. 952, Table 44.23)
30. A (p. 956, column 2)
31. C (p. 957, column 2)

CHAPTER 45

1. C (p. 964, column 1)
2. A (p. 964, column 1)
3. B (p. 964, column 2)
4. A (p. 965, column 2)
5. A (p. 965, column 1)
6. B (p. 965, column 2)
7. D (p. 966, column 2)
8. D (p. 967, column 2)
9. B (p. 968, column 1)
10. C (p. 968, column 1)
11. C (p. 968, column 1)
12. D (p. 968, column 2)
13. A (p. 968, column 2)
14. A (p. 969, column 1)
15. B (p. 969, column 1)
16. C (p. 969, column 2)
17. D (p. 969, column 2)
18. A (p. 970, column 2)
19. D (p. 970, column 2)
20. A (p. 970, column 2)
21. C (p. 971, column 1)
22. B (p. 972, column 1)
23. B (p. 972, column 2)
24. C (p. 973, Table 45.2)
25. D (p. 973, Table 45.3)

26. A (p. 973, column 2)
27. B (p. 974, column 2)
28. A (p. 975, Table 45.6)
29. C (p. 975, Table 45.7)
30. B (p. 976, column 2)
31. B (p. 976, column 2)
32. C (p. 977, column 1)
33. D (p. 977, column 2)
34. D (p. 978, Fig. 45.15)
35. A (p. 978, Fig. 45.15)
36. B (p. 978, Fig. 45.15)
37. C (p. 978, Fig. 45.15)
38. A (p. 978, Table 45.8)
39. C (p. 980, column 2)
40. D (p. 981, column 1)
41. D (p. 981, column 1)

CHAPTER 46

1. B (p. 987, column 2)
2. D (p. 989, Table 46.1)
3. E (p. 989, Table 46.1)
4. C (p. 989, Table 46.1)
5. A (p. 989, Table 46.1)
6. B (p. 989, Table 46.1)
7. A (p. 990, Table 46.2)
8. B (p. 990, column 1)
9. B (p. 990, column 2)
10. B (p. 993, column 1)
11. D (p. 994, column 1)
12. C (p. 994, Table 46.3)
13. C (p. 995, Table 46.4)
14. A (p. 995, Table 46.5)
15. C (p. 996, column 1)
16. A (p. 996, column 1)
17. B (p. 996, column 2)
18. D (p. 997, column 2)
19. B (p. 999, Table 46.6)
20. A (p. 999, column 2)
21. C (p. 999, column 2)
22. D (p. 1000, Table 46.7)
23. A (p. 1000, Table 46.7)
24. B (p. 1000, Table 46.7)
25. C (p. 1000, Table 46.7)
26. B (p. 1002, Table 46.9)
27. A (p. 1002, Table 46.9)
28. D (p. 1002, Table 46.9)
29. C (p. 1002, Table 46.9)
30. D (p. 1003, Table 46.10)
31. B (p. 1003, Table 46.10)
32. A (p. 1003, Table 46.10)
33. C (p. 1003, Table 46.10)
34. D (p. 1006, column 2)

CHAPTER 47

1. C (p. 1010, column 2)
2. C (p. 1011, column 2)
3. A (p. 1013, column 2)
4. D (p. 1013, column 2)
5. A (p. 1015, Table 47.2)
6. C (p. 1015, Table 47.2)
7. B (p. 1015, Table 47.2)
8. D (p. 1015, Table 47.2)
9. D (p. 1017, column 1)
10. A (p. 1018, column 1)
11. C (p. 1020, column 1)
12. B (p. 1020, column 2)
13. C (p. 1021, column 2)
14. B (p. 1025, column 1)
15. B (p. 1025, Table 47.8)
16. A (p. 1025, Table 47.8)
17. A (p. 1025, Table 47.8)
18. A (p. 1025, Table 47.8)
19. B (p. 1025, Table 47.8)
20. A (p. 1026, column 1)
21. A (p. 1026, column 1)
22. B (p. 1026, column 2)
23. C (p. 1026, column 2)
24. A (p. 1026, column 2)
25. A (p. 1027, column 1)
26. B (p. 1027, column 1)
27. A (p. 1027, column 1)
28. A (p. 1027, column 1)
29. B (p. 1027, column 1)
30. C (p. 1027, column 1)

CHAPTER 48

1. D (p. 1033, column 1)
2. B (p. 1034, column 2)
3. B (p. 1036, column 1)
4. C (p. 1036, column 2)
5. A (p. 1037, column 1)
6. B (p. 1037, column 2)
7. D (p. 1040, column 1)
8. C (p. 1040, column 1)
9. A (p. 1041, column 2)
10. C (p. 1043, column 1)
11. D (p. 1045, column 1)
12. A (p. 1045, column 2)
13. A (p. 1045, column 2)
14. C (p. 1045, column 2)
15. C (p. 1045, column 2)
16. B (p. 1045, column 2)
17. C (p. 1048, Table 48.12)

CHAPTER 49

1. A (p. 1050, column 1)
2. B (p. 1051, column 1)
3. B (p. 1052, column 1)
4. D (p. 1052, column 2)
5. C (p. 1052, column 2)
6. A (p. 1050, column 1)
7. C (p. 1052, column 2)
8. B (p. 1051, column 1)
9. A (p. 1054, column 4)

CHAPTER 50

1. D (p. 1059, column 2)
2. D (p. 1060, Table 50.2)
3. T (p. 1060, column 2)
4. T (p. 1061, column 1)
5. B (p. 1062, Table 50.4)
6. C (p. 1062, Table 50.5)
7. T (p. 1062, column 2)
8. T (p. 1063, column 1)
9. T (p. 1063, column 2)
10. T (p. 1064, column 2)
11. T (p. 1065, column 1)
12. T (p. 1065, column 2)
13. D (p. 1066, column 1)
14. T (p. 1067, column 1)
15. T (p. 1067, column 1)
16. T (p. 1067, column 2)
17. E (p. 1068, column 1)
18. T (p. 1068, column 1)
19. T (p. 1069, column 1)
20. T (p. 1070, column 1)
21. D (p. 1071, column 1)
22. E (p. 1072, column 1)

TABLE 50.2. SPECIMENS NOT ROUTINELY ACCEPTED FOR ANAEROBIC CULTURE

Throat, nasopharyngeal, or gingival swabs
Sputa
Bronchial wash, lavage, or brush (except when collected with a protected double-lumen catheter)
Gastric and bowel contents
Ileostomy and colostomy effluent
Voided or catheterized urine
Female genital tract specimens collected through the vagina
Surface swabs of ulcers, wounds, and abscesses

CHAPTER 51

1. E (p. 1074, column 2)
2. B (p. 1075, column 1)
3. T (p. 1077, column 2)
4. T (p. 1077, column 2)
5. T (p. 1077, column 2)
6. D (p. 1078, column 2)
7. T (p. 1080, column 1, Fig. 51.2)
8. D (p. 1081, column 1)
9. C (p. 1082, column 1, Fig. 51.4)
10. T (p. 1082, column 2)
11. E (p. 1082, column 2)
12. F (p. 1083, column 2, Fig. 51.4)
13. D (p. 1085, column 1)
14. D (p. 1085, column 2, Fig. 51.6)
15. D (p. 1086, column 1)
16. T (p. 1086, column 2)
17. T (p. 1093, column 2)
18. T (p. 1094, column 2)
19. E (p. 1095, column 1)
20. D (p. 1096, column 1)
21. T (1097, column 2)
22. T (p. 1098, column 2)
23. E (p. 1099, column 2)
24. C (p. 1101, column 2)
25. E (p. 1101, column 2)
26. T (p. 1103, column 2)
27. C (p. 1104, column 1)
28. F (p. 1104, column 1)
29. E (p. 1105, column 1)
30. T (p. 1106, (column 2)
31. D (p. 1107, column 1)
32. D (p. 1109, column 1)
33. E (p. 1111, column 1)
34. D (p. 1111, column 1)
35. T (p. 1112, column 2)
36. T (p. 1114, column 2)
37. B (p. 1115, Table 51.26)
38. T (p. 1116, column 2, Fig. 51.17)
39. D (p. 1118, column 2)
40. F (p. 1119, column 2)
41. D (p. 1121, column 1)
42. E (p. 1121, column 2)

CHAPTER 52

1. T (p. 1125, column 2)
2. D (p. 1125, column 2)
3. D (p. 1126, column 1)
4. D (p. 1126, column 2)
5. D (p. 1128, column 1)
6. D (p. 1129, column 2)
7. F (p. 1130, column 1)

TABLE 52.6. AGENTS OF OPPORTUNISTIC MYCOSES[a]

I. *Candida* and other opportunistic yeasts
   Candida albicans
   Candida glabrata
   Candida tropicalis
   Candida parapsilosis
   Candida krusei
   Candida lusitaniae
   Candida dubliniensis
   Cryptococus neoformans
   Malassezia sp
   Rhodotorula sp
   Saccharomyces cerevisiae
   Trichosporon sp
II. Agents of hyalohyphomycosis
   Aspergillus sp
   Fusarium sp
   Pseudallescheria boydii
   Scedosporium prolificans
   Scopulariopsis sp
III. Agents of zygomycosis
   Absidia sp
   Mucor sp
   Rhizomucor sp
   Rhizopus sp
IV. Agents of pheohyphomycosis
   Alternaria sp
   Bipolaris sp
   Curvularia sp
   Exserohilum sp
V. *Pneumocystis carinii*

[a]List is not all inclusive.

8. E (p. 1131, column 1)
9. B (p. 1132, column 1, Fig. 52.7)
10. E (p. 1133, column 1)
11. C (p. 1133, column 2, Fig. 52.9)
12. E (p. 1134, column 2)
13. C (p. 1135, column 2)
14. E (p. 1136, column 2, Table 52.6)
15. T (p. 1137, column 2)
16. E (p. 1138, column 1, Fig. 52.15)
17. T (p. 1140, column 1)
18. T (p. 1141, column 2, Fig. 52.19)
19. T (p. 1145, column 2)
20. T (p. 1146, column 2)
21. B (p. 1147, column 1)

CHAPTER 53

1. T (p. 1158, column 1)
2. T (p. 1158, column 2)
3. D (p. 1159, column 2)
4. T (p. 1166, column 1)
5. T (p. 1167, column 1)
6. T (p. 1168, column 1)

TABLE 54.1. SELECTED DIFFERENTIAL CHARACTERISTICS OF AEROBIC ACTINOMYCETES ENCOUNTERED IN CLINICAL SPECIMENS[a]

Characteristic or Feature	Genus							
	Actinomadura	*Gordona*	*Nocardia*	*Nocardiopsis*	*Oerskovia*	*Rhodococcus*	*Streptomyces*	*Tsukamurella*
DAP isomer type	*meso*	*meso*	*meso*	*meso*	None	*meso*	L	*meso*
Cell wall sugars[b]	Mad	Arab, Gal	Arab, Gal	None	Gal	Arab, Gal	None	Arab, Gal
Size of mycolic acid (no. of carbons)	None	48–66	44–60	None	None	34–64	None	64–78
Acid fastness (weak)[c]	No	Yes	Yes	No	No	Yes	No	Yes
Lysozyme resistance	No	Variable	Yes	No	Yes	Variable	No	Yes
Aerial filament growth	Variable	No	Yes	Yes	No	No	Yes	No
Hyphal fragmentation	No		Yes	No	Yes (motile)	Yes	Variable	

[a]*Mycobacterium* and *Dermatophilus* are not listed because the former is characterized in Table 47.4, and the latter is easily differentiated and rarely encountered in clinical specimens.
[b]Arab, arabinose; Gal, galactose; Mad, madurose.
[c]Acid fastness: weak, 0.5% to 1% sulfuric acid in decolorizer; strong, 3% hydrochloric acid in decolorizer. Compiled from references 1 and 4.

7. A (p. 1169, column 2)
8. E (p. 1170, column 2)
9. D (p. 1171, column 1)
10. T (p. 1171, column 1)
11. A (p. 1176, column 1)
12. D (p. 1181, column 1)
13. T (p. 1181, column 1)
14. T (p. 1183, column 2)
15. B (p. 1184, column 2)
16. T (p. 1185, column 1)
17. C (p. 1188, column 1)
18. D (p. 1190, column 2)
19. A (p. 1191, column 2)

CHAPTER 54

1. B (p. 1201, column 1)
2. D (p. 1202, column 1, Table 54.1)
3. C (p. 1204, column 1)
4. A (p. 1204, column 1)

TABLE 55.1. LABORATORY RESPONSIBILITIES FOR PERFORMING ANTIMICROBIAL SUSCEPTIBILITY TESTS

Select isolates to be tested
Select antimicrobics to test
Perform tests using standardized procedures whenever possible
Assist with interpretation of nonstandardized tests
Report results
  Accurately
  Timely
  Selectively

5. D (p. 1204, column 1)
6. D (p. 1206, column 2)
7. C (p. 1206, column 2)
8. A (p. 1207, column 1)
9. C (p. 1209, column 2)
10. B (p. 1210, column 2)
11. B (p. 1210, column 2)
12. A (p. 1214, column 1)
13. A (p. 1215, column 2)
14. D (p. 1216, column 1)
15. C (p. 1218, column 1)
16. T (p. 1202, column 2)
17. F (p. 1207, column 1)
18. T (p. 1210, column 2)
19. F (p. 1210, column 2)
20. T (p. 1217, column 1)

CHAPTER 55

1. C (p. 1222, column 1, Table 55.1)
2. C (p. 1222, column 1, Table 55.2)

TABLE 55.2. FREQUENTLY USED IN VITRO SUSCEPTIBILITY TESTS

Dilution tests
  Broth microdilution
  Agar
  Semiautomated
Diffusion tests
  Disk (Kirby Bauer)
  Fixed gradient (Etest or epsilometer)
  Spot tests (e.g., β-lactamase)

3. A (p. 1222, column 2)
4. B (p. 1223, column 1)
5. C (p. 1223, column 2)
6. D (p. 1223, column 2)
7. C (p. 1224, column 2)
8. B (p. 1224, column 2)
9. D (p. 1225, column 2)
10. C (p. 1228, column 1)
11. B (p. 1228, column 1)
12. C (p. 1231, column 1)
13. A (p. 1231, column 2)
14. A (p. 1231, column 2)
15. C (p. 1232, column 1, Fig. 55.9)
16. T (p. 1224, column 2)
17. T (p. 1229, column 1)
18. T (p. 1229, column 2)
19. T (p. 1232, column 2)
20. T (p. 1233, column 1)

CHAPTER 56

1. B (p. 1236, column 1)
2. C (p. 1237, column 2)
3. A (p. 1238, column 1)
4. B (p. 1238, column 2)
5. D (p. 1240, column 1)
6. B (p. 1241, column 2)
7. C (p. 1242, column 1, Table 56.2)
8. C (p. 1242, column 2)
9. C (p. 1242, column 1)
10. C (p. 1244, column 1)
11. T (p. 1236, column 2)
12. F (p. 1238, column 1)
13. T (p. 1239, column 1)
14. T (p. 1241, column 2)
15. T (p. 1242, column 2)

TABLE 56.2. EXAMPLES OF HUMAN PATHOGENS FIRST IDENTIFIED FROM CLINICAL SPECIMENS USING MOLECULAR APPROACHES

Disease	Pathogen	Reference
Non-A, non-B hepatitis	Hepatitis C virus	67
Bacillary angiomatosis	*Bartonella henselae*	68
Whipple disease	*Tropheryma whippelii*	46
Hantavirus pulmonary syndrome	Sin nombre virus	69
Kaposi sarcoma	Human herpes virus 8	70

Adapted from reference 47.

CHAPTER 57

1. A (p. 1247, column 1)
2. B (p. 1247, column 2)
3. B (p. 1250, column 1)
4. C (p. 1253, Table 57.5)
5. A (p. 1253, Table 57.5)
6. D (p. 1253, Table 57.5)
7. B (p. 1253, Table 57.5)

CHAPTER 58

1. C (p. 1256, column 2)
2. A (p. 1258, column 1)
3. D (p. 1258, column 2)
4. B (p. 1258, column 2)
5. B (p. 1258, column 2)
6. A (p. 1259, column 1)
7. D (p. 1259, Table 58.2)
8. A (p. 1259, Table 58.2)
9. C (p. 1259, Table 58.2)
10. B (p. 1259, Table 58.2)
11. B (p. 1260, Table 58.3)
12. A (p. 1260, Table 58.3)
13. E (p. 1260, Table 58.3)
14. C (p. 1260, Table 58.3)
15. D (p. 1260, Table 58.3)

CHAPTER 59

1. B (p. 1268, column 1)
2. E (p. 1269, column 2)
3. E (p. 1270, column 2)
4. T (p. 1273, column 2, Table 59.4)
5. D (p. 1274, column 2)
6. T (p. 1275, column 2)
7. T (p. 1278, column 2)
8. C (p. 1278, column 2)
9. A (p. 1279, column 1)
10. T (p. 1281, column 2)

CHAPTER 60

1. E (p. 1291, column 2)
2. C (p. 1282, column 1)
3. F (p. 1292, column 2, Figure 60.2)
4. D (p. 1282, column 1, Table 60.1)

TABLE 57.5. CULTURE OF POTENTIAL SOURCES OF CROSS-INFECTION IN NOSOCOMIAL INFECTION OUTBREAK[a]

Source	Culture Method	Comment
Blood products	Broth culture incubated aerobically and anaerobically at 30°–32°C for 10 days	Following transfusion reaction; obtain simultaneous blood cultures by venipuncture
Parenteral fluids and intravenous devices	Broth or membrane filter method	Culture needle, catheter, administration set, fluid, closure; obtain blood culture
Environmental surfaces	Swab-rinse or impression plate	No evidence that any particular level of contamination correlates with nosocomial infection
Tubes and containers	Broth-rinse or swab-rinse with semiquantitative plating	At least two colonies of each morphologic type should be picked for identification
Disinfectants and antiseptics	Plating of serial dilutions of the product with and without specific neutralizers	Organisms usually nonfermenting Gram-negative aerobic bacilli
Respiratory therapy equipment	Broth-rinse or swab-rinse	Only in situations of high endemic or epidemic levels of nosocomial respiratory infection
Air	Mechanical air sampler (preferred); settling plates (poor)	No uniform agreement on acceptable levels of contamination; lack of correlation with infection
Water and ice	Membrane filter	Poor correlation of culture findings with illness
Hands of personnel	Broth-bag: 10–20 mL nutrient broth in sterile plastic bag. Wash hands in broth and plate semiquantitatively	May confirm the mechanism of cross-infection; impress the importance of hand washing

[a]Cultures to be performed only if clearly indicated by epidemiologic data.
From reference 62.

5. T (p. 1294, column 2)
6. F (p. 1295, column 2)
7. D (p. 1296, column 1)
8. B (p. 1298, column 2)
9. C (p. 1300, column 1)
10. C (p. 1301, column 1)
11. A (p. 1302, column 2)
12. T (p. 1305, column 1)
13. T (p. 1305, column 2)
14. A (p. 1307, column 2)
15. B (p. 1308, column 2)
16. T (p. 1311, column 1)
17. A (p. 1312, column 2)
18. F (p. 1313, column 2)
19. F (p. 1315, column 2)
20. T (p. 1317, column 2)
21. D (p. 1320, column 2)
22. B (p. 1321, column 2)
23. B (p. 1323, column 2)
24. T (p. 1324, column 2)
25. T (p. 1325, column 1)
26. T (p. 1326, column 2)
27. T (p. 1327, column 2)
28. T (p. 1329, column 2)
29. T (p. 1331, column 2)
30. T (p. 1332, column 1)
31. T (p. 1334, column 1)
32. T (p. 1334, column 2)
33. D (p. 1335, column 2)
34. T (p. 1338, column 1)
35. F (p. 1340, column 2)
36. T (p. 1341, column 2)

CHAPTER 61

1. E (p. 1348, column 1)
2. T (p. 1349, column 2)
3. T (p. 1351, column 2)
4. T (p. 1352, column 1)
5. E (p. 1356, column 1)
6. T (p. 1356, column 2)
7. T (p. 1359, column 2, Figure 61.9)
8. T (p. 1359, column 2)
9. T (p. 1363, column 2)
10. E (p. 1379, column 2)
11. C (p. 1381, column 1)
12. T (p. 1382, column 2)
13. C (p. 1389, column 2)
14. E (p. 1390, column 2)
15. F (p. 1392, column 2)

CHAPTER 62

1. D (p. 1402, Table 62.1)
2. E (p. 1402, Table 62.1)
3. B (p. 1402, Table 62.1)
4. A (p. 1402, Table 62.1)
5. C (p. 1402, Table 62.1)

TABLE 59.4. MOST RAPID, EXPEDIENT, SENSITIVE, AND SPECIFIC TEST FOR VIRAL DIAGNOSIS

Virus Group	Diagnose Acute Infection			Determine Immunity[b]	Comments
	Specimen	Test	Time[a]		
Herpesviruses					
Herpes simplex virus	Vesicle/ulcer/eye/ NP/mouth swab, WBCs, tissue biopsy	Culture in shell vial	16 hr	ELISA FA	Encephalitis—nucleic acid detection becoming standard
	CSF	Nucleic acid detection	6–8 hr		
Cytomegalovirus	Urine, BAL; NP aspirate, tissue biopsy	Culture in shell vial	24–48 hr to 10 d	ELISA FA	Asymptomatic shedding vs. infection
	WBCs	Antigenemia	4–5 hr		
	CSF	Nucleic acid detection	6–8 hr		
Epstein-Barr virus	Serum	Monospot, VCA IgM	1–2 d	VCA	May need to repeat test
Varicella-zoster virus	Vesicle/ulcer swab	Antigen detection by FA	2–4 hr	ELISA, FAMA	CF antibody low
		Culture in shell vial	3 d		sensitivity to
Human herpes virus type 6 (HHV-6)	Serum	Anti–HHV-6 IgM	1–3 d	ELISA	determine immunity
Human herpes virus type 7 (HHV-7)	Serum	Anti–HHV-7 IgM	1–3 d	ELISA	
Human herpes virus type 8 (HHV-8)	Tissue	Histopath			
Respiratory viruses					
Respiratory syncytial virus	NP aspirate	Antigen ELISA	4 hr	ELISA	
	Trach aspirate	DFA			
	Throat swab	Culture	6 d		
Influenza A, B	NP aspirate	Antigen	3 hr	ELISA	
	Trach aspirate	DFA		HI	Multiplex PcR assay
	Throat swab	Culture	7 d		available as RUO assay
Parainfluenza 1, 2, 3	NP aspirate	Antigen	3 hr	ELISA	(Hexoplex; Prodesse,
	Trach aspirate	DFA		HI	Inc. Way Kesha, WI)
	Throat swab	Culture	7 d		
Adenovirus	NP aspirate	Culture	7 d	ELISA	
	Trach aspirate	Antigen	3 hr		
	Throat/eye swab	DFA, ELISA			
Hepatitis viruses					
Hepatitis A (HAV)	Serum	Anti-HAV	2 d	Anti-HAV IgG	Culture not available
Hepatitis B (HBV)	Serum	HBsAG, anti-HBc IgM	2 d	Anti-HBVs	
Hepatitis C (HCV)	Serum	Anti-HCV, ELISA, confirmatory immunoblot	2 d		Quantitative RT-PCR and genotyping useful in patient management
	Serum, EDTA-plasma	RT-PCR	2–5 d		
Hepatitis D (HDV)	Serum	HDV antigen Anti-HDV IgM	2 d		
Hepatitis E (HEV)	Serum	Anti-HEV IgM ELISA			No antibody tests licensed in U.S.
Gastroenteritis viruses					
Rotavirus	Stool	Antigen, ELISA latex	3 hr		Culture not available
Enteric adenovirus	Stool	Antigen, ELISA	3 hr		
Norwalk (SRSV)	Stool	EM	days		
		EM, research ELISA available in some centers			
Astroviruses	Stool	EM	days		EM only available in some centers
Enteroviruses					
Coxsackie	NP/throat swab, stool WBCs, CSF	Culture	3–5 d	Neutral antibody	
Echo					
Polio		RT-PCR	6–8 hr		
Measles	Serum	Anti-measles IgM, IgG	2 d	ELISA, IFA	Culture available but time consuming
Rubella	Serum	Anti-rubella IgM, IgG	2 d	ELISA, IFA	Culture difficult, time consuming
Mumps	Serum	Anti-mumps IgM, IgG	2 d	ELISA, IFA	Culture available but time consuming
Human immunodeficiency virus (HIV)	Serum	Anti-HIV ELISA	2 d		PCR for proviral DNA, p24 antigen useful for acute disease and neonatal evaluation
		Western immunoblot	2 d		
	EDTA-plasma	RT-PCR quantitative (viral load)	2–3 d		

(continued)

TABLE 59.4. *(continued)*

Virus Group	Diagnose Acute Infection			Determine Immunity[b]	Comments
	Specimen	Test	Time[a]		
Arbovirus	Serum	Antibody CF	2–5 d	IFA, CF	Paired acute and convalescent sera required; PCR available in some centers
Colorado tick fever	Blood clot	Culture: mouse inoculation	2 wk	Research	Available in state labs; culture is most sensitive; serology, DFA on blood smears less sensitive
		IgG paired sera	2–3 d		
Parvovirus B19	Serum	Anti-parvo IgM	2–3 d	ELISA, RIAAQ3	
	Peripheral WBCs	PCR			
Hantavirus	Serum	IgM, IgG	1–2 d		Available in most state labs

[a]Mean time from receipt of specimen in the lab to positive result.
[b]Serum specimen for IgG antibody, using the test method indicated.
BAL, bronchoalveolar lavage; CF, complement fixation; CSF, cerebrospinal fluid; EDTA, ethylenediamine tetraacetic acid, anticoagulated peripheral blood for culture of white cells (buffy coat); ELISA, enzyme-linked immunosorbent assay; EM, electron microscopy; FA, immunofluorescence assay (DFA, direct FA; IFA, indirect FA); FAMA, immunofluorescence assay against membrane antigen; HBc, hepatitis B core; HBsAg, hepatitis B surface antigen; HI, hemagglutination inhibition; Ig, immunoglobulin; NP, nasopharyngeal; PCR, reverse transcriptase polymerase chain reaction; RT-SRSV, small round structured viruses; VCA, viral capsid antigen; WBCs, peripheral white blood cells.

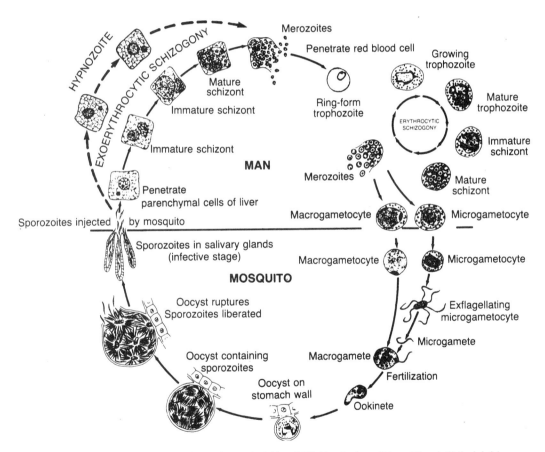

FIGURE 60.2. Life cycle of malaria. (From Strickland GT. *Tropical medicine,* 7th ed. Philadelphia: WB Saunders, with permission.)

TABLE 60.1. CLASSIFICATION OF HUMAN PARASITES

Protozoa
  Amoebas
    Entamoeba histolytica
    Entamoeba dispar
    Entamoeba coli
    Entamoeba polecki
    Entamoeba hartmanni
    Endolimax nana
    Blastocystis hominis
    Iodamoeba butschlii
    Naegleria fowleri
    Acanthamoeba culbertsoni
  Flagellates
    Giardia lamblia
    Chilomastix mesnili
    Dientamoeba fragilis
    Trichomonas hominis
    Trichomonas vaginalis
    Leishmania tropica
    Leishmania mexicana
    Leishmania braziliensis
    Leishmania donovani
    Trypanosoma gambiense
    Trypanosoma rhodesiense
    Trypanosoma cruzi
  Ciliates
    Balantidium coli
  Sporozoa
    Plasmodium vivax
    Plasmodium malariae
    Plasmodium ovale
    Plasmodium falciparum
    Babesia microti
  Coccidia
    Cryptosporidium sp.
    Cyclospora cayetanensis
    Isospora belli
    Sarcocystis sp.
    Toxoplasma gondii
  Microsporidia
    Encephalitozoon
    Nosema
    Pleistophora
    Enterocytozoon
    Trachipleistophora
Nematodes
    Ascaris lumbricoides
    Enterobius vermicularis
    Ancylostoma duodenale
    Necator americanus
    Strongyloides stercoralis
    Trichuris trichiura
    Trichinella spiralis
    Toxocara canis
    Ancylostoma braziliense
    Wuchereria bancrofti
    Brugia malayi
    Loa loa
    Onchocerca volvulus
    Mansonella ozzardi
    Mansonella streptocerca
    Mansonella perstans
    Dirofilaria sp.
Trematodes
    Fasciolopsis buski
    Heterophyes heterophyes
    Metagonimus vokogawai
    Opisthorchis sinensis
    Opisthorchis viverrini
    Fasciola hepatica
    Paragonimus westermani
    Schistosoma mansoni
    Schistosoma japonicum
    Schistosoma haematobium
Cestodes
    Diphyllobothrium latum
    Diphylidium caninum
    Hymenolepsis nana
    Hymenolepsis diminuta
    Taenia solium
    Taenia saginata
    Echinococcus granulosus
    Echinococcus multilocularis
    Multiceps multiceps

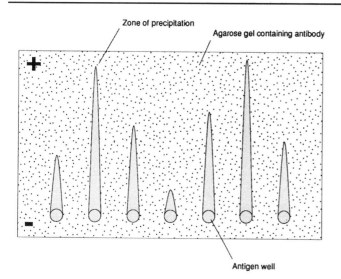

FIGURE 61.9. Principle of rocket immunoelectrophoresis.

6. C (p. 1407, Table 62.2)
7. D (p. 1407, Table 62.2)
8. A (p. 1407, Table 62.3)
9. B (p. 1407, column 2)
10. C (p. 1408, Table 62.4)
11. D (p. 1408, Table 62.4)
12. A (p. 1408, Table 62.4)
13. B (p. 1408, Table 62.5)
14. B (p. 1408, Table 62.5)
15. C (p. 1408, Table 62.5)
16. A (p. 1408, Table 62.5)
17. D (p. 1411, column 1)
18. A (p. 1412, column 2)
19. B (p. 1413, column 1)
20. B (p. 1413, Fig. 62.3)
21. D (p. 1413, Fig. 62.3)
22. C (p. 1413, Fig. 62.3)
23. A (p. 1413, Fig. 62.3)
24. B (p. 1414, column 1)
25. A (p. 1415, column 1)
26. C (p. 1415, column 2)
27. B (p. 1419, column 2)

CHAPTER 63

1. C (p. 1426, column 1)
2. A (p. 1426, column 1)
3. D (p. 1426, column 1)
4. B (p. 1426, column 1)
5. B (p. 1427, column 1)
6. C (p. 1427, column 1)
7. A (p. 1427, column 1)
8. B (p. 1427, column 1)
9. A (p. 1427, column 1)
10. D (p. 1427, column 1)
11. C (p. 1427, column 1)
12. A (p. 1427, column 1)
13. B (p. 1427, column 1)
14. B (p. 1428, column 2)
15. B (p. 1428, column 2)
16. D (p. 1430, column 1)
17. D (p. 1431, column 2)
18. C (p. 1432, column 1)
19. B (p. 1434, column 1)
20. D (p. 1434, column 1)
21. C (p. 1434, column 1)
22. B (p. 1434, column 1)
23. A (p. 1434, column 1)
24. C (p. 1436, column 2)
25. A (p. 1436, column 2)
26. C (p. 1438, Table 63.4)
27. D (p. 1438, Table 63.4)
28. B (p. 1438, Table 63.4)
29. A (p. 1438, Table 63.4)
30. D (p. 1442, column 2)
31. C (p. 1443, Fig. 63.7)
32. A (p. 1445, column 1)
33. C (p. 1446, column 1)

CHAPTER 64

1. C (p. 1449, Table 64.2)
2. D (p. 1449, Table 64.2)
3. A (p. 1449, Table 64.2)
4. B (p. 1449, Table 64.2)
5. B (p. 1449, column 1)
6. A (p. 1450, column 1)
7. A (p. 1450, column 2)
8. C (p. 1451, column 1)
9. D (p. 1452, column 1)
10. C (p. 1452, column 1)
11. D (p. 1453, column 1)
12. A (p. 1453, column 2)
13. B (p. 1454, column 1)
14. B (p. 1454, column 2)

CHAPTER 65

1. D (p. 1458, column 2)
2. B (p. 1458, column 2)
3. B (p. 1459, column 1)
4. A (p. 1460, column 1)
5. B (p. 1460, column 2)
6. C (p. 1460, column 2)
7. B (p. 1461, column 1)
8. C (p. 1461, column 2)
9. B (p. 1462, column 2)
10. C (p. 1464, column 1)
11. D (p. 1464, column 2)
12. B (p. 1467, column 2, Table 65.4)
13. D (p. 1468, column 2)
14. A (p. 1469, column 1)
15. C (p. 1469, column 1)
16. T (p. 1459, column 2)
17. F (p. 1460, column 1)
18. F (p. 1463, column 1)
19. T (p. 1464, column 1)
20. T (p. 1464, column 2)
21. T (p. 1465, column 2)
22. F (p. 1467, column 1)
23. T (p. 1467, column 2)
24. F (p. 1468, column 2)
25. F (p. 1469, column 1)

CHAPTER 66

1. A (p. 1471, column 1, Table 66.1)
2. B (p. 1471, column 1, Table 66.1)
3. A (p. 1471, column 2)
4. D (p. 1472, column 1)
5. A (p. 1473, column 1)
6. C (p. 1473, column 2)
7. D (p. 1473, column 2)
8. B (p. 1474, column 2)
9. C (p. 1474, column 2)
10. D (p. 1475, column 1)
11. A (p. 1476, column 1, Table 66.2)
12. D (p. 1476, column 2)
13. D (p. 1477, column 1)
14. C (p. 1478, column 1)
15. A (p. 1478, column 2, Fig. 66.1)
16. F (p. 1473, column 1)
17. T (p. 1474, column 1)
18. F (p. 1480, column 2)
19. F (p. 1482, column 2)
20. F (p. 1485, column 1)

CHAPTER 67

1. D (p. 1486, column 2)
2. A (p. 1486, column 2)
3. B (p. 1487, column 1)
4. A (p. 1437, column 2)
5. C (p. 1489, column 1)
6. B (p. 1489, column 2)
7. C (p. 1493, column 2)
8. A (p. 1494, column 1)
9. C (p. 1494, column 2)
10. A (p. 1495, column 1)
11. B (p. 1496, column 2)
12. C (p. 1497, column 1)
13. D (p. 1498, column 1)
14. C (p. 1499, column 2)
15. C (p. 1502, column 2)
16. D (p. 1502, column 2)
17. B (p. 1503, column 2)
18. D (p. 1504, column 2)
19. D (p. 1506, column 1)
20. B (p. 1508, column 1)
21. F (p. 1486, column 2)
22. T (p. 1496, column 2)
23. T (p. 1502, column 2)
24. T (p. 1505, column 1)
25. F (p. 1508, column 1)

CHAPTER 68

1. A (p. 1518, column 1)
2. C (p. 1518, column 2)
3. B (p. 1518, column 2)
4. A (p. 1519, column 1)
5. D (p. 1519, column 2)
6. B (p. 1519, column 2)
7. A (p. 1520, column 1)
8. D (p. 1520, column 2)
9. T (p. 1517, column 2)
10. T (p. 1517, column 2)
11. F (p. 1518, column 1)
12. T (p. 1519, column 1)
13. T (p. 1519, column 1)
14. T (p. 1519, column 2)
15. T (p. 1519, column 2)
16. T (p. 1519, column 1)
17. F (p. 1520, column 2)
18. T (p. 1520, column 2)
19. F (p. 1520, column 2)
20. T (p. 1521, column 1)

CHAPTER 69

1. C (p. 1522, column 1)
2. B (p. 1522, column 2)
3. D (p. 1523, column 1)
4. A (p. 1523, column 1)
5. C (p. 1523, column 1)
6. B (p. 1523, column 2)
7. C (p. 1524, column 1)
8. A (p. 1524, column 2)
9. A (p. 1524, column 2)
10. C (p. 1526, column 1)
11. B (p. 1527, column 1, Table 69.1)
12. C (p. 1528, column 1)
13. C (p. 1528, column 1)
14. A (p. 1528, column 2)
15. B (p. 1529, column 2)
16. D (p. 1529, column 2)
17. C (p. 1530, column 1)
18. C (p. 1530, column 2)
19. A (p. 1531, column 2)
20. A (p. 1532, column 1)
21. T (p. 1522, column 2)
22. F (p. 1522, column 2)
23. T (p. 1523, column 2)
24. F (p. 1525, column 2)
25. T (p. 1526, column 2)

26. T (p. 1528, column 1)
27. T (p. 1529, column 2)
28. F (p. 1530, column 1)
29. T (p. 1530, column 2)
30. T (p. 1531, column 2)

CHAPTER 70

1. C (p. 1533, column 1, Table 70.1)
2. A (p. 1534, column 2)
3. D (p. 1534, column 2)
4. D (p. 1534, column 2)
5. A (p. 1536, column 1)
6. B (p. 1537, column 1, Table 70.5)
7. A (p. 1537, column 1)
8. C (p. 1538, column 1)
9. D (p. 1538, column 2)
10. A (p. 1538, column 2)
11. C (p. 1540, column 1, Fig. 70.4)
12. A (p. 1541, column 1, Fig. 70.5)
13. B (p. 1542, column 1)
14. D (p. 1542, column 1)
15. B (p. 1543, column 1)
16. T (p. 1533, column 1)
17. T (p. 1536, column 2)
18. F (p. 1537, column 2)
19. F (p. 1539, column 1)
20. T (p. 1539, column 2)
21. T (p. 1542, column 1)
22. F (p. 1542, column 2)
23. T (p. 1543, column 2)
24. T (p. 1544, column 1)
25. T (p. 1544, column 1)

CHAPTER 71

1. C (p. 1546, column 1)
2. D (p. 1546, column 2)
3. D (p. 1547, column 1)
4. B (p. 1547, column 2)
5. C (p. 1547, column 2)
6. A (p. 1548, column 2)
7. B (p. 1549, column 2)
8. C (p. 1549, column 2)
9. B (p. 1550, column 2)
10. D (p. 1550, column 2)
11. D (p. 1551, column 1)
12. A (p. 1552, column 2)
13. A (p. 1552, column 2)

14. C (p. 1552, column 2)
15. D (p. 1552, column 2)
16. B (p. 1553, column 1)
17. B (p. 1554, column 1)
18. B (p. 1554, column 1)
19. A (p. 1554, column 2)
20. C (p. 1560, column 1)
21. C (p. 1560, column 1)
22. T (p. 1558, column 1)
23. T (p. 1558, column 2)
24. T (p. 1559, column 1)
25. F (p. 1560, column 2)
26. T (p. 1561, column 1)
27. F (p. 1561, column 1)
28. T (p. 1561, column 2)
29. T (p. 1561, column 2)
30. F (p. 1562, column 1)

CHAPTER 72

1. D (P. 1568, Column 1)
2. B (p. 1568, column 2)
3. A (p. 1573, column 1)
4. D (p. 1574, column 1, Table 72.4)
5. D (p. 1575, column 2)
6. B (p. 1575, column 2)
7. D (p. 1576, column 2)
8. C (p. 1581, column 1)
9. D (p. 1582, column 1)
10. C (p. 1582, column 2)
11. B (p. 1585, column 2)
12. B (p. 1587, column 2)
13. C (p. 1587, column 2)
14. D (p. 1593, column 1)
15. A (p. 1593, column 1)
16. F (p. 1568, column 1)
17. T (p. 1569, column 2)
18. T (p. 1578, column 2)
19. F (p. 1578, column 2)
20. T (p. 1579, column 2)
21. T (p. 1580, column 1)
22. T (p. 1580, column 2)
23. F (p. 1585, column 1)
24. F (p. 1589, column 2, Table 72.9)
25. F (p. 1592, column 1)

CHAPTER 73

1. B (p. 1603, column 2)
2. D (p. 1605, column 2)

3. C (p. 1605, column 2)
4. A (p. 1606, column 1)
5. B (p. 1606, column 1)
6. B (p. 1606, column 2)
7. C (p. 1607, column 2)
8. C (p. 1607, column 2)
9. D (p. 1609, column 1)
10. B (p. 1611, column 2)
11. T (p. 1602, column 2)
12. F (p. 1602, column 2)
13. T (p. 1605, column 1)
14. T (p. 1605, column 2)
15. F (p. 1605, column 1)
16. F (p. 1609, column 1)
17. F (p. 1610, column 1)
18. T (p. 1611, column 1)
19. F (p. 1612, column 2)
20. F (p. 1612, column 2)

CHAPTER 74

1. B (p. 1616, column 1)
2. C (p. 1617, column 2, Fig. 74.1)
3. C (p. 1618, column 2)
4. D (p. 1619, column 1)
5. A (p. 1620, column 1)
6. B (p. 1620, column 1)
7. C (p. 1622, column 1)
8. D (p. 1624, column 1)
9. C (p. 1625, column 2)
10. A (p. 1626, column 2, Table 74.4)
11. F (p. 1617, column 1)
12. T (p. 1618, column 2)
13. F (p. 1619, column 1)
14. T (p. 1623, column 1)

15. F (p. 1623, column 1)
16. T (p. 1625, column 1)
17. F (p. 1627, column 1)
18. T (p. 1627, column 2, Table 74.4)
19. F (p. 1628, column 1)
20. T (p. 1631, column 1)

CHAPTER 75

1. D (p. 1634, column 1)
2. B (p. 1635, column 1)
3. C (p. 1637, column 1)
4. A (p. 1637, column 2)
5. D (p. 1638, column 1, Table 75.2)
6. B (p. 1638, column 2)
7. D (p. 1638, column 2)
8. C (p. 1640, column 1)
9. A (p. 1641, column 1)
10. C (p. 1642, column 1, Table 75.4)
11. B (p. 1643, column 1)
12. B (p. 1643, column 2)
13. C (p. 1644, column 1)
14. B (p. 1644, column 1)
15. B (p. 1644, column 1)
16. F (p. 1633, column 1)
17. F (p. 1635, column 1)
18. T (p. 1635, column 1)
19. F (p. 1636, column 1)
20. F (p. 1636, column 1)
21. F (p. 1640, column 1)
22. F (p. 1642, column 2)
23. T (p. 1643, column 1)
24. T (p. 1643, column 1)
25. F (p. 1644, column 2)